BREAST CANCER: ORIGINS, DETECTION, AND TREATMENT

DEVELOPMENTS IN ONCOLOGY

K. Hellmann, P. Hilgard and S. Eccles, eds.: Metastasis: Clinical and Experimental Aspects. 90-247-2424-4.
H.F. Seigler, ed.: Clinical Management of Melanoma. 90-247-2584-4.
P. Correa and W. Haenszel, eds.: Epidemiology of Cancer of the Digestive Tract. 90-247-2601-8.
L.A. Liotta and I.R. Hart, eds.: Tumour Invasion and Metastasis. 90-247-2611-5.
J. Banoczy, ed.: Oral Leukoplakia. 90-247-2655-7.
C. Tijssen, M. Halprin and L. Endtz, eds.: Familial Brain Tumours. 90-247-2691-3.
F.M. Muggia, C.W. Young and S.K. Carter, eds.: Anthracycline Antibiotics in Cancer. 90-247-2711-1.
B.W. Hancock, ed.: Assessment of Tumour Response. 90-247-2712-X.
D.E. Peterson, ed.: Oral Complications of Cancer Chemotherapy. 0-89838-563-6.
R. Mastrangelo, D.G. Poplack and R. Riccardi, eds.: Central Nervous System Leukemia. Prevention and Treatment. 0-89838-570-9.
A. Polliack, ed.: Human Leukemias. Cytochemical and Ultrastructural Techniques in Diagnosis and Research. 0-89838-585-7.
W. Davis, C. Maltoni and S. Tanneberger, eds.: The Control of Tumor Growth and its Biological Bases. 0-89838-603-9.
A.P.M. Heintz, C. Th. Griffiths and J.B. Trimbos, eds.: Surgery in Gynecological Oncology. 0-89838-604-7.
M.P. Hacker, E.B. Double and I. Krakoff, eds.: Platinum Coordination Complexes in Cancer Chemotherapy. 0-89838-619-5.
M.J. van Zwieten. The Rat as Animal Model in Breast Cancer Research: A Histopathological Study of Radiation- and Hormone-Induced Rat Mammary Tumors. 0-89838-624-1.
B. Lowenberg and A. Hogenbeck, eds.: Minimal Residual Disease in Acute Leukemia. 0-89838-630-6.
I. van der Waal and G.B. Snow, eds.: Oral Oncology. 0-89838-631-4.
B.W. Hancock and A.M. Ward, eds.: Immunological Aspects of Cancer. 0-89838-664-0.
K.V. Honn and B.F. Sloane, eds.: Hemostatic Mechanisms and Metastasis. 0-89838-667-5.
K.R. Harrap, W. Davis and A.N. Calvert, eds.: Cancer Chemotherapy and Selective Drug Development. 0-89838-673-X.
V.D. Velde, J.H. Cornelis and P.H. Sugarbaker, eds.: Liver Metastasis. 0-89838-648-5.
D.J. Ruiter, K. Welvaart and S. Ferrone, eds.: Cutaneous Melanoma and Precursor Lesions. 0-89838-689-6.
S.B. Howell, ed.: Intra-Arterial and Intracavitary Cancer Chemotherapy. 0-89838-691-8.
D.L. Kisner and J.F. Smyth, eds.: Interferon Alpha-2: Pre-Clinical and Clinical Evaluation. 0-89838-701-9.
P. Furmanski, J.C. Hager and M.A. Rich, eds.: RNA Tumor Viruses, Oncogenes, Human Cancer and Aids: On the Frontiers of Understanding. 0-89838-703-5.
J.E. Talmadge, I.J. Fidler and R.K. Oldham: Screening for Biological Response Modifiers: Methods and Rationale. 0-89838-712-4.
J.C. Bottino, R.W. Opfell and F.M. Muggia, eds.: Liver Cancer. 0-89838-713-2.
P.K. Pattengale, R.J. Lukes and C.R. Taylor, eds.: Lymphoproliferative Diseases: Pathogenesis, Diagnosis, Therapy. 0-89838-725-6.
F. Cavalli, G. Bonadonna and M. Rozencweig, eds.: Malignant Lymphomas and Hodgkin's Disease. 0-89838-727-2.
L. Baker, F. Valeriote and V. Ratanatharathorn, eds.: Biology and Therapy of Acute Leukemia. 0-89838-728-0.
J. Russo, ed.: Immunocytochemistry in Tumor Diagnosis. 0-89838-737-X.
R.L. Ceriani, ed.: Monoclonal Antibodies and Breast Cancer. 0-89838-739-6.
D.E. Peterson, G.E. Elias and S.T. Sonis, eds.: Head and Neck Management of the Cancer Patient. 0-89838-747-7.
D.M. Green: Diagnosis and management of Malignant Solid Tumors in Infants and Children. 0-89838-750-7.
K.A. Foon and A.C. Morgan, Jr., eds.: Monoclonal Antibody Therapy of Human Cancer. 0-89838-754-X.
J.G. McVie, et al, eds., Clinical and Experimental Pathology of Lung Cancer. 0-89838-764-7.
K.V. Honn, W.E. Powers and B.F. Sloane, eds.: Mechanisms of Cancer Metastasis. 0-89838-765-5.
K. Lapis, L.A. Liotta and A.S. Rabson, eds.: Biochemistry and Molecular Genetics of Cancer Metastasis. 0-89838-785-X.
A.J. Mastromarino, ed.: Biology and Treatment of Colorectal Cancer Metastasis. 0–89838–786–8.

BREAST CANCER: ORIGINS, DETECTION, AND TREATMENT

Proceedings of the
International Breast Cancer Research Conference
London, United Kingdom — March 24–28, 1985

edited by

Marvin A. Rich
AMC Cancer Research Center
Denver, Colorado, USA

Jean Carol Hager
AMC Cancer Research Center
Denver, Colorado, USA

Joyce Taylor-Papadimitriou
Imperial Cancer Research Fund
London, UNITED KINGDOM

Martinus Nijhoff Publishing
a member of the Kluwer Academic Publishers Group
Boston / Dordrecht / Lancaster

Distributors for North America:
Kluwer Academic Publishers
190 Old Derby Street
Hingham, Massachusetts 02043, USA

Distributors for the UK and Ireland:
Kluwer Academic Publishers
MTP Press Limited
Falcon House, Queen Square
Lancaster LA1 1RN, UNITED KINGDOM

Distributors for all other countries:
Kluwer Academic Publishers Group
Distribution Centre
Post Office Box 322
3300 AH Dordrecht, THE NETHERLANDS

Library of Congress Cataloging-in-Publication Data

International Breast Cancer Research Conference
  (1985 : London, England)
  Breast cancer.

  (Developments in oncology)
  Includes bibliographies and index.
    1. Breast—Cancer—Congresses. I. Rich, Marvin A.
II. Hager, Jean Carol, 1943–   . III. Taylor-
Papadimitriou, Joyce. IV. Title. V. Series.
[DNLM: 1. Breast Neoplasms—congresses.
W1 DE998N / WP 870 I5804b 1985]
RC280.B8I56 1985   616.99′449   85–32008
ISBN 0-89838-792-2

Printed in the United States of America

CONTENTS

NEW PERSPECTIVES FOR CLINICAL
CONTROL OF HUMAN BREAST CANCER

CONTRIBUTORS

NIKI J. AGNANTIS, Hellenic Anticancer Institute,
Athens, Greece

IQBAL ALI, Laboratory of Tumor Immunology and Biology,
National Cancer Institute, National Institutes of Health,
Bethesda, Maryland 20205

D S ALLEN, Clinical Endocrinology Laboratory, Imperial Cancer
Research Fund, London WC2A 3PX, Breast Unit, Guy's Hospital,
London, UK

ANNE-CATHERINE ANDRES, Ludwig Institute for Cancer Research,
Bern Branch, CH-3010 Bern Switzerland

GERT AUER, Karolinska Institute, Stockholm, Sweden

ROLAND BALL, Ludwig Institute for Cancer Research, Bern
Branch, CH-3010 Bern Switzerland

G BANDYOPADHYAY, Cancer Research Laboratory, University of
California, Berkeley, California 94720

MOZEENA BANO, Laboratory of Tumor Immunology and Biology,
National Cancer Institute, National Institutes of Health,
Bethesda, Maryland 20205

DIANA M. BARNES, Clinical Research Laboratories, Christie
Hospital & Holt Radium Institute, Manchester M20 9BX, UK

JIRI BARTEK, Imperial Cancer Research Fund, London WC2A 3PX,
UK; and Research Institute of Clinical and Exp. Oncology, Brno,
Czechoslovakia

RICHARD D. BULBROOK, Clinical Endocrinology Laboratory,
Imperial Cancer Research Fund, London WC2A 3PX, UK

K BUSER, Ludwig Institute for Cancer Research, Bern Branch,
3010 Bern Switzerland

JANET S. BUTEL, Department of Virology and Epidemiology,
Baylor College of Medicine, Houston, Texas 77030

ROBERT CALLAHAN, Laboratory of Tumor Immunology and Biology,
National Cancer Institute, National Institutes of Health,
Bethesda, Maryland 20205

FRANCOISE CAPONY, Unite d'Endocrinologie Cellulaire et Moleculaire, U 148 INSERM, 34100 Montpellier, France

ROBERT D. CARDIFF, Department of Pathology, University of California Medical School, Davis, California 95616

GHISLAINE CAVALIE-BARTHEZ, Unite d'Endocrinologie Cellulaire et Moleculaire, U 148 INSERM, 34100 Montpellier, France

ROBERTO CERIANI, John Muir Cancer and Aging Research Institute, Walnut Creek, California 94596

MONIQUE CHAMBON, Unite d'Endocrinologie Cellulaire et Moleculaire, U 148 INSERM, 34100 Montpellier, France

SIDNEY E. CHANG, Marie Curie Memorial Foundation, Research Institute, Oxted, Surrey, RH8 OTL, UK

A I COFFER, Hormone Biochemistry Department, Imperial Cancer Research Fund, London WC2A 3PX, UK

HEIDI DIGGELMANN, Swiss Institute For Experimental Cancer Research, 1066 Epalinges, Switzerland

ELISA M. DURBAN, The University of Texas, Dental Branch, Department of Microbiology, Houston, Texas 77225

JACQUELINE D. FETHERSTON, Laboratory of Tumor Immunology and Biology, National Cancer Institute, National Institutes of Health, Bethesda, Maryland 20205

BERNARD FISHER, Department of Surgery, University of Pittsburgh, School of Medicine, Pittsburgh, Pennsylvania 15261

MARCEL GARCIA, Unite d'Endocrinologie Cellulaire et Moleculaire, U 148 INSERM, 34100 Montpellier, France

BERND GRONER, Ludwig Institute for Cancer Research, Bern Branch, CH-3010 Bern, Switzerland

WALTER GUNZBURG, Ludwig Institute for Cancer Research, Bern Branch, CH-3010 Bern Switzerland

ADELINE J. HACKETT, Peralta Cancer Research Institute, Oakland, California 94609

PHILOMENA HAGEMAN, Division of Clinical Oncology and Department of Pathology, The Netherlands Cancer Institute, Amsterdam, The Netherlands

RICHARD HALLOWES, Tissue Cell Relationships Laboratory, Imperial Cancer Research Fund, London WC2A 3PX, UK

IAN HART, Imperial Cancer Research Fund, London WC2A 3PX; Royal Marsden Hospital, Sutton Surrey, SM2 5PX, UK

JOHN L. HAYWARD, Imperial Cancer Research Fund, London WC2A 3PX, Breast Unit, Guy's Hospital, London, UK

GLORIA HEPPNER, Department of Immunology, Michigan Cancer Foundation, Detroit, Michigan 48201

TOBY HORN, Laboratory of Tumor Immunology and Biology, National Cancer Institute, National Institutes of Health, Bethesda, Maryland 20205

ANTHONY HOWELL, Department of Medical Oncology, Christie Hospital & Holt Radium Institute, Manchester M20 9BX, UK

NANCY E. HYNES, Ludwig Institute for Cancer Research, Bern Branch, CH-3010 Bern, Switzerland

WALTER IMAGAWA, Cancer Research Laboratory, University of California, Berkeley, California 94720

CLEMENT IP, Department of Breast Surgery, Roswell Park Memorial Institute, Buffalo, New York 14263

ROLF JAGGI, Ludwig Institute for Cancer Research, Bern Branch, CH-3010 Bern Switzerland

MARY JONES, Christie Hospital & Holt Radium Institute, Manchester M20 9BX, UK

WILLIAM R. KIDWELL, Laboratory of Tumor Immunology and Biology, National Cancer Institute, National Institutes of Health, Bethesda, Maryland 20205

MARY-CLAIRE KING, School of Public Health, University of California, Berkeley, California, 94720

ROGER J.B. KING, Hormone Biochemistry Department, Imperial Cancer Research Fund, London WC2A 3PX, UK

SARA KOZMA, Ludwig Institute for Cancer Research, Bern Branch, CH-3010 Bern, Switzerland

KLAUS KRATOCHWIL, Institute of Molecular Biology, Austrian Academy of Sciences, A-5020 Salzburg, Austria

HONG GIOK KWA, The Netherlands Cancer Institute, 1066 CX Amsterdam, The Netherlands

JONATHON LI, Medical Research Laboratories, V.A. Medical Center, Minneapolis, Minnesota 55417

DIANA M. LOPEZ, Department of Microbiology and Immunology, University of Miami School of Medicine and the Comprehensive Cancer Center for the State of Florida, Miami, Florida 33101

RENATO MARIANI-COSTANTINI, Laboratory of Tumor Immunology and Biology, National Cancer Institute, National Institutes of Health, Bethesda, Maryland 20205

O MASSOT, Unite d'Endocrinologie Cellulaire et Moleculaire, U 148 INSERM, 34100 Montpellier, France

JOHN W. MOORE, Clinical Endocrinology Laboratory, Imperial Cancer Research Fund, London WC2A 3PX, UK

M MORISSET, Unite d'Endocrinologie Cellulaire et Moleculaire, U 148 INSERM, 34100 Montpellier, France

DAVID W. MORRIS, Department of Pathology, University of California Medical School, Davis, California 95616

HENNING T. MOURIDSEN, Department of Oncology I, Finsen Institute, 2100 Copenhagen O, Denmark

SATYABRATA NANDI, Cancer Research Laboratory, University of California, Berkeley, California 94720

ROELAND NUSSE, Department of Molecular Biology, The Netherlands Cancer Institute, 1066 CX Amsterdam, The Netherlands

J L PETERSE, Division of Clinical Oncology and Department of Pathology, Netherlands Cancer Institute, Amsterdam, The Netherlands

SHELAGH REDMOND, Ludwig Institute for Cancer Research, Bern Branch, CH-3010 Bern, Switzerland

ERNST REICHMANN, Ludwig Institute for Cancer Research, Bern Branch, CH-3010 Bern Switzerland

G G RIBEIRO, Christie Hospital & Holt Radium Institute, Manchester 20, UK

F RIJSEWIJK, Department of Molecular Biology, The Netherlands Cancer Institute, 1066 CX Amsterdam, The Netherlands

HENRI ROCHEFORT, Unite d'Endocrinologie Cellulaire et Moleculaire, U 148 INSERM, 34100 Montpellier, France

BRIAN SALMONS, Ludwig Institute for Cancer Research, Bern Branch, CH-3010 Bern Switzerland

DAVID SALOMON, Laboratory of Tumor Immunology and Biology, National Cancer Institute, National Institutes of Health, Bethesda, Maryland 20205

JEFFREY SCHLOM, Laboratory of Tumor Immunology and Biology, National Cancer Institute, National Institutes of Health, Bethesda, Maryland 20205

E SCHUURING, Department of Molecular Biology, The Netherlands Cancer Institute, 1066 CX Amsterdam, The Netherlands

HELENE S. SMITH, Peralta Cancer Research Institute, Oakland, California 94609

DEMETRIOUS A. SPANDIDOS, Beatson Institute for Cancer Research, Bearsden, Glasgow G61 1BD; and Hellenic Institute Pasteur, Athens, Greece

M SPENCER, Laboratory of Growth & Development of Children's Hospital, San Francisco, California 94118

FRANCESCO SQUARTINI, Istituto di Anatomia e Istologia Patologica, Scuola Medica, Universita degli Studi, 56100 Pisa, Italy

MARTHA STAMPFER, Lawrence Berkeley Laboratory, Berkeley, California, 94720

ROBERT STRANGE, Department of Pathology, University of California Medical School, Davis, California 95616

JOYCE TAYLOR-PAPADIMITRIOU, Imperial Cancer Research Fund, London WC2A 3PX, UK

BRIAN S. THOMAS, Clinical Endocrinology Laboratory, Imperial Cancer Research Fund, London WC2A 3PX, UK

ZOLTAN A. TOKES, Department of Biochemistry, Comprehensive Cancer Center, University of Southern California, School of Medicine, Los Angeles, California 90033

IYVAN TOUITOU, Unite d'Endocrinologie Cellulaire et Moleculaire, U 148 INSERM, 34100 Montpellier, France

M VAN LOHUIZEN, Department of Molecular Biology, The
Netherlands Cancer Institute 1066 CX Amsterdam, The Netherlands

ALBERT VAN OOYEN, Department of Molecular Biology, The
Netherlands Cancer Institute 1066 CX Amsterdam, The Netherlands

FRANCOISE VIGNON, Unite d'Endocrinologie Cellulaire et
Moleculaire, U 148 INSERM, 34100 Montpellier, France

DENNIS Y. WANG, Clinical Endocrinology Laboratory, Imperial
Cancer Research Fund, London WC2X 3PX, UK

BRUCE WESTLEY, Unite d'Endocrinologie Cellulaire et
Moleculaire, U 148 INSERM, 34100 Montpellier, France

SANDRA R. WOLMAN, Cytogenetics Laboratory, Department of
Pathology, New York University, School of Medicine, New York,
New York 10016

LAWRENCE J.T. YOUNG, Department of Pathology, University of
California Medical School, Davis, California 95616

PREFACE

The control of breast cancer, a leading cause of cancer death in women, will depend ultimately on our understanding of the disease--its origin, and progression which in turn will permit the effective management of its treatment, its detection, and perhaps even its prevention. It is for a better understanding of this spectrum of biological processes crossing back and forth across scientific and clinical disciplines that this volume strives.

Several broad topics have been addressed in organizing a large mass of work representing state of the art updates from many of the major breast cancer research groups around the world. The chapters in the first section speak to the factors affecting the growth and development of normal and malignant mammary epithelium. Special emphasis is placed on insights drawn from developmental biology, the cellular interactions that occur in the mammary gland during growth and differentiation; and the study of hormones and growth factors in the regulation of growth and differentiation of normal and malignant breast tissues.

In the section on the biology of breast cancer, there is a characterization of relevant model systems for the study of breast cancer and their contribution to our understanding of preneoplasia and progression in mammary cancer. Included as well is the current status of major studies on the immunological aspects of breast cancer and the latest efforts in the development of markers for metastasis in breast cancer.

The past several years have seen an explosion of activity in molecular biology with a very significant portion of the work relevant to oncology occurring in the area of mammary cancer. The section on the molecular basis of mammary carcinogenesis encompasses a broad range of topics from the molecular biology of preneoplasia and carcinogenesis to the identification of genes associated with inherited and environmentally-induced breast cancer.

The fourth section addressing perspectives for the clinical control of human breast cancer includes research updates on such topics as the dietary influences in breast cancer risk and the factors important to the diagnosis and prognosis of breast cancer. The clinician, and perhaps to even a greater extent, the breast cancer scientist faces an enormous body of data arising from clinical trials and reports on new options for the management of breast cancer. It is toward the characterization, the rationalization and the placing of these clinical results in context of what we know of the biology of breast cancer that this section of the book is aimed.

Special emphasis has been placed on the interaction between laboratory and clinical research in breast cancer. It is likely that the complete conquest of breast cancer will ultimately arise from the discoveries of the laboratory that have been well integrated with the clinical awareness that comes from managing the disease. Be it prevention, detection, diagnosis or treatment, true success will directly depend on the flow of knowledge from both the laboratory and the clinic and their pragmatic fusion. The clinician must be aware of new findings and of changes and progress in our concepts of the breast cancer's natural history. At least equally important, is the fact that the malignant transformation of a cell is not cancer, and the laboratory scientist through focusing on one or another of the facets of the disease, must be guided by an awareness of all of the pathophysiological entities that constitute the totality of the disease. It is our hope that this volume will contribute to the accomplishment of this process.

This work has its origins in the formal presentations, the workshops and the discussions at the 1985 biennial conference of the International Association for Breast Cancer Research held in London, England, and is accordingly dedicated to all of the participants.

The editors are grateful to their own institutions, the AMC Cancer Research Center in Denver, and the Imperial Cancer Research Fund in London for their generous support and to the National Institutes of Health (Grant CA 40043) as well. We acknowledge the excellent assistance of Carol Rains in preparing the manuscript.

Dr. Marvin A. Rich
Dr. Jean Carol Hager
Dr. Joyce Taylor-Papadimitriou

BREAST CANCER: ORIGINS, DETECTION, AND TREATMENT

1

THE IMPORTANCE OF EPITHELIAL-STROMAL INTERACTION IN MAMMARY
GLAND DEVELOPMENT

K. KRATOCHWIL

Institute of Molecular Biology, Austrian Academy of Sciences,
Salzburg, Austria

INTRODUCTION

The fact that two dissimilar tissues influence each other in
their developmental behaviour is known to embryologists for a long
time. The first experiments of Spemann, eventually establishing
the phenomenon of "embryonic induction" were done some 80 years
ago (1). Originally, the term was coined for events when two
dissimilar tissues or blastemas come into close contact and, when
as a result of this association, at least one of the two partners
becomes determined for a new developmental pathway. A large number
of such inductive events has been discovered since but, quite
disappointingly, despite much effort not one system so far has
yielded a biochemical or molecular factor that could be identified
as mediator of induction.

Much later, in the fifties, the use of the term "inductive
tissue interaction" was extended to include also the developmental
interaction of already committed tissues, as it occurs during
organogenesis. Especially through the work of Grobstein and his
associates (for reviews see refs. 2, 3) we have learnt that the
different tissues building an organ (e.g. a glandular epithelium
and its investing mesenchyme) are truly interdependent in their
development, and we are now aware that this continuing interaction,
a characteristic feature of the vertebrate embryo, allows the
fine tuning required for constructing the complex architecture of
our organs (4).

Although evidence is much more difficult to obtain from
static systems, we are basically convinced that processes identical
or very similar to those governing the formation of organs in the
embryo, may also be responsible for maintaining organ architecture

and tissue differentiation in the adult. But even in the adult organism there are instances of more dynamic developmental changes. One of them is represented by organs that undergo growth and morphogenesis primarily in postnatal life, most prominently the mammary gland. Other examples may be seen in pathological processes associated with inflammation and wound healing, in hyperplasia and, most conspicuously, in infiltrating and metastasizing cancer. Because of their possible relevance for these processes, I shall very briefly review embryonic epithelial-mesenchymal interactions and then discuss some of our own experiments relating to the question of how these interactions may be affected by hormones.

EPITHELIAL-MESENCHYMAL INTERACTION IN EMBRYONIC ORGANOGENESIS

With very few exceptions, the epithelial component of an organ always develops in a bed of investing mesenchyme. Usually the two tissues associate only secondarily during development - which makes the embryologist's recombination experiments look less artificial ! In experimental situations, the interdependence of the tissues can be demonstrated by their separation, by subsequent recombination, and by exchanging one partner tissue by another. Most isolated epithelia cannot continue their development (the one exception is pancreas epithelium - ref. 5) unless recombined with mesenchyme. The requirement for organ-specific mesenchyme varies with the rudiment; most epithelia are dependent on the presence of mesenchyme from the same organ whereas species or even class (mammalian-avian) differences seem to be of little or no importance.

A great variety of heterologous experimental associations have shown that it is the mesenchymal component which determines the development of the composite explant. This is most clearly seen in (avian) skin: In "heterotopic" combinations of dermis and epidermis from feather-forming, scale-forming, or featherless areas, the appendages formed correspond to the source of the dermis (for review see ref. 6). Correspondingly, mesenchymes from the male or female genital tract specify epithelial morphogenesis and cytodifferentiation, as seen in reciprocal combination,

and urogenital sinus mesenchyme can even induce bladder
epithelium to form prostatic structures (reviewed in 7).
The mesenchymal tooth papilla induces the formation of an enamel
organ in foot epidermis (8). Even within the same organ, the
mesenchymal control of epithelial branching activity can be
demonstrated; exchanging a piece of mesenchyme from the actively
growing broncheal tree with a piece from the (quiescent) trachea
resulted in arrest of bronchial branching on one hand, and in a
supernumerary tracheal bud on the other (9, 10). Combining epithelia and mesenchymes from organs exhibiting characteristically
different epithelial branching patterns, such as mammary and
salivary gland, revealed that epithelial branching morphogenesis
is determined by the mesenchyme (11) even when it retains its
original differentiation (12).

The mechanism of these epithelial-mesenchymal interactions
so far remains enigmatic. Except for pancreas epithelium, the
growth and differentiation of which can be supported in vitro by
a poorly defined "mesenchymal factor" that is neither species nor
tissue-specific (13), epithelial development in culture depends on
the presence of living mesenchymal cells. Very characteristic is
the short-range, non-systemic effect of interaction, and in
contrast to earlier assumptions (2), there is now reasonable evidence that at least in kidney (14) and tooth (15), developmental
interaction may in fact depend on physical cell contact. Although
the dependence of epithelial growth on homotypic mesenchyme
could be explained by assuming organ-specific growth factors, it
is more difficult to visualize how the mesenchyme actually
controls the epithelial branching pattern. A model has been
proposed by Bernfield (16, 17) implicating the extracellular
matrix (ECM) as a mediator of this mesenchymal effect. The ECM
at the tissue interface shows a very characteristic structure,
and a number of its components have become known at the molecular
level (for reviews see 18, 19, 20). The basal surface of the
epithelium is lined by a basal lamina containing type IV collagen,
laminin, entactin, hyaluronate and basal lamina proteoglycans
(the composition may vary; embryonic laminae, though similar to
the adult structure under the electron microscope, are apparently

richer in glycosaminoglycans - (ref. 21). This lamina is under-
laid by fibrillar collagen of mesenchymal origin, the acellular
"reticular membrane". During epithelial growth and branching
activity, these interface ECM structures need to be constantly
remodelled, and it was in fact shown that basal lamina glycosaminoglycans turn over more rapidly at the growing tips of epithelial adenomeres than in the clefts between them or in inactive
areas (stalk) (ref. 22). The model by Bernfield (16, 17)
proposes that this differential stability of the basal lamina
constitutes a morphogenetic and growth signal to the epithelium.
The mesenchyme is assumed to degrade basal lamina constituents
in growth areas while stabilizing the lamina in other regions,
mainly through the deposition of fibrillar collagen. The
conspicuous association of collagen fibers with morphogenetically
inactive regions of an epithelium (clefts and stalk of the
salivary gland - ref. 23; trachea and primary bronchi in the
lung - ref.10) had been noted before and treatment of explants
with collagenase (23, 24) or with inhibitors of collagen synthesis
or cross-linking (25) in fact resulted in "depatterning" of the
epithelium.

EPITHELIAL-STROMAL INTERACTION IN POSTNATAL LIFE

Unlike comparable organs, mammary gland develops much later
and epithelial growth is most active in puberty. At that stage,
the mesenchymal component is represented by the fat pad. Whereas
epithelium and mesenchyme of the salivary gland, for instance,
evolve together to produce the characteristic organ structure,
mammary epithelium has to sprout into a preexisting resistant
stroma and it is hard to imagine that it can penetrate without
degrading stromal matrix components - a potentially dangerous
capacity. Adult mammary epithelium is still responsive to stromal
influences as seen in its inability to grow into non-fat mesoderm.
This responsiveness was even more clearly demonstrated by Sakakura
who implanted pieces of fetal mammary or salivary mesenchyme into
the fat pad of an adult gland (reviewed in ref. 26). The gland
epithelium invading these implants not only showed a characteristically altered growth and branching pattern but also showed

increased inclination to develop tumors. Cunha's experiments on
the reproductive tract (reviewed in 7) have also shown responsiveness of the epithelia (e.g. bladder) to heterotypic mesenchyme
to persist into postnatal periods.

Another line of evidence for the dependence of adult epithelium on stromal products may be seen in the beneficial effects
of collagen gels on growth and differentiation of mammary
epithelial cell lines (reviewed by Durban et al., this volume).
Interestingly, collagen substrata also stabilize the extracellular
matrix produced by these epithelia, suggesting again that its
effect may be mediated by the basal lamina (27, 28) in an analogous manner as had been proposed for embryonic organogenesis
(16, 17).

It is impossible to review here all the experiments and
observations that have contributed to our notion that epithelial-
-mesenchymal tissue interactions, which are so conspicuously
involved in embryonic organ formation, continue to be important
for maintaining organ structure and cellular differentiation in
the adult. Pathological processes, notably invasive cancer, are
characterized by a break-down of the normal tissue relationship,
by a destruction of the tissue interface and the stromal matrix,
and eventually, in case of a metastasis, new "heterotypic"
epithelial-stromal associations are created. Even if it is not
the primary cause for cancer, this disturbed tissue interrelation
conceivably could contribute to faster progression of the tumor
and reduced responsiveness to controlling influences.

HORMONES AND EPITHELIAL-MESENCHYMAL INTERACTIONS

As mentioned, experiments on a variety of embryonic organ
rudiments have established that it is the mesenchyme which directs
epithelial morphogenesis. On the other hand, there is equally
convincing evidence that in the mammary gland, growth and morphogenesis of the epithelium is under the control of hormones. This
apparent discrepancy could be reconciled if it were found that
hormones can influence tissue interaction. Our own experiments
on the embryonic mammary rudiment of the mouse have in fact
revealed an interdependence of hormone action and tissue

interaction by showing that (i) hormone effects are mediated
by tissue interaction and, further, (ii) that tissue interaction
is a prerequisite for the development of hormone responsiveness.

The Androgen Response of the Mouse Mammary Rudiment – A Case of Hormone-Induced Tissue Interaction

Mammary gland development in the mouse is sexually dimorphic
already in fetal life (which is not typical for mammals in
general). Originally, mammary buds form in both sexes on day
11 to 12, their development is identical until late on day 13,
but during day 14 the rudiments of male fetuses are destroyed
by the action of testicular hormones (29). Testosterone acts
directly on the gland as shown in organ culture (30) and both
tissues of the rudiment are visibly involved in the process.
The mesenchyme forms a conspicuous condensation around the epithelial bud, this bud separates from the epidermis and eventually
all or most of the gland epithelium becomes necrotic and disappears
(29). By tissue combination experiments, utilizing the androgen-
insensitive Tfm-mutant ("testicular feminization" – ref. 31) we
could show that testosterone acts only on the mesenchyme.
Experimental combinations of normal mesenchyme with androgen-
insensitive epithelium were responsive, whereas the reciprocal
combination (normal epithelium with mutant mesenchyme) was not
(32). The testosterone-induced destruction of the epithelial bud
is, thus, not caused by the hormone directly; the effect of
testosterone is mediated by the mesenchyme and the hormone quite
dramatically interferes in the process of tissue interaction.
Morphologically, the destruction of the mammary bud is so
reminiscent of the destruction of the Müllerian ducts (33) as
to suggest a similar mechanism for both hormone-induced processes.
Although morphogenetic cell death is a common feature in vertebrate development, destruction of one tissue may certainly seem
an odd instance of epithelial-mesenchymal interaction. It is
therefore important that Cunha (34) subsequently found the same
situation to prevail in the urogenital sinus. Using the same
experimental design (Tfm - wild-type tissue combinations) he showed
that testosterone acts on the mesenchyme which then induces even

androgen-insensitive epithelium to form prostatic acini. This case is the more interesting as prostatic epithelium itself later develops androgen receptors allowing direct hormonal control of its secretory activity. During embryonic sexual differentiation, however, the hormone addresses the mesenchyme which, as mentioned, is the dominant tissue during organogenetic morphogenesis. It is also interesting to note that the autoradiographs of Stumpf and collaborators (35, 36) revealed mesenchymal localization of sex steroid receptors in embryos, especially in areas subject to sexual dimorphism, which is quite different from the situation found in adult organs.

Development of Steroid Receptors as a Consequence of Epithelial-Mesenchymal Interaction

Using explanted mammary rudiments we could show that the organ is not sensitive to testosterone during the first two days of its development (37). Hormone responsiveness is acquired late on day 13 and, surprisingly, soon lost again on day 15. The testosterone-sensitive "window" in the development of the mammary gland lasts for only about 30 hrs. Quite interestingly, explanted glands become hormone-responsive in vitro, and then insensitive again, and both developmental changes occur precisely on schedule. Therefore, whatever controls the mammary rudiment's development (and loss) of testosterone responsiveness, it must be found in the gland itself.

We have followed the appearance of testosterone receptors during the entire prenatal development of the gland (38): The first binding sites become detectable on day 12 (earliest bud stage), their number increases to about 90 to 100 x 10^6 per gland on day 14 (the responsive stage) and, then, when the gland has become insensitive again, receptors persist at high levels at least until birth (day 19). While the development of hormone responsiveness from day 12 to day 14 is correlated with a sharp increase in receptor number, loss of responsiveness is not reflected in loss or decline of receptors, the gland exhibits "receptor-positive hormone resistance".

We knew from the Tfm - wild-type tissue combinations (32)
that the receptors must be found in the mesenchyme of the gland.
Although these experiments had established the mesenchyme as the
sole target tissue for testosterone, we were puzzled to find that
mammary mesenchyme, experimentally deprived of the epithelial
bud, never showed any reaction to the addition of the hormone.
Mouse mammary epithelium could successfully be replaced by
mammary epithelia from other species (rat, even from the rabbit -
a species whose glands do not show a testosterone response),
but not by epithelia from other (mouse) organs, such as salivary
gland, pancreas (39). Finally, the role played by mammary epithelium in the mesenchyme's reaction to testosterone became
quite apparent from ^{3}H-testosterone autoradiographs, as shown in
Fig. 1 (ref. 40): Androgen receptors were localized in the
mesenchyme as expected, however, they were restricted to few
layers of mesenchymal cells surrounding each epithelial bud. This
finding immediately suggested that mammary epithelium induces
formation of testosterone receptors in adjacent mesenchyme and
this was then demonstrated again by tissue combination experiments (Fig. 3) (ref. 40). The short range of the inductive
influence, its organ specificity, the lack of species specificity,
all suggest that receptor induction represents a classical
instance of inductive tissue interaction. This is the first
system in which we know the cause for receptor formation and it
shows that epithelial-mesenchymal interaction is also involved
in the development of hormone responsiveness (which is, of course,
a differentiative function).

Estrogen Receptors and Estrogen Response of the Mammary Rudiment
The early mammary anlage is also affected by estrogens.
These hormones play no physiological role at this stage, experimentally administered they cause nipple malformation and arrest
of mammary development(41, and our own unpublished observations).
We have found that the gland possesses estrogen receptors distinct
from androgen receptors, and both types of receptors appear and
develop at the same time (in preparation). Again, ^{3}H-estradiol
is bound only by the few mesenchymal cells lining each epithelial

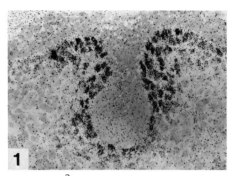 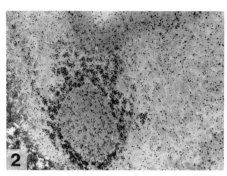

Fig. 1: ³H-Dihydrotestosterone autoradiograph of a 14-day mammary rudiment. Only the few mesenchymal cells around the gland bud and its stalk possess androgen receptors, suggesting that receptor formation had been induced by the epithelium (from ref. 40).

Fig. 2: ³H-Estradiol autoradiograph of a 14-day mammary rudiment (oblique section not showing the stalk of the gland). Distribution of estrogen receptor-containing cells in the mesenchyme is similar to the distribution of androgen receptor-possessing cells shown in Fig. 1.

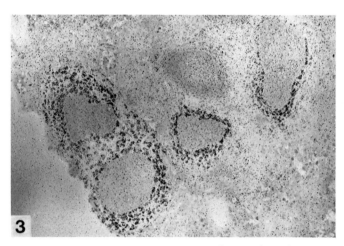

Fig. 3: Induction of androgen receptor formation in mesenchyme experimentally combined with several pieces of mammary epithelium. After 3 days in culture, each epithelial sphere has become surrounded by a halo of mesenchymal cells containing androgen receptors, as shown in this ³H-testosterone autoradiograph (from ref. 40).

bud (Fig. 2) and it thus appears that both receptors are present in the same cell. Epithelial-mesenchymal combination experiments have shown that the estrogen-receptor is induced by mammary epithelium in the same way as is the androgen receptor. Since the effect of the hormone, which acts on the mesenchyme, is to prevent outgrowth of the epithelial sprout, it is shown again that the action of estrogens on mammary gland development is mediated through the mesenchyme.

A Model for the Interplay Between Hormone Action and Tissue Interaction in the Mammary Rudiment

According to our present understanding, hormone action and epithelial-mesenchymal interaction are linked in two ways: the development of hormone responsiveness, as well as the eventual action of the hormones, both depend on specific tissue interaction (Fig. 4). First, the newly formed epithelial bud induces

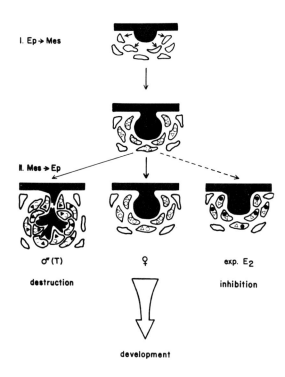

Fig. 4

neighboring mesenchymal cells to form receptors for androgens as well as estrogens. Then, this mesenchyme decides the further fate of the gland depending on its exposure to hormones. In the male (left), under the influence of testosterone, this mesenchyme causes the destruction of the epithelial bud. Experimentally applied estrogen (right) causes the mesenchyme to inhibit outgrowth of the primary epithelial sprout. In both cases, the effect of the hormones on gland development are mediated by the mesenchyme. It is only in the absence of either sex steroid that the gland is allowed to proceed in its development (center), as it does in the female fetus.

ACKNOWLEDGMENT

Parts of the original work reported here were supported by NCI Contract NO1-CB-33883, and by the Austrian Fonds zur Förderung der Wissenschaftlichen Forschung, project P 5015. I thank E. Gurtner and I. Gmachl for their help in preparing the manuscript.

REFERENCES

1. Spemann, H. Verh.Anat.Ges. 15: 61-79, 1901.
2. Grobstein, C. Nat.Cancer Inst.Monogr. 26: 279-299, 1967.
3. Wessells, N.K. Tissue Interactions and Development. W.A. Benjamin, Menlo Park, CA, 1977.
4. Kratochwil, K. In: Cell Interactions and Development: Molecular Mechanisms (Ed. K.M. Yamada) J.Wiley and Sons, New York, 1983, pp. 99-122.
5. Rutter, W.J., Wessells, N.K. and Grobstein, C. Nat.Cancer Inst.Monogr. 13: 51-64, 1964.
6. Sengel, P. Morphogenesis of Skin. Cambridge Univ.Press, Cambridge, 1976.
7. Cunha, G.R., Chung, L.W.K., Shannon, J.M., Taguchi, O. and Fujii, H. Rec.Progr. in Hormone Res. vol. 39: 559-598, 1983.
8. Kollar, E.J. and Baird, G.R. J.Embryol.Exp.Morphol. 24: 173-186, 1970.
9. Alescio, T. and Cassini, A. J.Exp.Zool. 150: 83-94, 1962.
10. Wessells, N.K. J.Exp.Zool. 175: 455-466, 1970.
11. Kratochwil, K. Develop.Biol. 20: 46-71, 1969.
12. Sakakura, T., Nishizuka, Y. and Dawe, C.J. Science 194: 1439-1441, 1976.
13. Rutter, W.J., Pictet, R.L., Harding, J.D., Chirgwin, J.M., MacDonald, R.J. and Przybyla, A.E. In: Molecular Control of Proliferation and Differentiation (Eds. J. Papaconstantinou and W.J. Rutter) Academic Press, New York, 1978, pp. 205-227.

12

14. Saxén, L., Lehtonen, E., Karkinen-Jääskeläinen, M.,
    Nordling, S. and Wartiovaara, J. Nature 259:
    662-663, 1976.
15. Thesleff, J., Lehtonen, E., Wartiovaara, J. and Saxén, L.
    Develop.Biol. 58: 197-203, 1977.
16. Bernfield, M.R. In: Morphogenesis and Pattern Formation:
    Implications for Normal and Abnormal Development.
    (Eds. L. Brinkley, B.M. Carlson and G. Connelly) Raven Press,
    New York, 1981, pp. 139-162.
17. Bernfield, M., Banerjee, S.D., Koda, J.E. and Rapraeger, A.C.
    In: Role of Extracellular Matrix in Development (Ed.
    R.L. Trelstad) Alan Liss, New York, 1984, pp. 545-572.
18. Hay, E.D. (Ed.) Cell Biology of Extracellular Matrix.
    Plenum Press, New York, 1981.
19. Piez, K.A. and Reddi, A.H. (Eds.) Extracellular Matrix
    Biochemistry. Elsevier, New York, 1984.
20. Trelstad, R.L. (ed.) The Role of Extracellular Matrix in
    Development. Alan R. Liss, New York, 1984.
21. Gordon, J. and Bernfield, M.R. Develop.Biol. 74:
    118-135, 1980.
22. Bernfield, M.R. and Banerjee, S.D. Develop.Biol. 90:
    291-305, 1982.
23. Grobstein, C. and Cohen, J. Science 150: 626-628, 1965.
24. Wessells, N.K. and Cohen, J.H. Develop.Biol. 18:
    294-309, 1968.
25. Spooner, B. and Faubion, J. Develop.Biol. 77: 84-102, 1980.
26. Sakakura, T. In: Understanding Breast Cancer. (Eds. M.A.
    Rich, J.C. Hager and P. Furmanski). Marcel Dekker, New York,
    1983, pp. 261-284.
27. David, G. and Bernfield, M.R. J.Cell Biol. 91: 281-286, 1981.
28. Parry, G., Lee, E.Y.-H., Farson, D., Koval, M. and Bissell,M.J.
    Exp.Cell Res. 156: 487-499, 1985.
29. Raynaud, A. In: Milk: The Mammary Gland and its Secretion.
    (Eds. S.K. Kon and A.T. Cowie) vol. 1, 3-46, Acad.Press,
    New York, 1961.
30. Kratochwil, K. J.Embryol.Exp.Morph. 25: 141-153, 1971.
31. Lyon, M.F. and Hawkes, S.G. Nature 227: 1217-1219, 1970.
32. Kratochwil, K. and Schwartz, P. Proc.Natl.Acad.Sci. USA
    73: 4041-4044.
33. Trelstad, R.L., Hayashi, A., Hayashi, K. and Donahoe, P.
    Develop.Biol. 92: 27-40, 1982.
34. Cunha, G.R. and Lung, B. J.Exp.Zool. 205: 181-194, 1978.
35. Stumpf, W.E., Narbaitz, R. and Sar, M. J. Steroid
    Biochem. 12: 55-64, 1980.
36. Gasc, J.-M. and Stumpf, W.E. J.Embryol.Exp.Morphol. 63:
    207-223 and 225-231, 1981.
37. Kratochwil, K. Develop.Biol. 61: 358-365, 1977.
38. Wasner, G., Hennermann, I. and Kratochwil, K.
    Endocrinology 113: 1771-1780, 1983.
39. Dürnberger, H. and Kratochwil, K. Cell 19: 465-471, 1980.
40. Heuberger, B., Fitzka, I., Wasner, G. and Kratochwil, K.
    Proc.Natl.Acad.Sci. USA 79: 2957-2961, 1982.
41. Raynaud, A. and Raynaud, J. J.Ann.Inst.Pasteur 90: 39-91
    and 187-219, 1956.

2

THE IMPORTANCE OF MATRIX INTERACTIONS AND TISSUE TOPOGRAPHY FOR THE GROWTH
AND DIFFERENTIATION OF MAMMARY EPITHELIAL CELLS IN VITRO

ELISA M. DURBAN[1],JANET S. BUTEL,JIRI BARTEK*[2],AND JOYCE TAYLOR-PAPADIMITRIOU*
Department of Virology and Epidemiology, Baylor College of Medicine, Houston
TX 77030 and *Imperial Cancer Research Fund, London, U.K.

INTRODUCTION

Mammary gland morphogenesis and mammary epithelial cell proliferation
and functional differentiation are processes which normally require various
interactions, such as those between different cells, between cells and
extracellular matrix components, and between cells, hormones, and growth
factors. How such interactions are coupled in vivo to bring about controlled
mammary cell growth and normal cell function remains to be established;
clearly, it is a problem that cannot be easily addressed experimentally in
the animal. The last few years have seen considerable progress in the
development of culture systems which permit an examination in vitro of
such interactions crucial either to normal cell behaviour or to transformed
cell characteristics. Thus, it is now possible to dissociate mammary cells
from the normal topological relationships that exist in vivo and provide
them with an in vitro environment which permits growth and reorganization
of individual cells and small units into structures with the proper tissue
topography which can express markers of epithelial cell function in response
to hormonal stimuli.

In this paper, we will review the studies on which we base our present
understanding of the conditions important for modulating the proliferative
and differentiated phenotypes of mammary epithelial cells in culture. We
will summarize and discuss data utilizing both murine and human mammary cell
systems from our own laboratories as well as others. Our discussion will
be limited to a consideration of recent studies relevant to interactions
between mammary cells and extracellular matrix components in vitro as well
as those bearing on topological relationships important for normal tissue

Present address: 1 The University of Texas, Dental Branch, Department of
                    Microbiology, Houston, TX 77225; 2 Research Institute
                    of Clinical and Exp. Oncology, Brno, Czechoslovakia

behaviour. The requirement of hormones and other soluble factors for
mammary cell growth and differentiation will be dealt with only as it
relates to the main emphasis of this discussion. For detailed descriptions
of the role of hormones in mammary gland function, the readers are referred
to recent reviews (1,2).

MAMMARY EPITHELIAL CELL BEHAVIOUR IN CULTURE
The influence of the culture substratum on mammary cell phenotype

Methods which permit limited growth of primary mammary epithelial
cells either on conventional plastic substrata (e.g. 3,4,5) or in organ-
type cultures (e.g. 6) have been available for almost two decades. Despite
the importance of these earlier studies, it is without argument that the
introduction by Emerman, Pitelka, and collaborators in 1977 (7,8) of
collagen type I as matrix for the culture of murine mammary epithelial
cells was a crucial step which prompted new approaches in the study of
synergistic interactions that regulate normal mammary cell behaviour.
A vast literature now exists which indicates that many different types
of cells can exhibit enhanced proliferative capacity and markers of
differentiation when collagen is used as the culture substratum (recently
reviewed by Yang and Nandi; 9). It is clear that the behaviour of
differentiated mammary epithelial cells can be markedly modulated by the
substrata upon which the cells are cultured (Table 1). Typically,
mammary cells expressing differentiated features in vivo lose this
phenotype when plated on a plastic surface, even in the presence of
lactogenic hormones (7,8,10,13,14). The same is true if the cells are
plated on attached collagen gels or on floating gels made inflexible
by glutaraldehyde crosslinking (7,10,11,12,15). On floating collagen
gels, however, a number of features of the differentiated phenotype are
maintained, such as cell polarization, microvilli, epithelial junctional
complexes, and lactose pools (7,10,11,14), and some functional markers
can be hormonally stimulated, such as the secretion and synthesis of the
milk proteins, the caseins (7,8,10,11,12). The potential usefulness of
collagen as substrata for culture is further illustrated by experiments
in which expression of the mammary differentiated phenotype could be
modulated by cycling the cells from plastic, where they had lost their
differentiated phenotype, onto floating collagen gels where reexpression
of differentiated markers was still possible (7,10). It should be noted

Table 1. The influence of the culture substratum on hormonally-responsive mammary cell phenotype.

Source of mammary tissue	Culture substratum	Lactogenic hormones	Expression of differentiation markers*	References
Midpregnant mice	plastic	(+ or -)	lost	7,8,10
	on attached collagen** gels	(+ or -)	lost	7,10,11
	on floating collagen gels crosslinked with glutaraldehyde	(+)	lost	11,12
	on floating collagen gels	(-)	some maintained for a short period	8,11
		(+)	maintained and enhanced	7,8,10,11,12
	plastic →floating collagen gels	(+)	reexpressed	7,10
Lactating mice dissociated cells	plastic	(+ or -)	lost	13,14
	floating collagen gels	(-)	some maintained for a short period	13,14
		(+)	maintained	14
alveoli	floating collagen gels	(+)	maintained; also induced synthesis and secretion of lactose	15

* at approximately 1 wk of plating
** rat tail collagen consisting primarily of collagen type I

that although lactose pools in dissociated mammary cells from lactating
mice can be maintained for short periods on floating collagen gels, the
ability to synthesize and secrete lactose becomes impaired in those cultures
(14). This late marker of secretory mammary function appears to require
maintenance of tissue architecture in culture, as lactose synthesis has only
been possible when the mammary tissue cultured on the collagen matrix
consisted of integral alveolar units (15).

Growth and morphogenesis within collagen gels

A modification of the culture system discussed above was introduced
by Yang et al. (16) who utilized the collagen as a 3-dimensional matrix.
By embedding dissociated or partially dissociated mammary tissue within
the collagen prior to its gelation, a culture environment results which
supports two unique features: (1) maintenance of the proliferative capacity
of mammary cells over an extended period of time in culture, and (2) ability
of dissociated cells and small tissue units to grow and rearrange themselves
into 3-dimensional duct-like structures with a morphology closely resembling
the topography of the intact mammary gland. Fig. 1 shows an example of
this type of growth when dissociated mammary cells from virgin mice are
embedded and maintained within attached collagen gels. Human mammary
organoids (epithelial multicellular structures) show a similar morphogenesis
when grown in collagen gels; however, the branching is more evident when
the gels are floated (17, 18).

Mammary cells from midpregnant and lactating mice behave similarly with
respect to the generation of 3-dimensional structures in collagen. The
overall efficiency of growth, however, is less when the cultures are
initiated using mouse mammary cells derived from fully functional lactating
glands (19) or cells isolated from human milk samples. This decreased
growth potential may reflect reduced proliferative capacity of cells that
have already initiated the program of terminal differentiation which leads
to gland involution in vivo.

To analyze morphogenesis in the collagen, human mammary organoids were
pulse-labelled with ^{3}H-thymidine and then sectioned and processed for
autoradiography. The 3-dimensional ductal pattern was found to occur by
random proliferation of cells throughout the growing structure (Fig. 2;
Bartek, Durban, Taylor-Papadimitriou, unpublished observations). That
tissue-like organization occurs within the collagen matrix is supported
by the generation of a lumen within many of the outgrowths. A representative

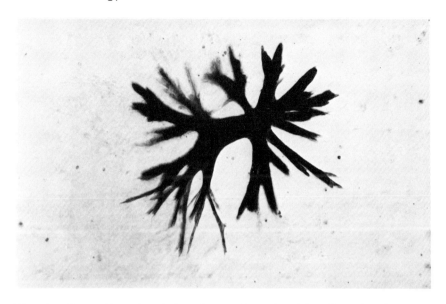

Fig. 1. Three-dimensional ductal growth produced by dissociated mammary epithelial cells from virgin mice within attached collagen gels. Cells shown after 2 wks of growth. X150.

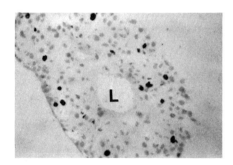

Fig. 2. Section through a human mammary organoid cultured within collagen for 6 days. The cells were labelled with ^{3}H-thymidine the last 3 days of culture. Lumen (L). X75.

electron micrograph of mammary cells from virgin mice after 2 wks of growth in collagen is shown in Fig. 3. A group of morphologically polarized cells exhibit numerous microvilli projecting towards a lumen. It is worth noting that with mammary cells derived from virgin mice this type of tissue-like growth is not dependent upon the addition of lactogenic hormones, in contrast to the hormonal requirement of the same cells under

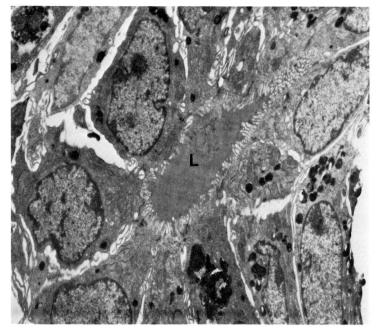

Fig. 3. Electron micrograph of a section through a 3-dimensional outgrowth produced by mammary epithelial cells from virgin mice within collagen illustrating lumen (L) formation and cell polarization. X7560.

those conditions for the expression of markers of cell function (see below).

The generation of lumina by human mammary organoids within free-floating collagen gels has been critically analyzed by Foster et al. (17). An important observation made by those investigators is that while the mammary organoids retain the proper tissue topography after collagenase digestion, dramatic changes in cell organization occur within 48-96 hr in collagen, resulting in partial loss of the proper topological relationships. Following cell growth and polarization of cytoplasmic organelles, however, cell migration occurs which leads both to formation of lumina and to restoration of topological organization (17).

Expression in collagen of markers representative of tissue topological relationships

The above observations concerning morphogenesis of the mammary outgrowths suggested to us that the environment provided by the 3-dimensional collagen culture system promotes cellular behaviour similar to that in

the mammary gland in vivo. It appears that the proper topological relationships are not merely maintained but can actually be generated in culture.
Thus, we addressed the question of whether the tissue-like organization
of the structures produced in collagen is an accurate reflection of the
cell phenotypes expressed in vivo. Our approach has been, first,to define
the cell types within the human mammary organoids grown in collagen using
well-characterized monoclonal antibodies to cytokeratins and to differentiation antigens, and second, to relate these findings to the cell phenotypes expressed in vivo as visualized in tissue sections of resting breast.
The resting breast tissue utilized in these studies was processed into
epithelial organoids of varying sizes according to the procedure of
Hallowes et al. (20). Based on differential filtration, this procedure
yields three fairly homogeneous fractions of mammary organoids: (1) large
ducts greater than 400 μ in size, (2) smaller ducts and ductules which are
retained by 200 μ filters, and (3) terminal duct lobular units which are
greater than 95 μ in size. The cell fraction remaining after filtration
consists primarily of fibroblasts which can be used as controls for the
in vitro assays of cell phenotypes. The isolated mammary organoids were
embedded in collagen using standard techniques (16,19,20) and maintained
for up to 1 month in serum-containing medium supplemented with insulin,
transferrin, epidermal growth factor, and hydrocortisone. In some
experiments, prolactin was also added to the culture medium. Control
cultures were maintained on plastic for the duration of the experiments.
After allowing for a period of growth and cell reorganization in collagen
(2-3 wks), cryostat sections were prepared from the embedded organoids,
the sections were reacted with the antibodies, and then processed either
for indirect immunofluorescence or immunoenzyme assay.

A description of the monoclonal antibodies utilized and the cell
types and cellular products recognized is summarized in Table 2. These
include monoclonal antibodies to the cytokeratins which, in the human
breast, allow discrimination between epithelial and stromal elements
(LP34; 21), between lumenal (secretory) and basal (myoepithelial) epithelial
cell populations (LE61; 22), between lumenal cells with different
proliferative capacities (BA16; 23 and Bartek et al., MS in preparation),
and between lumenal cells undergoing different pathways of differentiation,
i.e., secretory vs squamous (RKSE-60; 24). Two monoclonal antibodies to
differentiation antigens present in the human milk fat globule, HMFG-1

and HMFG-2, were utilized as a measure of secretory activity by the cultured cells. The epitopes recognized by the HMFG antibodies are heterogeneously expressed in resting breast. The HMFG-1 epitope, however, is strongly expressed in lactating epithelial cells while the epitope recognized by the HMFG-2 antibody is expressed only weakly in normal lactating tissue (25). Whatever the physiological state, both these epitopes are expressed exclusively by the lumenal epithelial cells. Lastly, we employed an antibody to cell-associated fibronectin (FN-3; 26) in an effort to follow deposition of a basement membrane.

Table 2. Monoclonal antibodies utilized to compare human mammary cell phenotypes in vitro and in vivo.

Antibody	Antigens Recognized	Cell populations distinguished	Ref.
LP34	all human epithelia	epithelial vs nonepithelial	21
LE61	all mammary lumenal epithelial cells	lumenal vs basal	22
BA16	some lumenal epithelial cells	subsets of lumenal cells	23
RKSE-60	suprabasal cells in skin (no reaction with normal breast	squamous vs secretory	24
HMFG-1	surface mucin (milk fat globule membrane)	secretory lumenal epithelia	25
HMFG-2	surface mucin	secretory lumenal epithelia	25
FN-3	cell-associated fibronectin	deposition of basement membrane	26

From the results summarized in Table 3, it is apparent that the growth and cell reorganization that takes place within the collagen matrix can generate the full complement and arrangement of mammary cell phenotypes detectable in sections of resting breast. The staining patterns observed with the keratin monoclonal antibodies LE61 and BA16 provide evidence of the in vitro expression of the lumenal and basal cell phenotypes. The

lack of staining with the marker of squamous differentiation, RKSE-60,
indicates that even after 1 month of culture within the collagen matrix
the mammary cells remain committed to the secretory pathway of differentiation. In addition, this interpretation is supported by the reactivity
obtained with antibodies against the differentiation markers, HMFG-1 and
HMFG-2. The staining with these latter antibodies is enhanced after
culture within collagen and is restricted to the lumenal epithelial cells
(Fig. 4, A and B). It should be noted that the expression of HMFG-1 and
HMFG-2 did not appear to be influenced by prolactin levels in the medium.
Further evidence of normal cell behaviour is suggested by the reactivity
obtained with the organoids in collagen (Fig. 4C), but not prior to
culture, with fibronectin antibodies that discriminated a structure
presumed to be a basement membrane.

Table 3. Staining patterns of monoclonal antibodies with human mammary
cells in vitro and in vivo.

| | Resting breast | | Mammary organoids* | | | |
| | | | prior to culture | | after culture in collagen** | |
Antibody	lumenal	basal	lumenal	basal	lumenal	basal
LP34	+++	+++	+++	+++	+++	+++
LE61	++	-	++	-	++	-
BA16	++	-	++	-	++	-
	-		-		-	
RKSE-60	-	-	-	-	-	-
HMFG-1	-/+	-	-/+	-	+	-
HMFG-2	-/+	-	-/+	-	++/+++	-

* these results apply to the 200 μ fraction of organoids
**expression at approximately 3 wks of culture

It is informative to compare the phenotypes of human mammary cells
grown on plastic with those grown in the collagen gels. It has been
shown that mammary epithelial cells from reduction mammoplasty organoids
can be grown and passaged in both serum-containing and defined media
(27, 28). The staining patterns we have obtained for human mammary cells
grown on plastic in serum-containing medium indicate that the topography-
specific expression of cell phenotypes is disrupted and the squamous
pathway of differentiation is favored even in the absence of cAMP elevating

22

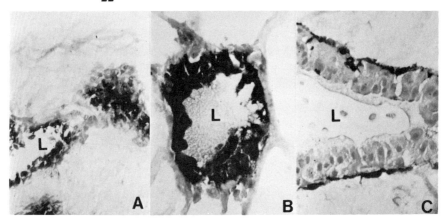

Fig. 4. Staining pattern of human mammary organoids (200 µ fraction) by immunoenzyme assay with monoclonal antibodies (A)HMFG-1, (B)HMFG-2, and (C)FN-3. Lumen (L). X85.

agents. These observations emphasize the potential that the combined approaches of 3-dimensional growth in collagen and well-characterized immunological cell markers introduce to the delineation of cell lineages in the mammary gland as well as to the examination of matrix and cell interactions in normal and abnormal processes.

A detailed examination of the cell phenotypes generated in collagen by mouse mammary cells, as described here for human cells, has not been undertaken to date. That some effort should be invested in such studies is illustrated by the popularity of the murine system for studies on the hormonal control of mammary cell growth and differentiation and on factors that influence the development of mammary tumors.

Maintenance vs induction of mammary-specific cell functions in culture

In studies of the expression of mammary cell-specific functions in culture, an important distinction to be made is between the maintenance of a function whose expression had been initiated in vivo and the induction of a function which requires that all steps crucial to bring about its expression be reproduced by the in vitro environment. Tonelli and Sorof (29) were the first investigators to clearly address this distinction in vitro utilizing the 3-dimensional collagen system and mammary cells from virgin mice. They showed that mammary cells from virgin mice can be induced to synthesize caseins, the major milk proteins, in response to hormonal stimuli if the cells are cultured under conditions that permit

3-dimensional growth. We extended these observations using cells from unprimed virgin BALB/c mice in two ways; we examined both qualitative and quantitative characteristics of casein synthesis in vitro and compared those to in vivo values, and we analyzed the influence of time of culture in collagen on the process of induction (19). Primary cultures of dissociated mammary cells from virgin mice were embedded in collagen and maintained in serum-containing medium supplemented with insulin for up to 4 wks. At various times, medium containing lactogenic hormones (prolactin, hydrocortisone, and aldosterone) was added and the behaviour of the cells was monitored every 3-7 days over a period of 8 wks with respect to casein synthesis and cell growth. Casein synthesis was assayed quantitatively by an ELISA competition assay and qualitatively by the immunoblot procedure for gel-purified proteins using specific antisera against purified mouse caseins. Our observations showed that mammary cell growth within the collagen matrix plateaus after 1 wk in culture, at which time morphological differentiation (illustrated in Fig. 3) and 3-dimensional organization (shown in Fig. 1) are clearly recognizable.

An unexpected finding was that the duration of culture within the collagen prior to hormonal stimulation influences the kinetics of casein synthesis (Table 4). Cells that had been cultured for only 1 wk in growth medium (i.e., medium without lactogenic hormones) did not accumulate detectable levels of casein until after 3 wks of exposure to lactogenic hormones, whereas cells cultured for either 2 or 4 wks responded by accumulating caseins after 2 wks and 3 days of induction, respectively. While the levels of total caseins that accumulated under optimal conditions on induction in culture were comparable to the levels found during lactation in vivo (19), the relative proportion of specific casein poly-peptides synthesized in culture was altered from α casein (43K) in favor of the β casein (30K) species as in the midpregnant state (Fig. 5). Addition of lactogenic hormones at the time of embedding did not alter the observed time response.

These results suggest that a period of culture within the collagen, independent of cell growth and morphological differentiation, is required to permit mammary epithelial cells from unprimed mammary glands to become responsive for hormone-induced differentiation. As discussed below, one possible explanation is that during growth within collagen the cells synthesize and deposit extracellular matrix components that are important

Table 4. Kinetics of casein accumulation in collagen by mammary epithelial cells from virgin mice in the presence and absence of lactogenic hormones.

Sample[a]	Time in growth medium (weeks)	Time in induction medium (weeks)	Total time in culture (weeks)	Cells/collagen Gel (X 10^{-6})	Detection of casein polypeptides by immunoblot assay[b]
Control	1	none	1	2.2	0
	2	none	2	4.0	0
	3	none	3	3.1	0
	4	none	4	1.3	0
	5	none	5	3.6	0
	7	none	7	3.3	0
Set 1	1	3 days	1 wk,3days	3.1	0
	1	1	2	3.0	0
	1	2	3	2.0	0
	1	3	4	2.0	+
	1	4	5	4.5	++
	1	6	7	4.5	+++ (10 ng/μg protein)[c]
Set 2	2	3 days	2 wk,3days	2.0	0
	2	1	3	1.4	0
	2	2	4	2.1	++
	2	3	5	3.4	++
	2	5	7	4.0	+++ (12 ng/μg protein)
Set 3	4	3 days	4 wk,3days	2.0	+++
	4	1	5	1.5	++
	4	3	7	3.0	++++(20 ng/μg protein)

a   5 x 10^5 cells were seeded per culture.

b   0=none detected; + to ++++ = relative intensity of casein bands in immunoblot assay.

c   amount of casein as determined in the competition ELISA assay.

in modulating the responsiveness of the cells to lactogenic hormones.

We have recently attempted to apply the knowledge gained from the studies with mammary cells from virgin mice to the human system. We directed our efforts at establishing conditions appropiate for inducing functional differentiation in culture with human mammary organoids from resting breast. As yet, efforts to induce expression of casein and/or α-lactalbumin by the human cells have been unsuccessful, despite evidence of both morphological differentiation and expression of differentiation antigens, HMFG-1 and HMFG-2 (see above; Fig. 4) by the cells.

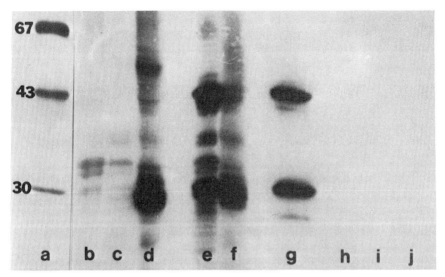

Fig. 5. Qualitative analysis of intracellular casein polypeptides in mouse mammary cell extracts by immunoblot detection using antiserum against total mouse caseins. Lane a, molecular weight markers; lane b, uncultured mammary cells from virgin mice; lane c, mammary cells from virgin mice cultured for 6 wks in collagen in the absence of lactogenic hormones; land d, same cells as in lane c but induced with lactogenic hormones the last 2 wks in culture; lane e, uncultured mammary cells from lactating mice; lane f, uncultured mammary cells from midpregnant mice; lane g, mouse caseins standard; lanes h-j, same samples as those in lanes b-d but reacted with preimmune serum. Bound antibodies were detected using 125I-labeled protein A. 75 μg protein were loaded per lane.

ELEMENTS OF THE INTERACTION BETWEEN THE COLLAGEN SUBSTRATUM AND MAMMARY CELLS THAT INFLUENCE EXPRESSION OF FUNCTIONAL MARKERS

The role of the collagen substratum on the modulation of mammary cell behaviour in culture has been addressed experimentally and theoretically (11,30,31,32,33,34). There are at least three elements of the cell-matrix interaction that appear to be important in the modulation of the mammary cell phenotype. First, the flexibility of the collagen matrix has marked effects on cell shape (7,11,13). Second, the culture substratum can modulate the synthesis and stability of cell-secreted extracellular matrix components (e.g., glycosaminoaglycans (GAG's), collagen type IV) which undoubtedly determine whether a recognizable basement membrane is deposited and assembled (33,35). Finally, the culture substratum can have an effect on the synthesis and stability of mammary-specific mRNA's and their protein products (32,36).

Acquisition of cell shape and orientation typical of mammary secretory cells appears to be a necessary step for the expression of morphological and functional markers of secretory cell differentiation in culture. This was illustrated (Table 1) by the loss of mammary differentiated features when the cells grow as flat monolayers on plastic, on attached collagen gels, or on inflexible glutaraldehyde-fixed gels. As discussed above, we observed that mammary cells not primed for differentiation in vivo appear to require a period of contact with the collagen matrix before they accumulated detectable levels of caseins (19). This time interval was greater than that required for changes in cell shape, organization into 3-dimensional structures, and expression of morphological differentiation. Thus, we speculated that during this time the cells secrete basement membrane components such as collagen type IV and GAG's which may be participants in the sequence of events that regulate gene expression (30).

Recently, Parry et al. (33) examined the influence of the culture substratum on the synthesis of GAG's by differentiated mouse mammary cells. Their findings indicate that the culture substratum influences both the relative amounts of GAG's produced by the cells and their extracellular fate. Cells grown under conditions permissive for functional differentiation (e.g., floating collagen gels) deposit an extracellular matrix rich in dermatan sulfate. In contrast, cells grown on plastic or on attached gels synthesize a GAG fraction rich in hyaluronic acid and low in dermatan sulfate and over 50% of this fraction is secreted into the culture medium rather than assembled into an extracellular matrix.

The generation of basement membrane-like structures by mouse (7,13,35) and human (36) mammary cells in vitro is dependent upon the culture substratum and correlates with the ability of the cells to express markers of differentiation. Interestingly, human milk cells, a rather homogeneous population of secretory cells, favor the pathway of squamous differentiation in collagen despite their capacity to generate 3-dimensional ductal structures. This observation is likely to reflect the lack of myoepithelial cells in the cell population and the inability of the secretory milk cells to deposit a basement membrane-like structure. Relevant to this, differentiated rat mammary epithelial cells degenerate on collagen type I matrices if maintained under conditions which prevent the myoepithelial components from producing collagen type IV (37).

Thus, in attempting to define the interaction between the collagenous substratum and mammary epithelial cells, the contribution of the interaction between different cell types should not be underestimated. Such consideration is particularly relevant to studies where the main source of biological material is provided by established cell lines, often consisting of a homogeneous population of cells, far removed from the original topography and physiology of the mammary gland. As a note of interest, in our experience to date, the only cell line that has exhibited inducibility for the synthesis of casein in collagen is the mouse mammary epithelial cell line, COMMA-1D (38; Durban, Medina, and Butel, unpublished observations). This cell line consists of a heterogeneous population of cells with potential for in vivo and in vitro morphogenesis (38; Medina and Oborn, MS submitted).

Lastly, it is now apparent that the collagen substratum can also affect the level of synthesis and stability of mammary-specific mRNA's and their protein products. For example, Lee et al. (32) recently showed that differentiated mouse mammary cells on floating collagen gels accumulate 3-10 fold more casein mRNA in response to lactogenic hormones than when cultured on plastic or on attached collagen gels. Importantly, mouse mammary cells on plastic do synthesize small amounts of caseins which are rapidly degraded intracellularly.

CONCLUSIONS

It is clear that the approaches and observations discussed here with cells in culture provide a framework for defining the events that regulate the synergistic interactions characteristic of normal mammary cell behaviour in vivo. It is our belief that the collagen culture system introduced by Nandi and collaborators (9) which permits the generation of 3-dimensional tissue-like structures is particularly useful in studies where the source of biological material is either established cell lines or mammary cells not primed for differentiation in vivo.

Two unique advantages of the 3-dimensional collagen system should be emphasized. First, the proliferative potential of the mammary cells is maintained in culture, thus, allowing the generation of sufficient cells under various conditions of growth and differentiation to carry out biochemical experiments. Second, the parameters of growth and differentiation can be dissociated in culture as the expression of markers of cell function can be modulated due to maintenance and/or induction of the hormonally-responsive phenotype.

As an example of the potential applications of this system, we have taken advantage of the ability to dissociate growth and differentiation in culture to study the expression of mouse mammary tumor virus proteins in the course of normal mammary cell growth and differentiation in collagen in comparison to normal mammary gland development in vivo. Results of those studies have provided evidence that normal mouse cells expressing the functional mammary cell phenotype have an enhanced permissiveness for processing viral structural proteins (Durban, Medina, and Butel, MS in preparation), an observation which may have implications in the development of the mammary preneoplastic and/or neoplastic phenotypes.

ACKNOWLEDGMENTS

From Baylor College of Medicine, we are grateful to Dr. Dan Medina for advice and support in work with mouse mammary cells, and Dr. Egon Durban for his help with the preparation of the mouse caseins antiserum. From the Imperial Cancer Research Fund, we are indebted to Dr. R.C. Hallowes for providing and processing the human mammary tissue and Dr. J. Burchell for help and advice concerning differentiation-antigen expression by human mammary cells. E.M.D. was a recipient of a National Service Award (CA 06984) from the National Institutes of Health. This work was supported in part by research grant CA 25215 from the National Institutes of Health to J.S.B.

REFERENCES

1. Vonderhaar, B.K. Hormones and Growth Factors in Mammary Gland Development. In: Control of Cell Growth and Proliferation, C.M. Venezrale (ed.), Van Nostrand, Reinhold and Co., 1984, pp 11-33.
2. Vonderhaar, B.K. and Bhattacharjee, M. The Mammary Gland: a Model for Hormonal Control of Differentiation and Preneoplasia. In: Biological Responses in Cancer: Progress Toward Potential Application, Vol III, E. Mihich (ed.), Plenum Publishing Co., N.Y. (in press).
3. Lasfargues, E. Y. Anat. Rec. 127: 117-130, 1957.
4. Daniel, C.W. and DeOme, K.B. Science 149: 634-636, 1965.
5. Buehring, G.C. J. Natl. Cancer Inst. 49: 1433-1434, 1972.
6. Topper, Y.J., Oka, T., Owens, I.S., and Vonderhaar, B.K. In Vitro 8:

228-234, 1972.
7. Emerman, J.T. and Pitelka, D. R. In Vitro 13: 316-328, 1977.
8. Emerman, J. T., Enami, J., Pitelka, D. R., and Nandi, S. Proc. Natl. Acad. Sci. USA 74: 4466-4470, 1977.
9. Yang, J. and Nandi, S. Int. Rev. Cyt. 81: 249-286, 1983.
10. Bissell, M. J. Int. Rev. Cyt. 70: 27-100, 1981.
11. Shannon, J. M. and Pitelka, D. R. In Vitro 17: 1016-1028, 1981.
12. Lee, E.Y.-H., Parry, G., and Bissell, M. J. J. Cell Bio. 98: 146-155, 1984.
13. Emerman, J. T., Burwen, S. J., and Pitelka, D. R. Tissue Cell 11: 109-119, 1979.
14. Burwen, S. J. and Pitelka, D. R. Exp. Cell Res. 126: 249-262, 1980.
15. Cline, P.R., Zamora, P.O., and Hosick, H.L. In Vitro 18: 694-702, 1982.
16. Yang, J., Richards, R. J., Bowman, P., Guzman, R., Enami, J., McCormick K., Hamamoto, S., Pitelka, D., and Nandi, S. Proc. Natl. Acad. Sci. USA 77: 2088-2092, 1979.
17. Foster, C.S., Smith, C. A., Dinsdale, E. A., Monaghan, P., and Neville A.M. Dev. Bio. 96: 197-216, 1983.
18. Taylor-Papadimitriou, J., Bartek, J., Durban, E. M., Burchell, J., Hallowes, R. C., Lane, E. B., and Millis, R. In: Monoclonal Antibodies and Breast Cancer, R. Ceriani (ed.), 1985 (in press).
19. Durban, E. M., Medina, D., and Butel, J. S. Dev. Bio., 1985 (in press).
20. Hallowes, R. C., Bone, E. J., and Jones, W. In: Tissue Culture in Medical Research, R. J. Richards, and K. T. Rajan (eds.), Pergamon Press, Oxford, Vol II, pp. 215-245, 1980.
21. Taylor-Papadimitriou, J., Lane, E. B., and Chang, S. E. In: Understanding Breast Cancer, M. A. Rich, J. C. Hager, and P. Furmanski (eds.), Marcel Dekker, Inc., pp. 215-245, 1983.
22. Lane, E. B. J. Cell Biol. 92: 665-673, 1982.
23. Bartek, J., Durban, E. M., Hallowes, R. C., and Taylor-Papadimitriou, J. J. Cell Science, 1985 (in press).
24. Ramaekers, F.C.S., Puts, J. J. G., Moesker, O., Kant, A., Huysmans, A., Haag, D., Jap, P.H.K., Herman, C. J., and Vooijs, G. P. Histochem. J. 15: 691-713, 1983.
25. Taylor-Papadimitriou, J., Peterson, J. A., Arklie, J., Burchell, J., Cerianin, R. L., and Bodmer, W. J. Int. J. Cancer 28: 17-21, 1981.
26. Keen J., Chang, S.E., and Taylor-Papadimitriou. J. Mol Biol. Med. 2: 15-27, 1984.
27. Stampfer, M., Hallowes, R. C., and Hackett, A. J. In Vitro 16: 415-425, 1980.
28. Hammond, S. L., Ham, R. G., and Stampfer, M. R. Proc. Natl. Acad. Sci. 81: 5435-5439, 1984.
29. Tonelli, Q.J., and Sorof, S. Differentiation 22: 195-200, 1982.
30. Bissell, M. J., Hall, H. G., and Parry, G. J. Theor. Biol. 99: 31-68, 1982.
31. Emerman, J. T., Bartley, J. C., and Bissell, M. J. Exp. Cell Res. 134: 241-250, 1981.
32. Lee, E.Y.-H., Lee, W.-H., Kaetzel, C.S., Parry, G., and Bissell, M.J. Proc. Natl. Acad. Sci. USA 82: 1419-1423, 1985.
33. Parry, G., Lee, E.Y.-H., Farson, D., Koval, M., and Bissell, M.J. Exp. Cell Res. 156: 487-499, 1985.
34. Haeuptle, M.-T., Suard, Y.L.M., Bogenmann, E., Reggio, H., Racine, L., and Kraehenbuhl, J.-P. J. Cell Biol. 96: 1425-1434, 1983.
35. David, G., and Bernfield, M. Proc. Natl. Acad. Sci. USA 76: 786-790, 1979.

36. Peachey, L. A. and Smolira, M. A. Histochem. J. 16: 819-834, 1984.
37. Wicha, M. S., Liotta, L. A., Vonderhaar, B. K., and Kidwell, W. R. Dev. Bio. 80: 253-266, 1980.
38. Danielson, K. G., Oborn, C. J., Durban, E. M., Butel, J. S., and Medina, D. Proc. Natil. Acad. Sci. USA 81: 3756-3760, 1984.

3

REGULATION OF MAMMARY EPITHELIAL CELL PROLIFERATION: AN IN VITRO MOUSE MAMMARY EPITHELIAL CELL MODEL SYSTEM

W. IMAGAWA[1], G. BANDYOPADHYAY[1], M. SPENCER[2], J. LI[3], S. NANDI[1]
[1]Cancer Research Laboratory, University of California, Berkeley, CA 94720;
[2]Lab. of Growth & Development of Children's Hospital, San Francisco, CA 94118;
[3]Medical Research Labs., V.A. Medical Center, Minneapolis, MN 55417 U.S.A.

INTRODUCTION

The fundamental challenge in cancer biology today is to understand the abnormal growth control of tumor cells. Undoubtedly, as recent work on cellular oncogenes has indicated (1), there can be multiple abnormalities in growth regulation. The complexity of abnormal growth regulation seems imposing but, perhaps, it will become less intimidating if normal growth control is better understood. It is probably true that an understanding of the variations in tumor growth control must rest upon a foundation built from sound knowledge of the growth regulation of normal cells.

We have developed a serum-free, collagen gel culture system for normal and tumor mouse mammary epithelial cells in which the cells grow when embedded within a collagen gel matrix. Most of the work has been directed toward the dissection of the growth regulation of normal cells. By normal cells, we mean epithelial cells placed into primary culture where their growth is dependent upon the immediate nutritional/hormonal milieu, unlike cell lines which have undergone adaptation and selection for growth in vitro. Primary culture allows the study of growth responses which the cells may be capable of in vivo although additional constraints or modifications of growth responses related to epithelial/stromal interactions, tissue architecture, and unknown soluble factors may exist as well in vivo.

It is this complexity inherent in the regulation of mammary gland growth and development in vivo (reviewed in 2) that has provided the impetus for developing cell culture systems in which the growth and differentiation of the cells can be studied under defined conditions. These systems could be used to examine the direct effects of hormones on growth and differentiaton and to identify and examine the relationships among newly discovered growth factors and known hormones or nutritional factors involved in the regulation of these events. In this way in vitro systems can be used to sort out the complex interplay among physiologically relevant regulatory factors. The ultimate goal of cell culture would be the complete recapitulation of a mammary epithelial tree in vitro under defined conditions representing strict fidelity in the appropriate cellular growth, morphogenetic, and differentiative programs. Taking a step in this direction, we have succeeded in culturing mouse mammary epithelial cells for up to two months and have demonstrated that their growth is directly stimulated in vitro by mammogenic hormones. Perhaps, most striking of all, we have been able to grow normal cells in a variety of serum-free media. These different culture systems may serve as models for illuminating different pathways involved in the growth regulation of these cells.

SERUM-FREE COLLAGEN GEL CULTURE MODEL SYSTEM

Mammary epithelial cells are obtained by collagenase digestion of minced BALB/c mouse mammary glands followed by filtration through 150 μ Nitex and enrichment for epithelial cells by Percoll gradient centrifugation. The epithelial cell clumps or organoids are then mixed into an isosmotic, neutralized rat tail collagen solution (kept liquefied at 4°C) and pipetted into the desired culture dish. The collagen, containing the cells within it, is allowed to gel at room temperature and the appropriate culture medium added (see 3 for details). A HEPES-buffered (20 mM) 1:1 mixture of Ham's F12:Dulbecco's modified Eagle's medium serves as the basal serum-free medium. Hormones, growth factors, lipids etc. are added to this medium as described. The original serum-free formulation contained insulin, epidermal growth factor (EGF), and bovine serum albumin (fraction V) as essential supplements for sustaining growth (4). These requirements have changed following subsequent work showing that liposomes constructed from crude soybean lecithin can substitute for EGF and albumin.

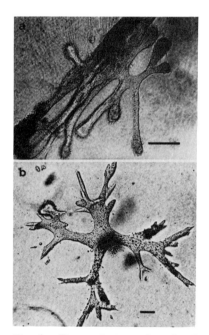

Fig. 1. Phase photographs of colonies growing in collagen gels. a) slowly growing colony exhibiting in vivo-like morphogenesis; b) faster growing colony than in (a) exhibiting a stellate morphogenesis. (bars = 100 μ)

There are two noteworthy features about this method of culturing mouse mammary epithelial cells. The first is that the cells can undergo prolonged and multifold colonial growth (not attainable when cells are cultured on plastic surfaces) and, second, the three-dimensional growth can produce a ductal-like morphogenesis. Fig. Ia shows a colony (originating from a single clump of cells seeded into the collagen) which has grown slowly forming long tubular arms and apparently undergoing branching morphogenesis. When growth is accelerated then the cell clumps form a more stellate morphology as seen in Fig. Ib. The epithelial nature of these cells has been demonstrated (5,6) and the cells are capable of Type IV collagen and laminin synthesis (7). Cells from mature virgin mice are capable of casein synthesis (unpublished observations) and by electron microscopy look secretory when stimulated by mammogenic hormones (6). These coordinate growth, morphogenetic, and differentiative responses of cells cultured in collagen gels are appealing in that they mimic more closely than culture systems using plastic substrata the normal developmental and hormonal responses seen in vivo.

FACTORS INFLUENCING MOUSE MAMMARY EPITHELIAL CELL GROWTH IN VITRO IN SERUM-FREE CULTURE

Insulin and somatomedin C.

When insulin was first tested in serum-free culture in the presence of cholera toxin, bovine serum albumin, and EGF it was found to be required for growth at an optimum concentration of 10 µg/ml (half-maximum was about 1 µg/ml) (4). This optimum concentration is high but can be reduced to 0.1 µg/ml if insulin is tested in medium containing liposomes of the appropriate composition. Further experience has shown that the strict requirement for insulin, probably reflecting insulin effects on cell viability, can be obviated only by somatomedin C (unpublished observation). Somatomedin C (50 ng/ml) can stimulate growth to the same extent as insulin (10 µg/ml) indicating that the requirement for a supraphysiological concentration of insulin to produce optimum growth may reflect, in part, the binding of insulin to somatomedin C receptors (8).

Epidermal growth factor.

Epidermal growth factor (EGF) is highly growth-stimulatory (1-10 ng/ml) to cells from virgin or midpregnant mice (6). The stimulatory effect occurs only if insulin or somatomedin C is also present in the medium. Although EGF is a potent growth promoter in vitro, mouse cells are not entirely dependent upon EGF for growth since EGF can be replaced by mammogenic hormones or phospholipids.

Mammogenic hormones.

In vivo, adrenal corticoids, prolactin or growth hormone, and ovarian steroids are known to stimulate mammary gland development (2). Table I lists

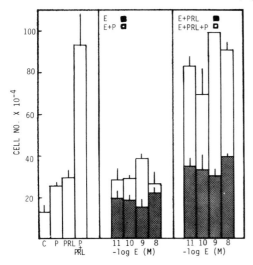

those mammogenic hormones which have been found to stimulate mouse mammary epithelial cell growth in serum-free collagen gel culture. Of these hormones, progesterone and prolactin are the most potent growth-stimulating hormones in vitro exhibiting a pronounced synergistic effect (6). Unlike EGF which is highly growth stimulatory to cells from virgin or midpregnant mice, mammogenic hormones are a more potent growth stimulant for cells from virgin mice (2- to 10-fold vs. at best 1.5- to 2-fold, for midpregnant mice).

Fig. 2. Cells from mature virgin BALB/c mice were cultured for 10 days in serum-free medium containing insulin (10 μg/ml) and liposomes (.01 μmole phosphate/ml). Hormones were added as indicated. C (control), P (progesterone, 10^{-7} M), PRL (ovine prolactin, 1 μg/ml), E (estrogen). At 10 days the cultures were terminated for DNA assay. Mean ± SD of 3 gels per combination is shown.

Notably absent from Table I is estrogen which is thought to be involved in ductal growth and lobuloalveolar development in mice. The effect of 17β-estradiol

Table I. In vivo mammogenic hormones that stimulate the growth of mouse mammary epithelial cells from virgin mice in vitro.

Hormone	Stimulate alone	Synergism with mammogenic hormones
progesterone (P)	yes	PRL
ovine, mouse prolactin (PRL)	yes	P,DOC,B,A
deoxycorticosterone (DOC)	yes	PRL
corticosterone (B)	no	PRL
aldosterone (A)	no	PRL
insulin	no	permissive requirement

Tested in serum-free medium containing insulin.

on growth was evaluated using cells from intact or ovariectomized mature virgin and midpregnant mice. It was tested alone or in combination with progesterone and/or prolactin in serum-free medium supplemented with EGF (10 ng/ml) or liposomes, and insulin (10 μg/ml). Fig. 2 shows the results of one experiment using cells from mature virgin mice cultured in medium containing liposomes and insulin (10 μg/ml). As can be seen, in this and other experiments, estradiol did not stimulate growth. Mouse mammary epithelial cells cultured in serum-free medium do contain a low level of estrogen receptors (50-200 fm/mg DNA) but they seem functional as demonstrated by estrogen-induced nuclear translocation and estrogen induction of progesterone receptors in culture (9).

We have undertaken an exhaustive series of experiments in which experimental conditions have been modified in attempts to determine if estrogen can directly stimulate growth. These experimental modifications are listed in Table 2. The effect of some of the other estrogens or estrogen metabolites tested for

growth-stimulating activity on cells from virgin mice are shown in Fig. 3. There was no stimulation of growth by estrogens in the absence or presence of mammogenic hormones in this experiment. Other experiments using different concentrations and combinations of progesterone and prolactin were also negative. In short, none of these modifications was capable of supporting a stimulatory effect of estrogen on growth. These negative results are not conclusive as yet since other conditions may yet be tested, particularly the

Table 2.   Modifications of the serum-free cell culture conditions under which estrogen was tested.

1.   Addition of relaxin or somatomedin C to look for synergistic or permissive effects.
2.   Changes in the cell dissociation procedure: low temperature (30°C vs. 37°C) collagenase digestion and deletion of pronase treatment in an attempt to raise the intracellular estrogen receptor concentration.
3.   Reduced insulin concentration (from 10 to 0.1 μg/ml) in the basal medium to suboptimal level and because a high insulin concentration may lower estrogen receptor levels (19).
4.   Inclusion of antiestrogens (tamoxifen and nafoxidine) in the medium to look for estradiol reversal of any antiestrogen-mediated inhibition of growth.
5.   Estrogens other than 17β-estradiol and estrogen metabolites were tested.
6.   Co-culture with mammary gland "stromal" cells or pieces of gland-free fat pads.

Estrogen was tested alone and in combination with different concentrations of progesterone and/or prolactin in serum-free medium containing insulin (10 μg/ml, except where noted) and liposomes (made from crude soybean lecithin) as essential components.

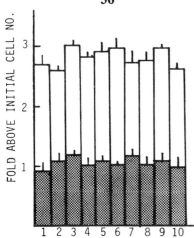

Fig. 3. Cells from mature virgin BALB/c mice were cultured for 10 days in serum-free medium with insulin (10 μg/ml) and liposomes (.01 μm phosphate/ml). Estrogen was added in the absence (shaded bars) or presence (open bars) of progesterone (10^{-7}M) and prolactin (1 μg/ml). Mean ± SD of 3 gels per combination is shown. (1) 4-hydroxy estrone dibenzoate, (2) 2-hydroxy estrone dibenzoate, (3) 11β-methoxy ethynyl estradiol, (4) hexestrol, (5) d-equilenin, (6) 16α-hydroxyestrone, (7) α-dienestrol, (8) DES, (9) 17β-estradiol, (10) no added estrogen control.

possible role of the stroma in mediating estrogen sensitivity of the epithelium. However, it is clear that estrogen does not stimulate growth under conditions where other mammogenic hormones show growth-stimulatory activity.

These results may mean that estrogen is not a direct mitogen for normal mammary epithelial cells. The observed stimulatory effects of estrogen on mammary gland growth in vivo may be due to its well known stimulation of progesterone receptors and prolactin secretion. Alternatively, estrogen may enhance growth indirectly by stimulating the production of growth factors or "estromedins" which then act upon the mammary gland (10).

Lipids.

The original serum-free system developed for mouse cells consisted of insulin (10 μg/ml), EGF (10 ng/ml), and bovine serum albumin (fraction V, 5 mg/ml). The deletion of any of these components inhibited growth. The albumin requirement was thought to reflect a lipid requirement for growth since delipidized albumin did not support growth (4). Further studies in medium containing delipidized albumin or in albumin-free media have shown that unsaturated fatty acids (oleic, linoleic, and arachidonic), and phospholipids, delivered as liposomes, are highly growth stimulatory.

Table 3 compares the effect of various fatty acids on growth. The optimum concentrations varied among experiments probably due to membrane damage during the collagenase dissociation. The stimulatory effect of soybean phospholipids on growth is shown in Table 4 where liposomes made from crude soybean

Table 3.   Effect of fatty acids on the growth of cells from midpregnant mice.

Fatty acid	Concentration (µg/ml)		
	5	10	20
Myristate (14:0)	84.8 ± 22	49.6 ± 38	108.8 ± 30
Palmitate (16:0)	214 ± 44	143 ± 71	64 ± 34
Linoleate (18:2)	296 ± 61	248 ± 57	326 ± 52
Oleate (18:1)	165 ± 38	206 ± 22	206 ± 36

Growth expressed as percent of control (no added fatty acid). Mean and standard deviation of 3 gels per combination are shown. Cells were cultured for 10 days before termination in serum-free medium containing insulin (10 µg/ml), EGF (.01 µg/ml), and delipidized albumin (5 mg/ml) with or without fatty acid (complexed to fatty acid-free albumin). The optimum concentration range (about 5-10 µg/ml) varies among experiments and among the fatty acids. Generally palmitate is not as growth stimulatory and more toxic than the unsaturated fatty acids. Cells from virgin mice respond similarly.

Table 4.   The effect of phospholipids on the growth of cells from virgin mice.

	*Concentration	Cell No. (x10^4)	Fold Control
Starting cell no.		11 ± 1	
Control		17 ± 1	1
Linoleate	10	62 ± 14	3.6
Crude PC:Choles (3:2)	.01	57 ± 9	3.4
	.05	58 ± 4	3.4
	0.1	95 ± 10	5.6
PE:PC:Choles (1:1:1)	.01	17 ± 2	1.0
	.05	30 ± 6	1.8
	0.1	34 ± 6	2.0
Sphingomyelin	.01	11 ± 1	0.6
(bovine brain)	.05	19 ± 10	1.1
	0.1	10 ± 2	0.6

Cells from virgin mice were cultured for 17-18 days in basal medium containing insulin (10 µg/ml), EGF (10 ng/ml) with or without lipids as indicated. PC, PE = phosphatidylcholine, -ethanolamine. Choles = cholesterol. Molar ratios indicated in parentheses. Mean ± SD of 3 gels per combination are shown. *For linoleate, µg/ml; for phospholipids and sphingomyelin, µmoles phosphate/ml.

(a complex lipid mixture composed primarily of phospholipids with neutral lipids comprising a lesser fraction) were compared to liposomes made from purified soybean phospholipids in medium containing EGF and insulin. Further work has shown that liposomes composed of crude soybean lecithin can also stimulate growth in the absence of EGF (or hormones) to the same extent as EGF (or hormones). Neither linoleic acid nor liposomes made from purified phosphatidylcholine had this latter effect (unpublished observations).

The effect of lipids on growth may result partly from increased prostaglandin synthesis since direct exposure of cultured cells to prostaglandins E_1, E_2, and arachidonate stimulates growth 2- to 5-fold above controls cultured in serum-free medium containing insulin (10 µg/ml) and EGF (10 ng/ml) (unpublished observations).

Cyclic adenosine 3',5'-monophosphate (cyclic AMP).

Cholera toxin which irreversibly stimulates endogenous cyclic AMP levels is highly stimulatory to the growth of mammary epithelial cells (11). This effect of cholera toxin can be demonstrated in serum-free medium containing only insulin (10 µg/ml). Exogenously added mono- or dibutyryl cyclic AMP can stimulate growth (5- to 10-fold) under the same conditions (unpublished observations).

Others.

The tumor promoter 12-0-tetradecanoylphorbol-13-acetate (TPA) stimulates growth in both serum-containing (12) and serum-free medium. Lithium (5 mM) stimulates the growth of normal cells but not cells from most BALB/cfC3H tumors in serum-free medium (13). The effect seems not to be due to an alteration in sodium transport by the cells. Both TPA and lithium can replace the EGF but not the insulin growth requirement.

DISCUSSION

The serum-free culture of mouse mammary epithelial cells has proved to be a fruitful model system useful for examining the growth regulation of mammary epithelial cells. For example, this model system has permitted the demonstration of the direct growth-stimulatory effects of mammogenic hormones on normal cells in vitro cultured under defined conditions. Using this system we can now begin to examine the mechanisms of action and interrelationships among the growth-promoting hormones and growth factors which affect mammary epithelial cells. Moreover, the differences in the sensitivity to hormones and growth factors exhibited by cells from virgin and midpregnant mice may be giving us some insight into physiologically relevant regulatory mechanisms. Of course, the physiological significance of EGF- or somatomedin C-stimulated growth remains to be evaluated, but cell culture has served a useful role in identifying new hormones or growth factors which may affect mammary gland growth.

The multiplicity of factors which affect the growth of mouse mammary epithelial cells in vitro are summarized in Table 5. Most of these factors stimulate growth in the absence of the others. However, insulin (0.1-10 μg/ml) is most usually required to be present in the basal medium; an exception is somatomedin C which stimulates growth in insulin's absence. These multiple factors may represent different or a few pathways involved in growth stimulation. The appropriate studies in which these factors can be combined to search for additive or synergistic effects can be done to help resolve this question. The opportunity these different culture systems offers is the means to seek a commonality in the growth-stimulatory actions of hormones, growth factors, and, of particular interest in mammary biology, lipids. Lipid involvement is very intriguing since there is evidence that the growth of mouse mammary tumors is stimulated by linoleate (14).

In fact, some of these results seem to suggest that lipid-dependent pathways are involved in the growth regulation of mammary epithelial cells. The ability of phospholipids, TPA (which activates kinase C (15), or lithium (which raises the level of intracellular phosphoinositides (16)), to stimulate growth seems to suggest that growth may be regulated by a pathway involving phosphatidylinositol hydrolysis and kinase C activation (17).

Table 5.   Factors which stimulate mouse mammary epithelial cell growth in serum-free collagen gel culture.

Classification	Permissive factors
Mammogenic hormones: progesterone, prolactin, corticosterone, aldosterone, deoxycorticosterone, insulin	insulin (for mammogenic (hormones) phospholipid
Growth factors: epidermal growth factor, somatomedin C	Insulin (for EGF)
Lipids: phospholipids, unsaturated fatty acids (prostaglandins)	EGF, insulin
Cyclic nucleotides: cyclic AMP (cholera toxin)	insulin
Others: TPA, lithium	insulin

In addition, since linoleate (a precursor to the prostaglandins), prostaglandins, and cyclic AMP, whose synthesis may be stimulated by prostaglandins (18), can stimulate growth, there is the possibility that cyclic AMP-mediated events such as protein kinase A activation are also involved in growth control. The challenge is to determine if mammogenic hormones or growth factors activate these pathways by generating lipid intermediates concomitantly with cell proliferation.

These insights gained in the study of the growth regulation of normal cells can, finally, be used in the dissection of tumor growth. Individual tumors may present defects in any one or more of the pathways involved in normal growth regulation. In this view, the growth regulation of normal cells in culture is representative of the entire cellular repertoire of responses to growth-stimulatory signals. Tumors would possess a subset of this repertoire. By comparing the growth regulation of tumor cells and their normal counterparts in vitro under defined conditions it should be possible to reach some understanding of the pathological changes occurring in normal growth regulatory pathways leading to neoplasia.

ACKNOWLEDGMENTS

This investigation was supported by Grants CA05388 and CA09041, awarded by the National Cancer Institute, DHHS.

REFERENCES

1. Shih, T.Y. and Weeks, M.O. Cancer Invest. 2:109-123, 1984.
2. Topper, Y.J. and Freeman, C.S. Physiol. Rev. 26:1049-1094, 1980.
3. Imagawa, W., Tomooka, Y., Yang, J., Guzman, R., Richards, J. and Nandi, S. In: Methods for Serum-free Culture of Cells of the Endocrine System, vol. 2 (Ed. D. Barnes), Alan R. Liss, NY, 1984, pp. 127-141.
4. Imagawa, W., Tomooka, Y. and Nandi, S. Proc. Natl. Acad. Sci. USA 79:4074-4077, 1982.
5. Yang, J., Richards, J., Guzman, R., Imagawa, W. and Nandi, S. Proc. Natl. Acad. Sci. USA 77:2088-2092.
6. Imagawa, W., Tomooka, Y., Hamamoto, S. and Nandi, S. Endocrinology (in press).
7. Richards, J., Pasco, D., Yang, J., Guzman, R. and Nandi, S. Exp. Cell Res. 146:1-14, 1983.
8. Clemmons, D.R. and Van Wyk, J.J. In: Handbook of Experimental Pharmacology, vol. 57 (Ed. R. Baserga), Springer-Verlag, 1981, pp. 161-208.
9. Edery, M., Imagawa, W., Larson, L. and Nandi, S. Endocrinology 116:105-112, 1984.
10. Sirbasku, D.A. Proc. Natl. Acad. Sci. USA 75:3786-3790, 1978.

11. Yang, J., Guzman, R., Richards, J., Imagawa, W., McCormick, K. and Nandi, S. Endocrinology 107:35-41, 1980.
12. Guzman, R.C., Osborn, R.C., Richards, J.E. and Nandi, S. J. Natl. Cancer Inst. 71:69-73, 1983.
13. Tomooka, Y., Imagawa, W., Nandi, S. and Bern, H.A. J. Cell. Physiol. 117:290-296, 1983.
14. Welsch, C.W. and Aylsworth, C.F. J. Natl. Cancer Inst. 70:215-221, 1983.
15. Castagna, M., Takai, Y., Kaibuchi, K., Sano, K., Kikkawa, U. and Nishizuka, Y. J. Biol. Chem. 257:7847-7851, 1982.
16. Berridge, M.J. and Irvine, R.F. Nature 312:315-321, 1984.
17. Michell, R.H. Cell Calcium 3:429-440, 1982.
18. Hassid, A. J. Cell. Physiol. 116:297-302, 1983.
19. Butler, W.B., Kelsey, W.H. and Goran, N. Cancer Res. 41:82-88, 1981.

4

POLYPEPTIDE GROWTH FACTORS AND THE GROWTH OF MAMMARY EPITHELIAL CELLS

D. SALOMON, M. BANO, and W. R. KIDWELL

Laboratory of Tumor Immunology and Biology, National Cancer Institute, National Institutes of Health, Bethesda, MD 20205 USA

INTRODUCTION

It is the goal of this chapter to provide a general yet comprehensive overview of some of the more well-defined growth factors that affect the proliferation of normal, preneoplastic, and malignant rodent and human mammary epithelial cells. In this context, we intend to focus only on those factors that directly stimulate the growth of mammary epithelial cells in vitro.

POLYPEPTIDE GROWTH FACTORS AFFECTING THE PROLIFERATION OF MAMMARY EPITHELIAL CELLS

A number of polypeptide growth factors that stimulate the proliferation of normal and neoplastic rodent and human mammary epithelial cells have been identified (Table 1). Although these growth factors have been demonstrated to affect mammary epithelial cell growth in vitro, their potential role in regulating the growth and/or differentiation of discrete cell types within the mammary gland in vivo is relatively unknown.
Epidermal growth factor (EGF).

EGF was first isolated from the submaxillary gland of male mice by Stanley Cohen and his associates (1-3). Mouse EGF is an acid and a heat stable, 53 amino acid peptide exhibiting a pI of 4.5 and a molecular weight of 6,045. EGF in serum and in certain tissues exists as a high molecular weight complex (Mr, 74,000) composed of two moles of EGF bound to two moles of an EGF-binding protein (Mr, 29,300; pI 5.4). The EGF-binding protein is an arginine esteropeptidase. Although the synthesis of EGF has only been demonstrated in the convoluted tubular cells of the submaxillary gland to date, EGF can be immunologically detected in a variety of other tissues and body fluids such as saliva, urine, and milk (4). Human EGF (urogastrone) exhibits a 70% amino acid sequence homology to mouse EGF, produces the same biological responses as mouse EGF in vivo and in vitro, and

Table 1. Characteristics of polypeptide growth factors that stimulate the growth of rodent and human mammary epithelial cells.

Growth factor	Source	Mammary target cells	Molecular weight (Mr)	Isoelectric point (pI)
EGF	Mouse submaxillary glands, human urine, milk	Rodent and human mammary epithelial cells	6,045	4.5
IGF-I IGF-II (MSA)	Human plasma, MCF-7, ZR-75-1 and T47-D cells, mouse mammary tumor cells	MCF-7, T47-D, and MDA-MB-231 cells	7,650 7,470	8.4 6.2
UDGF (estromedin)	Sheep and rodent uterus	MTW9/PL rat mammary tumor cells	4,200	7.3
MSF (somatomedin)	Porcine serum	Normal and tumor mouse mammary epithelial cells	10,000	5.5 - 6.0
MTF (TGF)	Primary DMBA and NMU rat mammary tumors	Rat and human mammary epithelial cells	6,000; 68,000	5.2
MDGF$_{II}$ (TGF)	Human mammary tumors, MCF-7 cells, human milk	MCF-7 cells, mouse mammary tumor cells	6,000; 30 - 40,000	4.0
CSSF	Primary DMBA and NMU rat mammary tumors	Rat mammary epithelial cells, whole organ explants of mouse mammary glands	68,000	5.9
MDGF$_I$	Human mammary tumors, MCF-7 cells, human milk	Mouse and rat mammary epithelial cells	62,000	4.8

EGF, epidermal growth factor; IGF, insulin-like growth factor; MSA, multiplication stimulating activity; UDGF, uterine-derived growth factor; MSF, mammary stimulating factor; MTF, mammary tumor factor; TGF, transforming growth factor; MDGF, mammary-derived growth factor; CSSF, collagen synthesis stimulating factor.

competes with mouse EGF for binding to identical, high affinity, specific membrane receptors (3). High molecular weight species of mouse and human EGF of 9,000 and 28,000 to 30,000 have been identified in the mouse sub-maxillary gland and human urine suggesting that the mature form of EGF in both species is probably derived by proteolytic processing from a larger precursor molecule by the arginine esterase, EGF-binding protein (1, 2, 4). Recently, the structure of the messenger RNA (mRNA) for mouse EGF has been determined from a series of overlapping complementary DNAs (cDNA) (5). The size of the mRNA (4.8 kilobases) indicates that this species is capable of encoding a preproEGF protein with a molecular weight of approximately 133,000. The sequence for mouse EGF is found within the carboxy-terminal portion of this precursor. Alignment of the cysteine residues within the amino-terminal region of preproEGF molecule with those present within EGF sequence suggests that there are at least seven cryptic, structurally related EGF peptides in this region. These peptides could be differen-tially processed from the precursor in specific tissues and at discrete developmental stages (6).

In vitro EGF is a potent mitogen for a variety of cell types (1, 2, 7). Specifically, EGF has been demonstrated to promote the growth of nor-mal and malignant rodent and human mammary epithelial cells in vitro (8-22). EGF (5 to 10 ng/ml) stimulates the growth of primary cultures of mouse mammary epithelial cells obtained from midpregnant or lactating mam-mary glands (22). Increased mammary epithelial cell growth is also ob-served in primary rodent and human mammary epithelial cell cultures propa-gated on tissue culture plastic, on type I collagen or collagen gels, or within type I collagen gels (10, 11, 14, 23). Mammary epithelial cells obtained from virgin mice are generally more sensitive to the mitogenic effects of EGF than are cells obtained from pregnant or lactating animals or from spontaneously occurring mouse mammary tumors (14). EGF has also been demonstrated to be required for the lobuloalveolar development of the mouse mammary gland in organ culture (20, 21). Under these culture condi-tions, glands obtained from 9-day estrogen- and progesterone-primed virgin mice will generally undergo a single round of development in serum-free medium containing insulin (I), glucocorticoids (H), prolactin (P), and aldosterone (A). Withdrawal of all hormones other than insulin results in the regression of the alveolar structures. However, addition of EGF in the presence of IHPA will initiate a second round of development following regression (20). EGF may also be involved in the first round of development since glands obtained from virgin mice primed for a minimum of 6 days will develop in the presence of EGF and IHPA but not in the presence of only IHPA (21).

Mammary epithelial cells obtained from normal rat mammary glands also respond to EGF (10-13). The mitogenic response induced by EGF in these mammary epithelial cell cultures is more pronounced when the cells are cultured on plastic or on type I collagen than when cultured on basement membrane type IV collagen, the species of collagen which these cells normally synthesize and rest upon (10-12). EGF can differentially increase the synthesis of type IV collagen in mammary epithelial cells when these cells are maintained on a foreign substratum (i.e., plastic and type I collagen). However, on type IV collagen the cells become refractory to the effects of EGF on collagen synthesis. These results suggest that EGF and possibly other hormones and growth factors may function as mitogens for mammary epithelial cells by their ability to enhance the synthesis of various components associated with the basement membrane (10).

Primary and secondary cultures of human mammary epithelial cells obtained from clostrum, milk, or reduction mammoplasties exhibit increased growth in response to EGF (15, 16, 23). EGF stimulates DNA synthesis in human mammary epithelial cells obtained from benign fibroadenomas (24). Under these conditions, the mitogenic effect of EGF is accentuated when the fibroadenoma cells are maintained on a feeder layer of fibroblasts in much the same manner as mouse or rat mammary epithelial cells become more responsive to EGF when embedded within a type I collagen gel (14, 23) or on type I collagen (10, 11), respectively. Further evidence that human mammary epithelial cells may be a possible target cell for EGF stems from the observations that the growth of some human breast cancer cell lines such as MCF-7 and T47-D is stimulated by EGF (25, 26). However, other human breast cancer cell lines possess EGF receptors yet fail to respond to this growth factor, suggesting that there is a lack of correlation between the expression of these two phenotypes (26).

A more comprehensive survey of the response of human breast cancer cells to EGF and EGF receptor expression on these cells has been undertaken by Fitzpatrick et al. (26). These authors examined 14 human breast cancer cell lines. All of the cell lines possessed EGF receptors. However, the number of EGF receptors varied from 200 binding sites per cell (MDA-MB-436) to 700,000 binding sites per cell (MDA-MB-231). Of four breast cell lines examined in detail, only two responded mitogenically to EGF (MCF-7 and T47-D), suggesting that the presence of the receptor is necessary but not entirely sufficient for eliciting a mitogenic response to EGF. These same authors (27) extended these studies to primary human breast cancer cells obtained from tumor biopsies. Specific binding of EGF of one femtomole or greater per mg of isolated tumor membranes was detected in 48% of 137 primary tumors and metastases examined. The presence of estrogen receptors (ER) and progesterone receptors (PgR) has been utilized as a prognostic indicator to select patients for adjuvant endocrine therapy. Tumor samples were therefore analyzed for possible correlations between the concentrations of these steroid receptors and the concentration of EGF receptors. Tumors with little or no ER and PgR, which accounted for approximately 20% of the total tumors, had the highest level of EGF binding in the individual tumor samples. Similar results were obtained by Perez et al. (28). This inverse correlation between high EGF binding and ER negativity may indicate that this class of tumors is less differentiated than those tumors which are ER positive and that EGF, or some EGF-related species, in contrast to estrogens, may regulate the growth of this former class of tumors.

Insulin and insulin-like growth factors (IGFs) - somatomedins.

A second major family of growth factors that are probably involved in regulating the proliferation of rodent and human mammary epithelial cells consists of insulin and the insulin-like growth factors (IGFs) or somatomedins (29, 30). IGFs are low molecular weight peptides (7,000 to 10,000) that are found in rodent and human sera. IGFs are primarily synthesized in the liver in response to growth hormone. The IGFs consist of two groups of peptides. The first group includes human IGF-I and rat somatomedin C (SM-C), which are basic peptides having isoelectric points greater than 7.5. The second group includes the more neutral and acidic peptides, human IGF-II and rat multiplication-stimulating activity (MSA). IGF-I exhibits extensive amino acid sequence homology to SM-C while IGF-II is virtually identical to MSA. Both IGF-I and IGF-II share partial amino acid sequence homology with each other and with the A and B chains of proinsulin. However, there is sufficient divergence of the sequences between the IGFs and insulin such that anti-insulin antibodies fail to recognize the IGFs. Like EGF, IGF-I and IGF-II are found in human serum (150 to 250 and 800 to 1,000 ng/ml, respectively) as high molecular weight proteins (125,000 to

200,000) due to their association with a 60,000 to 70,000 molecular weight binding protein which tends to aggregate under isotonic or neutral conditions. Following acid extraction, the carrier protein can be dissociated from the smaller IGF peptides.

In vivo and in vitro the IGFs share many of the same biological activities with insulin (29, 30). IGFs are extremely potent mitogens for rodent and human fibroblasts in vitro and are members of a larger functionally related class of growth factors called progression factors, which include EGF and transferrin (31, 32). The ability of the IGFs to stimulate DNA synthesis and cell growth is mediated through their interaction with specific, high affinity, cell surface receptors (29, 30, 32). Distinct classes of receptors exist for IGF-I, IGF-II, and insulin. Insulin has also been demonstrated to stimulate the growth of a variety of cells in vitro at relatively high concentrations (5 to 10 μg/ml) (7). The mitogenic effects of insulin are apparently in part due to the result of insulin binding to the IGF-I and IGF-II receptors at high concentrations (29, 30, 32).

Until recently, the biologic effects of IGFs on mammary epithelial cells have not been fully studied. Ptashne et al. (33) first demonstrated that crude preparations of rat somatomedin C, MSA (3 to 10 μg/ml), or a porcine serum somatomedin, mammary stimulating factor (MSF), could stimulate DNA synthesis in primary cultures of mouse mammary epithelial cells obtained from midpregnant mice. Subsequently, Kidwell et al. (10) showed a similar effect of purified MSA (1-50 ng/ml) on the growth of primary rat mammary epithelial cells. Furlanetto and DiCarlo (34) examined the ability of human IGF-I (pI 8.2) and insulin to stimulate DNA synthesis in four human breast cell lines (MCF-7, T47-D, MDA-MB-231, and HBL-100) following serum starvation. In all four cell lines, IGF-I (10 to 100 ng/ml) stimulated DNA synthesis. Insulin was also found to stimulate cell growth but at concentrations 10- to 1000-fold higher than IGF-I. Furthermore, all four cell lines were found to possess IGF-I receptors to which insulin was capable of binding at high concentrations suggesting that the mitogenic effects of this hormone were being mediated via its interaction with the IGF-I receptor. Myal et al. (35) also observed that IGF-I could stimulate the serum-free growth of T47-D cells. In addition, rat MSA (IGF-II) at 1 μg/ml was found to be more potent in stimulating the growth of these cells than either IGF-I or insulin. Furthermore, when T47-D cells were propagated on type I collagen gels in serum-free medium, the mitogenic response to IGF-I and IGF-II was increased by approximately 2- to 3-fold. The mitogenic response to each of these IGF peptides was correlated with the occupancy of specific IGF-I and IGF-II receptors on these cells. At high concentrations insulin was found to compete equally for binding to both classes of IGF receptors.

The elaboration of a spectrum of growth factors by tumor cells may be involved in maintaining the transformed state of these cells and/or in providing these cells with a selective growth advantage over their normal, nontransformed counterparts (36-38). Knauer et al. (39) have shown that the conditioned medium (CM) from chemically induced mouse mammary tumor cells contains IGF-II-like peptides (Mr, 7,000 to 20,000) which compete with rat MSA for binding to IGF-II receptors on chick embryo fibroblasts (CEF) and which like MSA stimulate DNA synthesis in CEF cells. Human mammary tumor cells may also be producing a series of IGFs. MCF-7, T47-D, MDA-MB-231, ZR-75-1, and HS578T cells contain immunoreactive IGF-I in their CM (34, 40). The serum-free CM levels of IGF-I ranged from 2.1 to 16.8 ng/ml and could only be detected by RIA after acid-ethanol extraction of the CM to remove interfering IGF-binding proteins. IGF-I can also be found in primary human mammary tumors. Biopsies (6 out of 6) of human mammary intraductal carcinomas exhibited positive staining for IGF-I following immunoperoxidase localization (41).

Uterine-derived growth factor (UDGF) - estromedins.

Attempts to demonstrate a direct mitogenic effect of estrogens in vitro on estrogen-responsive normal and malignant mammary epithelial cells have been equivocal. It has been suggested by Sirbasku (42, 43) that this lack of response to estrogens in vitro in cell types that are normally estrogen-dependent for growth in vivo may be due to the ability of estrogens to induce the production and/or secretion of growth factors (estromedins) in other estrogen-responsive target tissues which would then enter the circulation and promote the subsequent growth of mammary epithelial cells. A uterine-derived growth factor (UDGF) which fulfilled the criteria of an estromedin was isolated from pregnant sheep uteri and was purified to apparent homogeneity (42). UDGF has an apparent molecular weight of approximately 4,200 and a pI of 7.3. UDGF is heat and acid stable and insensitive to reduction with respect to its biologic activity. UDGF stimulates the growth of rat mammary MTW9/PL tumor cells (optimally at 5 to 10 ng/ml) in serum-free medium yet does not stimulate the growth of primary cultures of rat fibroblasts or other estrogen-nonresponsive cell types. A number of growth factors including EGF, FGF, MSA, IGF-I, and insulin could not replace the UDGF requirement for the growth of MTW9/PL cells in serum-free medium. Sheep pituitaries also contain an estrogen-inducible growth factor similar to UDGF which could stimulate the growth of rat MTW9/PL and human T47-D mammary tumor cells (43).

Transforming growth factors (TGFs).

Transformation of mesenchymal or epithelial cells with acutely transforming retroviruses, DNA tumor viruses, or chemical carcinogens generally results in a partial or complete relaxation in the growth factor(s) requirements for the anchorage-dependent proliferation of these transformed cells in vitro (36). The total loss of dependence upon a particular mitogenic peptide may be due to the constitutive production of the growth factor and/or other related peptides by the tumor cells. One such class of growth factors which are elaborated by tumor cells are transforming growth factors (TGFs) (37, 38). TGFs reversibly confer upon normal nontransformed cells, particularly immortalized fibroblasts such as normal rat kidney (NRK) cells, several properties associated with the transformed phenotype. These properties include the anchorage-independent growth (AIG) of cells in soft agar, a decreased serum and growth factor requirement for anchorage-dependent cell growth, and a loss of contact inhibition of cell growth. TGFs consist of a family of peptides (Table 2) which have been identified and partially purified from the CM and the acid-ethanol cellular extracts of chemically transformed rat and mouse cells, from several human tumor cell lines, and from solid rodent and human tumors (37, 38). However, the presence of TGFs in a variety of nonneoplastic tissues suggests that this class of growth factors may perform a more generalized function in such processes as embryogenesis, wound healing, bone resorption, and tissue stem cell proliferation (2, 37). Therefore, the nomenclature for this class of growth factors may be a misnomer and is generally used to operationally describe these activities rather than to ascribe any particular functional significance to them.

The potential function(s) or role of TGFs in regulating mammary epithelial cell growth and transformation is just starting to be defined. CM from Dimethylbenze-α-anthracene (DMBA)-induced rat mammary tumor cells or the acid-ethanol extracts prepared from primary DMBA or Nitrosomethylurea

(NMU)-induced rat mammary tumors contain a factor, mammary tumor factor (MTF), which exhibits αTGF activity (44). MTF inhibits the binding of EGF but not insulin to mouse embryonal carcinoma cells. MTF is mitogenic for rat and human mammary epithelial cells, NRK, Balbc/3T3, and CEF cells in low serum but not for the DMBA tumor cells. In addition, MTF is capable of inducing the AIG of NRK and 3T3 cells in soft agar. MTF is a heat-labile protein that exhibits a pI of 5.2 and exists in two molecular forms of 6,000 to 10,000 and 65,000 to 75,000 following gel filtration chromatography. In contrast to the primary tumors, transplantable DMBA or NMU rat mammary tumors lack any detectable MTF activity. This difference in MTF activity in the primary and transplantable tumors may reflect the relative hormone dependence or degree of differentiation between these two classes of tumors. The primary tumors are generally more differentiated and estrogen responsive than the transplantable tumors.

We have determined whether human mammary tumor cells produce a comparable activity(ies) (45). The concentrated, acid-treated CM from MCF-7 cells and 10 individual clones derived from these cells contain a growth factor(s), mammary-derived growth factor-II ($MDGF_{II}$), which like rat MTF is able to stimulate the growth of NRK cells in soft agar as colonies and is able to compete with ^{125}I-EGF for binding to EGF receptors. The AIG-conferring activity associated with $MDGF_{II}$ is heat stable unlike rat MTF but, like MTF, it is inactivated by prior treatment with dithiothreitol. The major species of $MDGF_{II}$ found in the CM of MCF-7 cells exhibit a molecular weight of approximately 6,000 following gel filtration chromatography and a pI of approximately 4.0 following isoelectric focusing (IEF).

$MDGF_{II}$ is not restricted to the CM of a human mammary tumor cell line since the acid-ethanol extracts prepared from human mammary tumor biopsies (46), from MCF-7 cells propagated in nude mice as tumors, or from two transplantable human mammary adenocarcinomas contain equivalent amounts of these two activities (EGF-competing and NRK colony-stimulating activities). However, due to the relatively poor recovery of these activities from either the CM of MCF-7 cells or from the tumors propagated in nude mice, it became apparent that an alternative source was necessary for obtaining sufficient quantities of these human TGF-like activities for further purification. We found that crude, delipidated human milk contains an abundant amount of TGF-like activity (46).

Following IEF, three major species of TGF that were capable of stimulating the AIG of NRK cells were detected at pH 4.0 to 4.2, 6.0 to 6.2, and 6.8 to 7.0 in both the crude human milk samples and in the human breast carcinoma biopsies. We have operationally designated the pI 4.0 TGF activity as $MDGF_{II}$ to distinguish it from a second biological activity found in human milk and breast tumors, $MDGF_I$ (50), and because this isoelectric variant is physiochemically and biologically similar to the major TGF species associated with the CM obtained from MCF-7 cells (45). Milk $MDGF_{II}$ (pI 4.0 TGF) is capable of stimulating the AIG of NRK cells, mouse mammary $Mm5mt/c_1$ C3H tumor cells, and certain clones of MCF-7 tumor cells in soft agar. $MDGF_{II}$ is also able to inhibit the binding of mouse EGF but not insulin to isolated A431 cell membranes suggesting that this growth factor may resemble an αTGF. In fact, the AIG-conferring activity of $MDGF_{II}$ for NRK cells and $Mm5mt/c_1$ cells is almost completely attenuated by an anti-EGF receptor mouse monoclonal antibody indicating that occupation of the EGF receptor is required for the AIG activity of $MDGF_{II}$. $MDGF_{II}$ is biologically and physiochemically distinct from the major species of human urinary EGF (pI 4.5). Petrides et al. (48) have also demonstrated that human milk contains three αTGF peptides (Mr ≈ 6,000) that compete with mouse EGF for human placental membrane receptor sites and which differ from the major species of human EGF, as well as from each other, by amino acid composition. All three peptides are potent mitogens for the anchorage-dependent growth of human fibroblasts and are able to promote the AIG of NRK cells. Noda et al. (49) have recently demonstrated the presence of βTGF species in human clostrum and milk.

Collagen synthesis stimulating factor (CSSF) and mammary-derived growth factor$_I$ ($MDGF_I$).

The growth and survival of normal mammary epithelial cells and differentiated tumor mammary epithelial cells requires the synthesis and deposition of and interaction with type IV collagen (9-12). Type IV collagen production in normal mammary epithelial cells is differentially stimulated by a number of mitogens such as EGF, MSA, embryonin, and α-fetoprotein (10). However, mammary tumor cells fail to respond to such growth factors as EGF apparently because these tumor cells are elaborating endogenous factors that differentially enhance the net production of collagen and are therefore relatively insensitive to exogenous growth factors that produce the same effect (47, 50). These mitogens are distinct from the TGF-like activities found in these same tumor cells and are apparently a unique set of growth factors.

Collagen synthesis stimulating factor (CSSF) has been partially purified from the acid-ethanol extracts prepared from primary DMBA- or NMU-induced rat mammary adenocarcinomas (47). CSSF is a heat and dithiothreitol-sensitive peptide having a molecular weight of approximately 68,000 and a pI of 5.9. Purified CSSF between 50 to 100 ng/ml differentially stimulates the synthesis of collagen by 2.5- to 10-fold in cultures of NRK cells, Balbc/3T3 cells, and in rat mammary epithelial cells, but not in cultures of DMBA tumor cells. CSSF stimulates the net production of collagen by differentially increasing the synthesis of collagen rather than by inhibiting collagen turnover. Moderate levels of CSSF are also found in extracts prepared from the transplantable MTW9/PL and MTW9A rat mammary tumors but not in the extracts prepared from transplantable DMBA or NMU tumors which fail to elaborate a basement membrane. A comparable biological activity, mammary-derived growth factor$_I$ (MDGF$_I$), has recently been isolated and purified to homogeneity from human mammary tumors and human milk (50). In contrast to rat CSSF, human MDGF$_I$ is insensitive to reduction and is heat stable. MDGF$_I$ has a molecular weight of 62,000 and a pI of 4.8. MDGF$_I$ stimulates the proliferation of normal rat and mouse mammary epithelial cells optimally between 5 to 10 ng/ml in serum-free medium. Preceeding any effect on cell growth, MDGF$_I$ produces a differential 4-fold increase in the net accumulation of type IV collagen in these cells and a 2-fold increase in laminin production. However, when normal mammary epithelial cells are propagated on an exogenous type IV collagen substratum, in contrast to type I collagen or plastic, they become refractory to the growth-promoting and collagen synthesis-stimulating effects of MDGF$_I$. These two biological responses are apparently mediated by the interaction of MDGF$_I$ with specific, high affinity ($K_D = 10^{-10}$ M) cell surface receptors for MDGF$_I$ on mammary epithelial cells and on other cell types, such as A431 and NRK cells, which respond to this growth factor. In NRK cells MDGF$_I$ differentially stimulates the synthesis of type I collagen by enhancing the levels of type I collagen mRNA. Using a cDNA probe against $\alpha I(I)$ collagen, NRK cells exposed to MDGF$_I$ for 2 days were found to have an approximately 4-fold higher amount of hybridizable type I collagen mRNA by cytoblot or dot-blot analysis than cells not exposed to MDGF$_I$.

CONCLUSIONS

It has been demonstrated that mammary epithelial cells respond to a variety of growth factors such as EGF, IGFs, and $MDGF_I$, and that the mitogenic response to these growth factors can be modified depending upon the composition of the extracellular substrate upon which these cells rest. Conversely, these growth factors may in turn function as mitogens for mammary epithelial cells by their ability to differentially modulate the net production of various components associated with the extracellular matrix such as type IV collagen and laminin. In contrast to normal mammary epithelial cells, malignant mammary epithelial cells are generally less selective or restrictive for their growth and/or survival on specific extracellular matrix proteins. This lack of substratum dependency is reflected in the relative growth autonomy or reduced dependency of rodent and human mammary tumor cells for or on specific mitogens such as EGF. Apparently, mammary tumor cells may be elaborating a spectrum of growth-promoting activities including IGFs, TGFs, and other MDGFs. These growth factors may be involved in maintaining the transformed phenotype of these tumor cells and in concomitantly stimulating the growth of these same cells or a different responding population of cells in an autocrine or paracrine manner, respectively. However, the presence of some of these same growth factors in nonneoplastic tissues and body fluids such as milk suggests that these activities may perform some other as of yet undefined physiological function(s) in normal mammary epithelial cells at certain developmental stages (e.g., during pregnancy or lactation). These growth factors could function as stem cell mitogens or morphogenic and/or survival factors in the normal mammary gland or in the neonatal gut epithelium.

Table 2. Biological and physiochemical properties of TGFs.

Properties	αTGF	βTGF[a]	γTGF
Molecular weight (Mr)	7,400(r)	25,000(μr) 12,500(r)	12,000(r)
Isoelectric point (pI)	6.8	~9.0	5.2-5.4
Heat stable	Yes	Yes	No
Acid stable	Yes	Yes	No
DTT stable	No	No	No
Amino acid sequence homology to EGF (mouse and human)	Yes	No	No
Competes with EGF for binding to EGF receptors	Yes	No[b]	No
Mitogenic for cells in monolayer (anchorage-dependent growth)	Yes	No (growth inhibitory)	Yes
Stimulates colony formation of cells in semisolid medium (anchorage-independent growth)	Yes	May require αTGF or EGF and PDGF	Yes

DTT, dithiothreitol;[a] analogous to GI chalone isolated from BSC-I African green monkey kidney cells;[b] distinct, high affinity receptors for βTGF have been identified on a variety of cell types.

REFERENCES

1. Carpenter, G. In: Handbook of Experimental Pharmacology. Tissue Growth Factors (Ed. R. Baserga), Vol. 57, Springer-Verlag, New York, 1981, pp. 89-132.
2. Burgess, A. and Nicola, N. In: Growth Factors and Stem Cells, Academic Press, New York, 1983, pp. 155-184.
3. Carpenter, G. Cell 37: 357-358, 1984.
4. Hirata, Y. and Orth, D.N. J. Clin. Endocrinol. 48: 673-679, 1979.
5. Scott, J., Urdea, M., Quiroga, M., Sanchez-Pescador, R., Fong, N., Selby, M., Rutter, W.J. and Bell, G.I. Science 221: 236-240, 1983.
6. Rall, L.B., Scott, J. and Bell, G.I. Nature (in press).
7. Barnes, D.W. and Sato, G. Anal. Biochem. 102: 255-270, 1980.
8. Rudland, P.S., Hallowes, B.C., Durbin, H. and Lewis, D. J. Cell Biol. 73: 561-577, 1977.
9. Kidwell, W.R., Wicha, M.S., Salomon, D.S. and Liotta, L.A. In: Control Mechanisms in Animal Cells (Eds. L. Jiminez de Asua, R. Levi-Montalcini, R. Shields and S. Icobelli), Raven Press, New York, 1980, pp. 333-340.
10. Kidwell, W.R., Bano, M. and Salomon, D.S. In: Cell Culture Methods for Molecular and Cell Biology. Methods for Serum-Free Culture of Cells of the Endocrine System (Eds. D.W. Barnes, D.A. Sirbasku and G.H. Sato), Vol. 2, Alan R. Liss Inc., New York, 1984, pp. 105-125.
11. Salomon, D.S., Liotta, L.A. and Kidwell, W.R. Proc. Natl. Acad. Sci. (U.S.A.) 78: 382-386, 1981.

12. Kidwell, W.R., Wicha, M.S., Salomon, D.S. and Liotta, L.A. In: Cell Biology of Breast Cancer (Eds. C.M. McGrath, M.J. Brennan and M.A. Rich), Academic Press, New York, 1980, pp. 17-33.
13. Smith, J.A., Winslow, D.P. and Rudland, P.S. J. Cell. Physiol. 119: 320-326, 1984.
14. Yang, J., Guzman, R., Richards, J., Imagawa, W., McCormick, K. and Nandi, S. Endocrinology 107: 35-41, 1980.
15. Stampfer, M., Hallowes, R.C. and Hackett, A.J. In Vitro 16: 415-425, 1980.
16. Hammond, S.L., Ham, R.G. and Stampfer, M.R. Proc. Natl. Acad. Sci. (U.S.A.) 81: 5435-5439, 1984.
17. Barnes, D.W. and Sato, G. Nature 281: 388-389, 1979.
18. Medina, D. and Oborn, C.J. Cancer Res. 40: 3982-3987, 1980.
19. Calvo, F., Brower, M. and Carney, D.N. Cancer Res. 44: 4553-4559, 1984.
20. Tonelli, Q.J. and Sorof, S. Differentiation 20: 253-259, 1981.
21. Vonderhaar, B.K. In: Control of Cell Growth and Differentiation (Ed. C.M. Veneziale), Van Nostrand Reinhold Co., New York, 1984, pp. 11-33.
22. Okamoto, S. and Oka, T. Proc. Natl. Acad. Sci. (U.S.A.) 81: 6059-6063, 1984.
23. Yang, J., Elias, J.J., Petrakis, N.L., Wellings, S.R. and Nandi, S. Cancer Res. 41: 1021-1027, 1981.
24. Taylor-Papadimitriou, J., Shearer, M. and Stoker, M.G.P. Int. J. Cancer 20: 903-913, 1977.
25. Imai, Y., Leung, C.K.H., Friesen, H.G. and Shiu, R.P.C. Cancer Res. 42: 4394-4398, 1982.
26. Fitzpatrick, S.L., LaChance, M.P. and Schultz, G.S. Cancer Res. 44: 3442-3447, 1984.
27. Fitzpatrick, S.L., Brightwell, J., Wiltliff, J.L., Barrows, G.H. and Schultz, G.S. Cancer Res. 44: 3448-3453, 1984.
28. Perez, R., Pascual, M., Macías, A. and Lage, A. Breast Cancer Res. and Treat. 4: 189-193, 1984.
29. Rechler, M.M. and Nissley, P.S. Nature 270: 665-666, 1977.
30. Phillips, L.S. and Vassilopoulou-Sellin, R. New Eng. J. Med. 302: 371-380, 1980.
31. Stiles, C.D., Capone, G.T., Scher, C.D., Antoniades, H.N., Van Wyk, J.J. and Pledger, W.J. Proc. Natl. Acad. Sci. (U.S.A.) 76: 1279-1283, 1979.
32. Burgess, A. and Nicola, N. In: Growth Factors and Stem Cells, Academic Press, New York, 1983, pp. 185-230.
33. Ptashne, K., Hsueh, H.W. and Stockdale, F.E. Biochem. 18: 3533-3539, 1979.
34. Furlanetto, R.W. and DiCarlo, J.N. Cancer Res. 44: 2122-2128, 1984.
35. Myal, Y., Shiu, R.P.C., Bhaumick, B. and Bala, M. Cancer Res. 44: 5486-5490, 1984.
36. Heldin, C-H. and Westermark, B. Cell 37: 9-20, 1984.
37. Brown, K.D. and Blakeley, D.M. Biochem. Soc. Trans. 12: 168-173, 1984.
38. Todaro, G.J., Marquardt, H., Twardzik, D.R., Reynolds, F.H. and Stephenson, J.R. In: Genes and Proteins in Oncogenesis (Eds. I.B. Weinstein and H.J. Vogel), Academic Press, New York, 1983, pp. 165-182.
39. Knauer, D.J., Iyer, A.P., Banerjee, M.R. and Smith, G.L. Cancer Res. 40: 4368-4372, 1980.

40. Huff, K.K., Lippman, M.E., Spencer, E.M. and Dickson, R.B. In: Abstracts, 7th International Congress of Endocrinology, Excerpta Medica, Princeton, New Jersey, 1984, pg. 728.
41. Spencer, E.M. and Bennington, J.L. In: Abstracts, 7th International Congress of Endocrinology, Excerpta Medica, Princeton, New Jersey, 1984, pg. 1524.
42. Ikeda, T. and Sirbasku, D.A. J. Biol. Chem. 259: 4049-4064, 1984.
43. Ikeda, T., Danielpour, D., Galle, P.R., Peter, R. and Sirbasku, D.A. In: Cell Culture Methods for Molecular and Cell Biology. Methods for Serum-Free Culture of Cells of the Endocrine System (Eds. D.W. Barnes, D.A. Sirbasku and G.H. Sato), Vol. 2, Alan R. Liss Inc., New York, 1984, pp. 217-242.
44. Zwiebel, J.A., Davis, H.R., Kohn, E., Salomon, D.S. and Kidwell, W.R. Cancer Res. 42: 5117-5125, 1982.
45. Salomon, D.S., Zwiebel, J.A., Bano, M., Losonczy, I., Fehnel, P. and Kidwell, W.R. Cancer Res. 44: 4069-4077, 1984.
46. Zwiebel, J.A., Bano, M., Nexo, E., Salomon, D.S. and Kidwell, W.R. Cancer Res. (in press).
47. Bano, M., Zwiebel, J.A., Salomon, D.S. and Kidwell, W.R. J. Biol. Chem. 258: 2729-2735, 1983.
48. Petrides, P.E., Hosang, M., Shooter, E.M. and Bohlen, P. In: Abstracts, 7th International Congress of Endocrinology, Excerpta Medica, Princeton, New Jersey, 1984, pg. 1757.
49. Noda, K., Umeda, M., and Ono, T. Gann 75: 109-112, 1984.
50. Bano, M., Salomon, D.S. and Kidwell, W.R. J. Biol. Chem. (in press).

5

ESTROGEN-REGULATED PROTEINS AND AUTOCRINE CONTROL OF CELL GROWTH IN BREAST CANCER

H. ROCHEFORT, F. CAPONY, G. CAVALIE-BARTHEZ, M. CHAMBON, M. GARCIA, O. MASSOT, M. MORISSET, I. TOUITOU, F. VIGNON and B. WESTLEY

Unité d'Endocrinologie Cellulaire et Moléculaire, U 148 INSERM, 60 Rue de Navacelles, 34100 Montpellier, France.

INTRODUCTION

Estrogens promote the development of breast cancer and stimulate the growth **in vitro** of some breast cancer cell lines (1)(2), but the mechanism of their cancerogenic and mitogenic action is unknown. We have used the hormone-responsive MCF_7 breast cancer cell line to analyse the mechanism by which estrogens regulate both the biosynthesis of specific proteins and cell proliferation. Estrogen-regulated proteins have been detected by a number of approaches in several metastatic breast cancer cell lines, mostly MCF_7 cells. These proteins are generally of unknown function (except for the progesterone receptor (RP)) and defined according to their molecular weight under denaturing conditions by SDS-gel polyacrylamide gel electrophoresis, e.g. 52 K (3), 28 K (4). More recently, an estrogen-regulated mRNA (pS2) coding for a secreted protein has also been described (5).

The estrogen-regulated proteins secreted by hormone-responsive cells appear to be particularly attractive for several reasons :

First, they may serve as potential circulating markers of hormone dependency in breast cancer as far as they can be released into the blood.

Second, some of these proteins or peptides released into the extracellular medium can totally modulate the growth of the producing cells (autocrine) (6), or neighbouring cells (paracrine). Therefore, they may serve as second messengers of steroid hormones for regulating a nonspecific mitogenic response.

Third, these proteins are relatively easy to detect and assay, contrary to cellular proteins (3).

The 52 K protein.

Six years ago, we found a protein of 52,000 mol wt (52 K) whose production in culture medium by estrogen-receptor-positive metastatic breast cancer cell lines is specifically increased by estrogens and inhibited by antiestrogens (3). The 52 K protein is a glycoprotein produced in small amounts (15 ng/ml of medium) by estrogen-treated MCF_7 cells, representing 20 to 40 % of total released proteins in the culture medium. On the basis of its high hormonal specificity (3), this protein can be used as a simple **in vitro** test to evaluate the estrogenic and antiestrogenic activity of a drug. The 52 K protein is more closely related to the control of cell proliferation by estrogen than the progesterone receptor, which is induced by Tamoxifen in cells whose growth is inhibited by this antiestrogen. However, its release into the medium is not stimulated by the other mitogens that have been tested (insulin, epithelial growth factor and charcoal-treated fetal calf serum (7)).

Due to its **rarity**, we used a three-step strategy to purify the 52 K protein and study its structure and function. First, we partially purified it from 22 l of conditioned medium from MCF_7 cells by Concanavalin A Sepharose. Second, we obtained several monoclonal antibodies. In collaboration with CLIN-MIDY Research Laboratory (Pr B. Pau), MAbs were raised, cloned and purified after fusion of lymphocytes from immunised high responder selected mice with the murine myeloma P3-X63-Ag8-653 (8). The 7 MAbs that were cloned and purified were all of the IgG1 isotype and their KD ranged from 0.35 to 2.3 nM. The antibodies specifically recognised the secreted 52 K protein and a cellular 52 K protein as evidenced by double immunoprecipitation and by immunoblotting after electrophoretic separation and transfer (9). In MCF_7 cell extracts, smaller processed forms of 48,000 and 34,000 mol wt were also immunoreactive. Double determinant immunoradiometric assay indicated that the 7 MAbs recognised three distinct regions of the Mr 52,000 protein and allowed the 52 K protein to be assayed in biological fluids such as culture media conditioned by cells, cytosol and mammary cyst fluid. Table 1 summarises recent results obtained on mammary cells lines indicating that the regulation of the 52 K protein by estradiol only occurs in estrogen and progesterone-receptor-positive cell lines. However, the production (at low levels) of immunoreactive 52 K protein was also observed in two receptor-negative cell lines (BT20, MDA-MB231) at the same constitutive level whether or not cells had been treated by estrogens. All tested cell lines containing estrogen receptors produce the protein, but to varying degrees. For instance, T47D (clone 11) cells have high concentrations of RP but produce low concentration of 52 K protein. In this cell line, other E_2-regulated proteins (e.g. 60 K) are more abundant.

Table 1. Distribution of the 52 K protein in different human mammary cell lines and comparison to other estrogen-regulated parameters.

	MARKERS OF RESPONSES TO ESTROGEN IN HUMAN CELL LINES						
	MCF_7	R_{27}	ZR_{75-1}	$T47D$ $Cl.11$	BT_{20}	MDA MB_{231}	HBL_{100}
R_E	+	+	+	+	−	−	−
R_P	+	+	+	++	−	−	−
52 K PROTEIN	++	++	++	+	+	+	−
E_2 ON CELL PROLIFERATION	+	+	+	+	−	−	−

RE= estrogen receptor. RP= progesterone receptor. The 4 receptor-positive cell lines responded to estradiol both by producing the 52 K protein and by increasing their growth. The receptor-negative cell lines produced the 52 K protein constitutively at the same level whether estradiol was present or not. HBL100 derived from human milk epithelial cells produced no detectable 52 K protein in the culture medium. The concentration of the 52 K protein in the medium measured by double determinant IRMA (8) varied between 0,5 to 5 ng per μg DNA per day (+) and 5 to 20 ng per ug DNA per day (++).
(From refs. 10, 29 and Garcia & Derocq, unpublished).

The identity and biological functions of the 52 K protein are presently unknown. The 52 K protein is not a major milk protein such as human casein or α-lactalbumin, which have different molecular weights. The relationship of the 52 K protein with other estrogen-regulated proteins, such as the 28 K protein (11), has been excluded in collaboration with McGuire et al., who provided their specific antibodies. The identification of the 52 K protein as a plasminogen activator was recently excluded after purification (12).

Finally, even though the molecular weight is similar to that of the MMTV gp52, it is most unlikely that the 52 K human protein is related to the protein which interacts with the antibodies to gp52. Our antibodies are, in fact, unable to interact with any protein of the C3H mouse mammary tumour, and in the sequence of the human MMTV-like clones, the envelope coding sequence gene does not appear to be expressed (13). The 52 K protein therefore does not seem to correspond to a known mammary protein.

We will not discuss the potential use of this protein and its antibodies as a marker in mammary pathology. This question has been addressed elsewhere (14)(15). The first clinical studies are in progress to correlate the concentration of this protein both with the receptor content of breast cancer tissue, and with the pathology of high and low-risk benign mastopathia. Instead, we address the question of the possible function of this protein in mediating the mitogenic activity of estrogens in epithelial breast cancer cells and the information provided by the study of its co and post-translational modifications.

Estrogen-regulated autocrine control of cell proliferation.

Several groups have reported the **in vitro** stimulatory effect of estrogens on the proliferation of estrogen-receptor-positive metastatic human mammary cancer cell lines (2)(16)(17), but not in primary cultures of normal rodent mammary tissue, which respond to estrogens with respect to progesterone receptor stimulation (18).

Human breast cell lines are therefore good systems for studying the mechanism by which estrogen stimulates their proliferation. We will show how two series of data obtained by endocrinologists and oncologists have led us to propose that estrogens may indirectly stimulate cell proliferation by inducing the synthesis and secretion of growth factors or mitogens into the medium. This mechanism was first proposed by Sirbasku (19) who anticipated that estrogens might act **via** endocrine-secreted estromedin, thus explaining why estradiol was more active **in vivo** than **in vitro.**

We then proposed an autocrine-type mechanism (10) and Vignon et al. (20) supported this hypothesis by showing that proteins from serum-free media conditioned by estrogen-stimulated MCF_7 cells increase the growth of resting MCF_7 cells. The mitogenic activity is retained by Con A Sepharose chromatography and eluted with the glycoprotein fraction. By contrast, the conditioned media from estrogen-withdrawn MCF_7 cells are inactive. Moreover, in the antiestrogen-resistant cell lines, R27, and RTx6, tamoxifen remains, as in the wild type MCF_7 cells, unable to stimulate the production of the estrogen-regulated 160 K secreted protein and of the pS2 mRNA (21) but became able, as an estrogen, to increase the production of the 52 K protein (22). These results also suggest that tamoxifen may decrease the production of estrogen-induced growth factor in antiestrogen-sensitive cells and increase this production in some antiestrogen-resistant cells (23).

More recently, we have purified to homogeneity a biologically active 52 K protein (24) and tested it on estrogen-deprived recipient MCF_7 cells. The basic of these experiments is indicated in Fig. 1. The 52 K protein produced by E_2-stimulated MCF_7 cells was purified by a two-step procedure (Con A-Sepharose + immunoaffinity chromatography) and its biological activity was tested on the same estrogen-withdrawn MCF_7 cells. The dose-dependent stimulation of cell growth, as evaluated by DNA assay, ranged from 120 % to 240 % (Table 2).

A mean stimulation of 170 % was obtained in the 7 experiments performed. This stimulation represented 40 % of the effect obtained by estradiol and was observed at 52 K protein concentrations similar to those released into the culture medium. The 52 K protein was also able to stimulate the number and length of microvilli at the cell surface, like estradiol, but earlier than the steroid hormone. This mitogenic activity of the purified 52 K protein could be due to a contaminant that we have not yet detected. However we have excluded, by ^{35}S cysteine-labelling experiments, the possibility that it contains TGFα, pS2-like proteins or Somatomedin C.

Fig. 1. Basis for studying the mitogenic activity of secreted proteins.

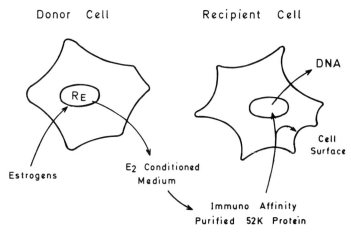

The donor cells are MCF$_7$ cells producing high levels of 52 K protein in the medium (20 ng per μg DNA per day) following estradiol stimulation with 10 nM. The recipient cells are MCF$_7$ cells deprived of estrogens for 4 days and growing slowly in 1 % charcoal-treated FCS. These cells produced less 52 K protein. The 52 K protein was purified to homogeneity by two successive affinity columns (Con A and MAb Sepharose) as described (9)(24).

Table 2. Mitogenic effects of estradiol, estradiol-conditioned medium and purified 52 K protein on MCF$_7$ cells.

	Estradiol		E$_2$ Cond. Medium	52 K Protein
% vs control	290 ± 100[a] (10)	530 ± 260[b] (7)	170 ± 40[a] (11)	170 ± 50[b] (7)
% vs E$_2$ stimulated	100	100	58	32
52 K Protein ng/ml			25–200	2,5–50

The stimulatory effect of these three treatments was evaluated on steroid-deprived MCF$_7$ cells by assaying cellular DNA. The concentration of 52 K protein was determined by IRMA. a and b are from 2 different series of experiment.
(Results are from (20) and Vignon et al. (24)).

Co and post-translational modifications of the protein.

We have recently characterised the co and post-translational modifications of the secreted 52 K protein by using several types of radio labelling, enzymatic digestions and double immunoprecipitation with the MAbs. The results are summarized in Fig. 2. The 52 K protein is N-glycosylated with at least two high-mannose or mixed oligosaccharide chains (25). Following deglycosylation with endoglycosidase H, an asialo protein of 48 K is still recognised by the antibodies and has the same molecular weight as after Tunicamycin inhibition of glycosylation. Moreover, the 52 K protein can be phosphorylated **in vivo** mostly on the high mannose oligosaccharide chains.

Fig. 2. Transit of the 52 K protein in MCF$_7$ cells.

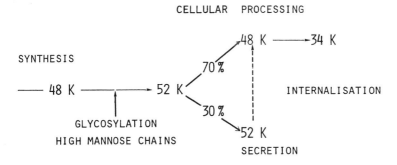

CELLULAR PROCESSING

A polypeptide chain of 48 K is co-translationally N-glycosylated with high-mannose chains to yield a 52 K cellular glycoprotein. This protein is also phosphorylated, mostly on high-mannose oligosaccharidic chains (26). In MCF$_7$ cells, this protein is mostly processed into smaller forms and accumulated as a 34 K protein, while the other part is secreted into the medium. Part of the secreted 52 K protein can be reinternalised by the same cells. The processing to lysosomes and the cellular uptake of the 52 K protein appears to be mediated by the mannose 6P receptor (27).

Preliminary evidence suggests that the phosphorylated sugar is mannose 6 phosphate, thus indicating that the 52 K protein may be internalised by interacting with mannose 6P receptors located on the cell membrane. This mechanism was first described for lysosomal hydrolases (27) which route **via** intracellular mannose 6P receptors and Golgi vesicles into lysosomes.

Under some conditions, these enzymes may be secreted and reinternalised through their interactions on mannose 6P receptors. Most of the related 52 K protein in MCF$_7$ cells is present in a processed form of

34 K (9) which appears to be located in lysosome-like vesicles, as seen by electron microscopic immunocytochemistry (Chambon et al., in preparation). These biochemical and ultrastructure studies also point to a mechanism by which the 52 K protein is able to bind and be internalised into the recipient MCF$_7$ cells. Part of the ^{35}S-labelled secreted 52 K protein has, in fact, been shown to be taken up and processed into a 34 K protein in MCF$_7$ recipient cells (24).

CONCLUSIONS

In human breast cancer cell lines, estrogens trigger two types of response, a specific one (estrogen-induced proteins) and a pleĩoreceptor and pleĩospecific one (stimulation of cell proliferation) as shown in Fig. 3. Among the estrogen-regulated proteins which have been described in MCF$_7$ cells, the secreted proteins are better candidates than the cellular proteins for mediating the effect of estrogens on cell proliferation and for acting as autocrine growth factors (Fig. 3 - Table 3). In addition to the 52 K protein, the pS2 protein (5), 160 K protein, TGFα (31) or other EGF related proteins (Lippman and Dickson, personal communication) have been shown to be secreted by MCF$_7$ cells and regulated by estrogens. It is conceivable that other proteins or peptides remain to be described. The pS2 and 52 K proteins are particularly interesting since they appear to be mostly produced by mammary tumors. However, the 52 K protein can also be produced by normal human mammary cells in culture, although in lower amounts than by MCF$_7$ cells, suggesting that it may also play a role in mammary carcinogenesis (28) (Cavalié, unpublished).

Fig. 3. The two types of response to estrogens and their relationship.

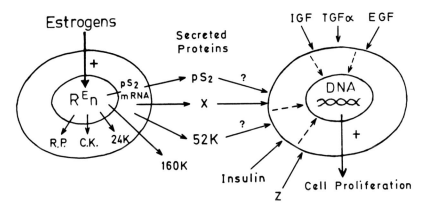

RE Specific Responses

Pleïoreceptor Responses

Estrogens induce several specific proteins (left) and stimulate cell proliferation (right). Other growth factors (IGF, TGFα, EGF, insulin) are also mitogens when added **in vitro** to hormone-responsive cell lines. Increased DNA synthesis and other pleïotypic responses are triggered by the activation of several types of receptors (pleïoreceptor responses). By contrast, estrogen-receptor-specific responses such as creatine kinase (C.K.), progesterone receptor (RP), 24 K, pS2 mRNA, are specifically regulated through activation of the nuclear estrogen receptor (R^E_n). Among them, we propose that some secreted proteins or peptides mediate (totally or partially) the mitogenic effect of estrogens, insofar their specific receptor are accessible at the surface of recipient cells.

Table 3. Estrogen-regulated proteins in breast cancer.

		Function	Localisation	Tissue Specificity
RP	(29)	Receptor	Cell	h. depd[t]
24–28 K	(4)	?	Cell + secr ?	h. depd[t]
30K	(30)	?	Cell	h. depd[t]
TGF	(31)	Growth Factor	Secreted	Transformed
pS2	(5)	?	Secreted	h. depd[t] + Transformed
52 K	(3)	Mitogen	Cell + secr ?	h. depd[t] + Transformed
160 K	(3,20)	?	Secreted	?

Characteristics of several estrogen-regulated proteins from the literature. References are in brackets. The first three are mostly cellular and appear to be more markers of differentiation linked to hormone responsiveness than regulators of cell proliferation. By contrast, some of the secreted proteins are candidates for mediating the proliferative effect of estrogens on the growth of breast cancer cells.

Taking an overview of recent progress in mammary cancer cell biology, it appears to us that the study of estrogen-regulated proteins in breast cancer by endocrinologists is converging with the results obtained by virologists and oncologists, who have described growth factors coded by oncogenes (32) and have introduced the concept of autocrine growth factors secreted by cancer cells (6). We propose that during earlier stages of mammary carcinogenesis and in hormone-dependent breast cancer, estrogens may increase the production of mitogens or growth factors coded or regulated by mammary oncogenes. Although there is some consensus among the investigators that estrogen-regulated proteins secreted by breast cancer cells are important in regulating the growth of these cells (28), the nature of the proteins involved is still controversial and is currently being studied in several laboratories.

In this short review, we report results favouring the 52 K protein as an estrogen-regulated autocrine mitogen. The 52 K glycoprotein, which is secreted under estrogen control in hormone-dependent breast cancer, and constitutively in other RE-negative breast cancers, has been probed by several monoclonal antibodies.

Basic studies of the structure and function of the protein indicate that it is a phosphoglycoprotein secreted into the medium, which can be rebound, internalised, and processed by the same MCF_7 cells. The protein is also a mitogen when added to recipient cells that produce little 52 K protein. However, the way in which the 52 K protein stimulates cell proliferation **in vitro** and its exact biological function **in vivo** are not yet understood. The study of the structure of this protein, the cloning of its cDNA and gene, and the selection of antibodies able to prevent its mitogenic activity may provide evidence to clarity these points.

ACKNOWLEDGEMENTS

We are grateful to the CLIN-MIDY/SANOFI Immunodiagnostic Laboratory (B. Pau) who have helped us to prepare the monoclonal antibodies, to E. Barrié for her skillful preparation of the manuscript, and to Mr Goodfellow for English language. We thank Drs M. Lippman, M. Rich, I. Keydar, and the Mason Research Institute, for their gifts of mammary cell lines and Pr P. Chambon for his gift of pS2 cDNA clone. This work was funded by INSERM grant (n°81039), the "Ligue Nationale Française de Lutte contre le Cancer" and the "Association pour le Développement de la Recherche sur le Cancer".

REFERENCES

1. Banbury Report. "Hormones and Breast Cancer" (Eds. M.C. Pike, P.K. Siiteri, C.W. Welsch), Cold Spring Harbor Laboratory, 1981.
2. Lippman, M.E., Bolan, G. and Huff, K. Cancer Res. **36**:4595-4601, 1976.
3. Westley, B. and Rochefort, H. Cell **20**:352-362, 1980.
4. Edwards, D.P., Adams, D.J., Savage, N., McGuire, W.L. Biochem. Biophys. Res. Commun. **93**:804-812, 1980.
5. Chambon, P., Dierich, A., Gaub, M.P., Jakowley, S., Jongstra, J., Krust, A., Lepennec, J.P., Oudet, P. and Reudelhuber, T. In: Recent Progress in Hormone Research (Ed. O. Greep), Academic Press, 1984, Vol. 40, pp. 1-42.
6. DeLarco, J.E. and Todaro, G.J. Proc. Natl. Acad. Sci. **75**:4001-4005, 1978.
7. Vignon, F., Capony, F., Chalbos, D., Garcia, M., Veith, F. Westley, B. and Rochefort, H. In: Hormones and Cancer 2, Progress in Cancer Research and Therapy (Eds. F.Bresciani, R.J.B. King, M.E. Lippman, M. Namer and J.P. Raynaud), Raven Press, New York, 1984, Vol. 31, pp. 147-160.
8. Garcia, M., Capony, F., Derocq, D., Simon, D., Pau, B. and Rochefort, H. Cancer Res. **45**:709-716.
9. Capony, F., Morisset, M., Garcia, M. and Rochefort, H. Submitted for publication.
10. Rochefort, H., Chalbos, D., Capony, F., Garcia, M., Veith, F., Vignon, F. and Westley, B. In: Hormones and Cancer (Eds. E. Gurpide, R. Calandra, C. Levy and R.J. Soto), Alan R. Liss, Inc., New York, 1984, Vol. 142, pp. 37-51.
11. Adams, D.J., Edwards, D.P. and McGuire, W.L. In: Biomembranes, 1983, Vol. 11, p. 389.
12. Massot, O., Capony, F., Garcia, M. and Rochefort, H. Mol. Cell. Endocrinol. **35**:167-175, 1984.
13. Callahan et al., 1985, this book.
14. Rochefort, H., Capony, F., Garcia, M., Morisset, M., Touïtou, I. and Vignon, F. In: Tumor Markers and Their Significance in the Management of Breast Cancer (Eds. C. Ip et al.) Alan R. Liss, Inc., New York, 1985, in press.
15. Garcia, M., Salazar-Retana, G., Richer, G., Domergue, J., Capony, F., Pujol, H., Laffargue, F., Pau, B. and Rochefort, H. J. Clin. Endocrin. Met. **59**:564-566, 1984.
16. Darbre, P., Yates, J., Curtis, S., King, R.J.B. Cancer Res. **43**:349-354, 1983.
17. Chalbos, D., Vignon, F., Keydar, I., Rochefort, H. J. Clin. Endocrin. Met. **55**:276-283, 1982.
18. Nandi, S., Imagawa, W., Tomooka, Y., McGrath, M.F. and Edery, M. Arch. Toxicol. **55**:91-96, 1984.
19. Sirbasku, D.A. and Benson, R.H. In: Hormones and Cell Culture (Eds. J.H. Soto and R. Ross), Cold Spring Harbor Laboratory, Cold Spring Harbor, 1979, Vol. 6, pp. 477-497.
20. Vignon, F., Derocq, D., Chambon, M. and Rochefort, H. C. R. Acad. Sci. (Paris) **296**:151-156, 1983.
21. Westley, B., May, F.E.B., Brown, A.M.C., Krust, A., Chambon, P., Lippman, M.E. and Rochefort, H. J. Biol. Chem. **259**:10030-10035, 1984.
22. Vignon, F., Lippman, M.E., Nawata, H., Derocq, D. and Rochefort, H. Cancer Res. **44**:2084-2088, 1984.

23. Rochefort, H., Vignon, F., Bardon, S., May, F.E.B. and Westley, B. In: Estrogen and Antiestrogen Action : Basic and Clinical Aspects (Ed. V.C. Jordan), University of Wisconsin Press, Madison, 1985, in press.

24. Vignon, F., Capony, F., Chambon, M., Garcia, M. and Rochefort, H. In preparation.

25. Touïtou, I., Garcia, M., Westley, B., Capony, F. and Rochefort, H. Submitted for publication.

26. Capony, F., Capony, J.P., Chalbos, D., Vignon, F. and Rochefort, H. In preparation.

27. Neufeld, E.G. and Cantz, M.J. Ann. N. Y. Acad. Sci. **179**:580, 1971.

28. Cavalié-Barthez, G., Chambon, M., Garcia, M., Hallowes, D, Veith, F., Vignon, F. and Rochefort, H. In: Annals of the New York Academy of Sciences, New York, in press, 1985.

29. McGuire, W.L. In: Recent Progress in Hormone Research, Academic Press, 1980, Vol. 36, pp. 135-156.

30. Hendler, F.J. and Yuan, D. Cancer Res. **45**:421-429, 1985.

31. Salomon, D.S., Zwiebel, J.A., Bano, M., Losonczy, I., Fehnel, P. and Kidwell, W.R. Cancer Res. **44**:4069-4077, 1984.

32. Heldin, C.H. and Westermark, B. Cell **37**:9-20, 1984.

33. Jakesz, R., Smith, C.A., Aitken, S., Huff, K., Schuette,W., Shackney, S. and Lippman, M. Cancer Res. **44**:619-625, 1984.

6

NEW CONCEPTS AND APPROACHES IN THE ANALYSIS OF MAMMARY PRENEOPLASIA AND TUMOR PROGRESSION

FRANCESCO SQUARTINI[1], AND IAN HART[2]

Istituto di Anatomia e Istologia Patologica, Scuola Medica, Università degli Studi, 56100 Pisa, Italy, and [2]Royal Marsden Hospital, Sutton Surrey, SM2 5PX, U.K.

In the evolution of research concerning the morphologic steps of breast carcinogenesis and their routes of progression the points of interest are so many that only a few can be focused and expanded at one time.

A first point of interest is that there are several, not a single one, pathways to breast carcinogenesis and that these pathways remarkably differ from each other in terms of target structure involved, hormones required for promotion, type of preneoplastic change if any, tumor behavior, etc. (1). Looking at the experimental and human models of breast tumorigenesis it appears that the focal preneoplastic changes are scattered at any level of the glandular tree and may be made of one or more structural components. In the mouse the hyperplastic alveolar nodules (HAN) are made up by alveoli and small terminal ducts, while the plaque-shaped pregnancy dependent tumors (P) are made up only by small terminal ducts with clavated ends or endbud-like structures radiating from a single center (2). It is apparent also an absolute prevalence of these early changes preceding mammary neoplasia in the functional part of the gland including extralobular terminal ducts and lobules with their subunits that are intralobular small terminal ducts and alveoli along them. In the human breast the terminal ductal lobular unit is the preferential site of focal proliferative changes (3,4).

A further point of interest to which special attention has been devoted in this volume, concerns the cells involved in breast carcinogenesis. The general belief is that there are three types of cells in the normal, mature mammary gland: alveolar epithelial (AE), ductal epithelial (DE) and myoepithelial (ME) cells. The existence of stem cells after glandular differentiation is disputed. The various cell types integrate to form structures. Alveoli are made up of AE (inner layer) and disconinuous ME cells, while ducts are made of DE+ME cells. The same is true for focal preoplastic changes. For instance, the HAN of mouse breast as well as the lobular carcinoma in situ of human breast are a mosaic of AE+ME cells. But the field is in rapid progress by the use of new, selected antibodies.

"Mammary gland cell types and their respective involvement in mouse mammary preoplasia and neoplasia" has been the topic of a presentation by Hilgers, Daams and Sonnenberg. Using antibodies against differentiation antigens, some of which had never been described before, five distinct cell types have been recognized in the developing mouse mammary gland, namely: basal or stem cells, developing either into myoepithelial cells or lumenal cell types called ductal type I, ductal type II and alveolar cells. Antigens included cell surface, cytoskeletal and basement membrane components. Mouse HAN were found to be very similar in structure and antigen patterns as the normal gland lobules consisting of ductal and alveolar-like components. On the other hand, in pregnancy dependent plaques or P tumors the antigen pattern was identical with that of the terminal end buds of young developing glands. Both basal and lumenal cell types were present. When P tumors undergo progression carcinomas tend to loose the basal markers, while the lumenal markers come up indicating development of acinar structures. From the presence of both basal and lumenal markers in these mammary tumors the conclusion was that they all originate from totipotent stem cells which, though transformed, have not lost the capacity to differentiate.

This conclusion looks somewhat different from that of previous experiments in which the cellular mosaicism of focal preoplastic changes was investigated by transplantation experiments (5). The transplant in hybrid mice of cell suspensions containing dissociated normal, preoplastic and tumor cells with different hystocompatibility markers in order to study the cellular composition of preoplastic changes has led to the conclusion that focal preoplasias are a mosaic of normal + transformed cells. For instance, HAN are a mosaic of transformed AE + normal ME cells. The back transplant in parents showed also that transformed AE cells of HAN do not survive without the support of normal ME cells (6). Therefore, survival of a preneoplastic change may depend on the presence of normal supporting cells. Conversely, progression to malignancy may occur when the transformed AE cells escape the control of normal ME cells or when the transformed AE cells become able to survive without support by the normal ME cells.

This point is crucial for the understanding of progression from preneoplasia to overt neoplasia. Therefore, Medina was asked to summarize the field talking on "Normal cell-transformed cell interactions in mouse mammary preneoplasia and tumor progression". In his experiments preneoplastic mammary nodules were enzymatically dissociated to produce yields of viable single cells and injected into the cleared mammary fat pads of syngeneic mice. All dissociated nodule cell lines showed a marked increase in tumorigenicity as compared to the same tissues transplanted as 1 mm^3 pieces. Addition of normal mammary cells to the nodule cells reversed the marked increase in tumorigenicity of enzymatically dissociated nodule cells to a level equal to or less than the tumorigenicity of control transplanted pieces. These results suggest that growth inhibitory effects of normal mammary cells may indeed prevent or delay tumor development by the committed preneoplastic cells (7) supporting the hypothesis previously reported.

But, is preneoplasia an integral part of breast cancer disease, or it is a different thing? To develop this not merely semantic question Cardiff was asked to report on the "Molecular aspects of mouse mammary preneoplasia and the concept of protoneoplasia". The mouse mammary tumor virus (MuMTV) has provided a window into the inner workings of the mammary epithelial cell at the earliest stages of neoplasia. Techniques of molecular biology have permitted to look through that window revealing a new biology which deserves consideration as a model for mammary tumorigenesis in all species. HAN cells, unlike normal mammary cells, are immortal and can be serially transplanted. HAN cells are also genetically altered as evidenced by the presence of acquired MuMTV restriction fragments in the DNA. The presence of acquired MuMTV provirus denotes an acquired genetic change in these somatic cells and implies that HAN are composed of clonal dominant populations. Clonal dominance implies in turn that these changes in the cell genotype are critical to the neoplastic process and probably responsible for the immortalization of the tissue. In addition, many facts strongly suggest that tumors are direct derivatives of the hyperplastic cells and this relationship makes the mouse mammary focal hyperplasias an integral and critical part of the neoplastic progression that ends in the malignant tumors. Therefore, HAN is clearly the first step of breast cancer disease although it is also clear that not all the cells in the HAN population are committed to malignant transformation. These evidences make the term preneoplasia inadequate and suggest "protoneoplasia" as a possible substitute for HAN and similar focal hyperplasias because this implies that they are the original, or first step in the neoplastic progression and that the protoneoplastic mammary hyperplasia is an integral though non obligate part of neoplastic progression (8).

However, not only the epithelial cells of mammary neoplasia are involved in tumor progression but, apparently, also other tumor associated cells. In this respect a new approach to the problem was presented by Heppner, Mahoney and Yamashiva reporting on "Relationship between tumor-associated macrophages (TAM) and expression of malignant behavior of mouse mammary cancers". TAM were isolated from primary tumor implants of a series of mouse mammary tumor lines previously characterized and differing in several characteristics including ability to metastasize (9). TAM characterization for functional, physical and biochemical properties indicated qualitative differences between TAM from metastatic versus nonmetastatic tumors and intratumoral heterogeneity of TAM populations. TAM from metastatic tumors are tumoricidal in vitro, whereas those from nonmetastatic tumors are less often cytotoxic. TAM from metastatic tumors are also larger and denser than those from nonmetastatic tumors. TAM from metastatic tumors have a high concentration of the ectoenzyme leucine aminopeptidase. Measuring the abilty of TAM to induce genetic mutations, both TAM from metastatic and nonmetastatic tumors appeared to be mutagenic but tumor cells of metastatic lines were more sensitive to induced mutation than were those from nonmetastatic tumors. These results, taken together, suggest an association between TAM and the expression or development of malignant behavior.

New data on the "Mechanisms of progression of mouse mammary tumors from pregnancy dependence to autonomy" were presented by Matsuzawa and Kaneko. The TPDM-4, a transplantable pregnancy dependent mammary tumor established in DDD mice, produces practically no growth behaving like a preneoplastic lesion in virgin mice. A study was conducted to investigate whether enzyme dissociation enhances progression of this tumor in virgins as observed with HAN. Tumors from early (F8), intermediate (F15) and late (F49) transplant generations were dissociated and injected into the fat pads of syngenic recipients which were then observed for tumor development. Significant outgrowths occurred in 43%, 60% and 89% of the transplanted mice respectively, but many of the early and intermediate generation outgrowths regressed. Tumors were also examined for ovarian dependence and estrogen and progesterone receptors. Ovarian dependence progressively decreased from early to late tumor generations. However, all the tumors examined contained significant levels of estrogen receptors regardless of their ovarian dependence, while only the dependent and responsive tumors also had progesterone receptors. In ovarian independent tumors progesterone receptors were not induced with estrogen in spite of the presence of estrogen receptors. No differences related to tumor progression were observed at different transplant generations in MuMTV DNA provirus and cell karyotype. Therefore, enzymatic dissociation enhances progression to autonomy of pregnancy dependent tumors but the unique detectable cell change associated with progression is the loss of progesterone receptors.

An approach to the human problem was finally presented by Bussolati, Gugliotta, Papotti and Botta reporting on "Morphologic markers in the definition of human mammary preneoplasia and its progression to cancer". Multiple duct papillomas and in situ lobular carcinomas are focal changes of the human breast whose preneoplastic potential has long been recognized. Evidence of progression in these changes may be visualized histologically using immunohistochemical methods. Anti-actin antibodies have been used to mark the actin-rich myoepithelial cells which form a continuous basal layer along the stalks of the benign papillomas while are absent from carcinomatous areas. Anti-CEA mono and polyclonal antibodies were found to bind selectively to the cytoplasm of the ductal in situ carcinomas. Several early carcinomatous CEA-positive actin-negative foci were detected thus confirming the direct transformation of benign lesions into carcinomas. Also in the lobular carcinoma in situ the behavior of myoepithelial cells may herald tumor progression. In fact, in situ associated with infiltrating lobular carcinoma show fewer myoepithelial cells which are mobilized from their basal position and mixed with the tumor cell populations within the alveolar lumina (10).

In the Poster Session connected with this Workshop there were many other interesting data which cannot be quoted because of the limitations of space alloted. The majority dealt with aspects of tumor cell progression which might be useful to predict malignancy or to identify tumor behaviors requiring possibly different treatments. The selected points discussed above provide a clue for their understanding.

REFERENCES

1. Squartini,F., Bistocchi,M., Sarnelli,R. and Basolo,F. Ann.N.Y.Acad.Sci. 383 , 1985 (in press).

2. Squartini,F. In: Pathology of Tumours in Laboratory Animals II (Ed. V. S.Turusov), IARC Scientific Publication No.7, Lyon, 1979, pp. 43-90 .

3. Wellings,S.R. Adv.Cancer Res. 31: 287-314, 1980.

4. Squartini,F. and Sarnelli,R. JNCI 67: 33-46, 1981.

5. Slemmer,G.L. J.Invest.Dermatol. 63: 27-47, 1974.

6. Slemmer,G.L. In: Cell Biology of Breast Cancer (Eds.C.M. MacGrath,M.A.Rich and M.J.Brennan), Academic Press, New York, 1980, pp. 93-143.

7. Medina,D., Shephard,F. and Gropp ,T. JNCI 60: 1121-1126, 1978.

8. Cardiff,R.D. Adv.Cancer Res. 42: 167-190, 1984.

9. Miller,F.R., Miller,B.E. and Heppner,G.G. Invasion Metastasis 3:22-31,1983.

10. Bussolati,G. Virchows Arch. B Cell Pathol. 32: 165-176, 1980.

7

CELL CULTURE STUDIES: A PERSPECTIVE ON MALIGNANT PROGRESSION OF HUMAN BREAST CANCER

H.S. SMITH[1], S.R. WOLMAN[2], G. AUER[3], A.J. HACKETT[1]

[1]Peralta Cancer Research Institute, 3023 Summit Street, Oakland, CA 94609, [2]Cytogenetics Laboratory, Department of Pathology, New York University School of Medicine, New York, New York 10016, [3]Karolinska Institute, Stockholm, Sweden

ABSTRACT

Primary breast cancers contain heterogeneous subpopulations which vary in the extent to which they are capable of aspects of metastatic spread. The conditions for cell isolation and culture, may select among differing populations. Using a system developed for culturing normal mammary epithelium, we have grown and characterized tumor-derived populations that appear to be partially transformed. The cells are invasive and show other characteristics distinguishing them from normal cells, but remain diploid. Because similar populations are not found in metastatic effusions, we hypothesize that the diploid cells represent an early stage of malignant progression. Such populations, which also have been isolated from hypodermal chest wall recurrences, have been used in a clonogenic assay for chemotherapeutic drug sensitivity, and the initial clinical correlations are promising.

Cultures derived from metastic effusions are highly variable in growth properties and usually do not clone with high efficiency. All are aneuploid. Unlike experimental models where metastases appear to be monoclonal (1), karyotypic polyclonality has been detected at first passage (2,3). Upon subculture, some effusions cease proliferation while others undergo crisis and develop into cell lines. In one case where the cells at first passage were polyclonal, the line that emerged subsequently was monoclonal indicating the degree of selection that can occur during the development of cell lines. Further studies to isolate and culture various populations from human breast cancers are needed because the cultured subsets can illustrate different links in the chain of events connecting biochemical and molecular studies on cell lines to studies of human cancer in vivo.

INTRODUCTION

Human specimens taken directly from the operating room have limited value for biochemical and molecular comparisons between tumor and normal tissues. In addition to the tumor cell types, these tissues contain varying amounts of other cells including lymphocytes, blood vessels, and stromal fibroblasts. When attempts are made to dissociate the tissue and isolate the tumor cells without contaminants, the result is often loss of tumor as well as stroma and too few cells are obtained for study. Culture is one approach to amplify the number of available cells. Unfortunately, only occasionally do tumor specimens develop into cell lines with infinite growth potential, while the vast majority of primary carcinomas and all normal tissues do not. Notable exceptions are the small cell lung cancers which are routinely established as cell lines (4); however, the normal counterpart of this malignant cell has not been cultured. Recently, some success has been reported in short term culturing of a variety of other tumor cell types (5).

The human mammary gland is a good system for studying malignant progression since specimens representing at least some stages of progression are readily available as discard material from surgical specimens. Reduction mammoplasties are an excellent source of normal epithelial cells since they usually show little or no pathology of the epithelial cells. Tissues peripheral to carcinomas in mastectomy specimens are another source of nonmalignant cells. Malignant lesions usually provide sufficient tissue beyond what is needed for pathologic diagnosis for the culture of carcinoma cells. Malignant effusions are a ready source of metastatic cells since effusions are often removed for the comfort of the patient.

Our laboratory has been involved in developing techniques for short term culture of human mammary epithelium (6-10). Our goal has been to isolate and culture with high efficiency and identify epithelial cells from every specimen regardless of stage in malignant progression. Here we describe our progress to date and illustrate how these cultures provide unique insights into the nature of malignant progression.

PROPERTIES OF CELLS CULTURED FROM PRIMARY CARCINOMAS

One of the problems with culturing breast carcinoma cells is
that tumors are quite desmoplastic. It is difficult to isolate the
tumor cells free from the reactive stroma. Some breast cancer cells
are only loosely attached to the stromal matrix so that they can be
dissociated mechanically. These cells represent a minority
population within the tumors, characterized by low viability
(11,12). The majority of breast carcinoma cells can only be
released after enzymatic digestion of the stromal matrix with
collagenase. With such treatment, part of the tumor is dissociated
to single cells but most remains as tightly associated cell clumps.
These conditions result in dissociation of the stromal fibroblasts
and blood vessels to single cells; the tumor clumps can then easily
be isolated free from fibroblasts by sedimentation at unit gravity
(13) or by filtration through nylon mesh filters (6). The tumor
cells proliferate to some degree in a variety of culture conditions
(14-18); however, recent media formulations have supported
considerably more proliferation in mass cultures (6,9) and have
permitted tumor cell growth in a highly efficient clonogenic assay
when cells are plated sparsely on a fibroblast feeder layer
(7,8,10). Most recently, a serum-free medium has been described
which allows clonal proliferation without fibroblast feeder cells
(19).

A number of criteria have been used to demonstrate the
epithelial nature of these cells. The cultured cells possess a
typical cubiodal morphology with the formation of secretory domes
and duct-like, three-dimensional ridges at confluence.
Ultrastructurally, the cells show junctional complexes and evidence
of secretory activity (6,13,20). The cells are positive for
cytokeratins (20-23), have a diminished punctate pattern of
cell-associated fibronectin (24,25) typical of epithelium and
express epithelial membrane antigens as defined by antibodies raised
to milk-fat globule (8,13,26).

There is some controversy as to whether the carcinoma-derived
cultures are bona fide tumor cells or nonmalignant cells originating
from tissue peripheral to the malignancy (17,27). Justification for
the belief that primary breast cancer cells are, in fact, being

cultured stems from scattered reports of consistent differences
between cultures derived from malignant and nonmalignant tissues.
Asaga et al., (28) reported a significant increase in multinucleated
cells after incubation of human mammary carcinoma cultures with
cytochalasin when compared with cultures derived from various benign
tissues. Similar results were reported for cultured rodent mammary
tissues (29). Carcinoma-derived cultures also showed increased
variability in surface antigen expression when compared to
nonmalignant tissue from the same donor (30). We have compared
tumor and nonmalignant cultures using a polyvalent antiserum
prepared by Edgington and colleagues (31,32) to a 19.5 kilodalton
glycoprotein reported to be tumor-specific. All tumor-derived
cultures were positive while all nonmalignant cultures tested were
negative (21). Unfortunately, this polyvalent antiserum can not be
used routinely to monitor tumor-derived cultures, since it is no
longer available. More recently, to obtain further evidence that
the cells cultured from primary carcinomas indeed represent
malignant cells, we investigated the phenotype of invasiveness,
probably the most important single criterion by which human solid
malignancies can be characterized (33). We employed an in vitro
assay for invasion utilizing denuded human amnions (34,35) and we
found that the tumor cells retained their malignant phenotype in
culture by being capable of invasive growth (Table 1).

There are two reasons why the malignant nature of the tumor
derived cells has been questioned. First, in earlier studies
(17,27), it had been observed that most of the carcinoma-derived
cultures were morphologically indistinguishable from non-malignant
cultured mammary cells. In 15 to 20% of cultures from primary
carcinomas, a cell type with unusually abnormal morphology was also
observed. The abnormal cell type, designated E', was thought to
resemble cells from some metastatic lesions, but unlike the cells
from metastases, it was unable to grow in culture. It was
hypothesized that E' cells were the tumor cells and that only
nonmalignant cells associated with cancers and not the actual tumor
cells were growing out in culture from the majority of primary
carcinomas. However, we have found that the normal as well as the

Table 1

Invasion of Human Amnions by Cultured
Normal and Malignant Epithelial Cells[1]

Specimen	Number Invasive / Total number tested
Nonmalignant Tissues (Short-Term Cultures)	
Reduction mammoplasties	0/5
Mastectomy tissue peripheral to carcinoma	0/2
Mastectomy tissue contralateral to carcinoma	0/1
Normal skin from cancerous breast	0/1
Total	0/9
Primary Carcinomas (Short-Term Cultures)	
Lobular	1/2
Infiltrating ductal	6/8
Inflamatory	1/1
Total	8/11
Established Cell Lines	2/3

[1] A portion of these data has been summarized from reference 33.

tumor cultures were reported as malignant, when coded samples were examined by a cytopathologist (unpublished observations). Since normal cells in culture can appear malignant, any morphological observation inferring normality or malignancy is likely to be invalid when considering cultured cells. Another reason for questioning the malignant origin of the cultured tumor cells is that we have found that the vast majority of cells in short-term cultures from 15 different primary breast carcinomas were completely diploid (23). Only an occasional cell within these cultures showed minimal and non-clonal karyotypic deviations from normality. Examples of the types of chromosomal aberrations seen are shown in Table 2.

However, similar (in some cases identical) short-term diploid
cultures of breast carcinoma retained their capacity for
invasiveness in the in vitro assay (Table 1). Nonmalignant cells,
similarly cultured, were not invasive in the same assay. These
observations provide strong evidence that the cells cultured from
primary carcinomas indeed represent malignant cells, and indicate
that at least some malignant populations need not have gross
karyotypic rearrangements.

Table 2

Typical Examples of Karyotypes of Epithelial Cells
Cultured from Primary Carcinomas[1]

Specimen	Total (banded)	46, XX or Random Loss	Aneuploid
Primary Carcinoma			
192T	11(11)	11	-
335T	10(10)	8	2(44,XX,-1, -15,-19,+M (?8p;7q)) (45,XX,4p-,-4, -13,-14,-22, +M1 (large submetacentric), +M2 (medium metacentric), +M3 (tiny metacentric))
407T	10(10)	10	-
469T	12(12)	10	1(46 XX, 14q+) 1(46 XX, 1q+)

[1]Data taken from reference 33.

We have also used cultured tumor-derived cells for evaluating
responses to the chemotherapeutic drug, adriamycin (7,36,37).
Utilizing a clonogenic assay (8), we found that the levels of
adriamycin required for 50% survival differed approximately 35-fold
among tumor specimens from donors who had had no prior therapy.

In contrast, specimens from donors who had failed prior chemotherapy regimens that contained adriamycin, had only a 5-fold range in drug sensitivity and the dose response curves clustered at the more resistant end of the spectrum (37). These results parallel the expected clinical response and suggest that the assay could be clinically relevant. The best way to determine the predictive value of the assay conclusively is to perform a prospective study using agents in a appropriate therapeutic context. The results presented here demonstrate that such a prospective study is both feasible and warranted. In collaboration with Dr. Marc Lippman (National Cancer Institute, Bethesda, MD), we plan to evaluate this clonogenic assay prospectively in a randomized clinical trial comparing the best drug chosen by the assay with vinblastin.

PROPERTIES OF CELLS CULTURED FROM METASTASES

To gain insight into the properties of cells representing later stages of malignant progression, we have begun to study malignant effusions. Almost all breast cancer cell lines in existence have been derived from pleural effusions (for reviews, see 38-40). Although it has been reported that the majority of metastatic specimens from pleural effusions can be cultured for a few population doublings (17), even under the best conditions only approximately 5 percent of these cultures develop into cell lines (38-41). In our experience, pleural effusions are much less predictable than primary carcinomas even when they are handled in an identical manner (42,43). Each pleural effusion seems to have a combination of properties in culture that deviate in a unique way from the uniform and predictable behavior of most primary carcinomas. Cellular morphology differs dramatically among pleural effusion specimens. In the samples we have studied, the cultures of malignant effusions grew very slowly and very few were able to clone on irradiated fibroblasts. Many malignant effusions grew better with medium M199 plus 10% fetal calf serum than with the medium formulation devised for normal mammary epithelium; occasionally the reverse was true.

In contrast to the primary carcinomas, the malignant effusion-derived cultures were aneuploid (Table 3) (33). We utilized flow cytometry to determine the DNA content of the slowly proliferating malignant effusion cultures. In one case (576M), aneuploidy was also verified karyotypically; the tumor cells had markers indicative of clonal origin with a modal value of 61 chromosomes (33). The specimen 600M which appeared diploid by flow cytometry was karyotypically abnormal with several marker chromosomes. The primary culture showed several distinct clones. Subsequently a cell line developed which represented selection in culture for one of the clones observed in primary passage (2). This tumor (600M) documents the rapid evolution which can occur from a

Table 3

DNA Content by Flow Cytometry of Cultured Mammary Epithelial Cells from Primary and Metastatic Carcinomas[1]

Specimen	Ploidy Value of G1 Peaks
Primary Carcinoma	
192T	2
343T	2
407T	2
469T	2
Effusion Metastases	
486M (ascites)	4.4
521M (ascites)	2.7, 2.9, 3.0[2]
522M (pleura)	no distinct peak
(broad	range from 2-4)
600M (pleura)	2.0, 2.0
576M (pleura)	2.4

[1]Data taken from reference 33.
[2]Assays done on three different cultures.

cytogenetically heterogeneous metastatic population to a culture representing only a portion of the original sample; it illustrates that extensive selection may influence the development of a cell line.

In contrast to the malignant effusions, cultures derived from skin metastases were similar to cultures derived from primary carcinomas. The majority of specimens grew and cloned readily in the enriched mammary medium. They were also predominantly diploid with some nonclonal aneuploid cells; only one of seven specimens was near-diploid with clonal rearrangements (23). The fact that skin metastases are more like primary carcinomas than other metastases is not surprising since it is known that hypodermal metastases have a more favorable prognosis.

RELATIONSHIP BETWEEN DNA CONTENT AND MALIGNANT PROGRESSION

The cells cultured from primary carcinomas are invasive, and show other characteristics which distinguish them from nonmalignant cells, even though they remain diploid. Because diploid populations were not found in metastatic effusions, we hypothesize that the diploid cells are "partially transformed" and represent an early stage of malignant progression. It is likely that the techniques we used for isolating and/or culturing the tumor cells are selective for the diploid, partially transformed cells. There is a large body of evidence indicating that over 50% of primary breast cancers in vivo contain aneuploid cells (for reviews, see 43,44). For example, from studies measuring DNA content by microspectrophotometry, approximately 50% of breast cancers are either diploid or tetraploid (possibly G2 phase) while the remainder contain aneuploid cells (45,46). Nearly all of the aneuploid tumors had DNA content in excess of the diploid value and most were between diploid and tetraploid. The presence of aneuploidy indicates a dire prognosis (45-49); therefore, aneuploidy is somehow associated with metastatic ability. Previously, it had been assumed that the diploid cells in tumors were nonmalignant in origin. However, even with microspectrophotometric techniques (45,47,50), where the invasive nature of the cell whose DNA content was being measured was verified directly, tumor cells with diploid values for DNA content were identified. Of course, the possibility can not be excluded that those tumors with diploid DNA contents actually contain cells with abnormal karyotypes.

Most of the karyotypic data on breast cancer tissues taken directly from surgery or after a few hours in culture indicate aneuploidy (for reviews see 51,52). For approximately 60% of breast cancers however, no mitotic spreads were available for study (53,54). Furthermore, those tumors with high thymidine labeling indices, which are more likely to yield cells in mitosis, are also the tumors most likely to be aneuploid in DNA content (55). Therefore, studies in which direct karyotypic analysis is successful may be biased toward aneuploidy.

Many aneuploid tumors also contain some diploid cells. For example, by microspectrophotometry, 30% of the aneuploid tumors also contain diploid malignant cells (for reviews, see 43,44). Of those tumors which were successfully karyotyped, approximately 60% contained at least some normal karyotypes (53) and in one report, 30% contained only diploid karyotypes (54). The percentage of diploid cells within the mixed tumors ranged from 2 to 75% (median value 9%). We suggest that these diploid tumor cells represent the "partially transformed" populations that we isolate after culture.

From examination of the original paraffin-embedded tissues, at least some of the specimens from which we have cultured diploid tumor cells originally contained aneuploid cells (Table 4). It is

Table 4
Comparison of Ploidy Levels of the Original Tumors With
Properties of Tumor-Derived Cells in Culture

Tumor Specimen	Ploidy of Original Tumor	Properties of Tumor-derived Cells in Culture		
		Diploid by Karyology	Diploid by Flow Cytometry	Invasion of Human Amnions
66T	Diploid	Yes	NT	NT
192T	Diploid	Yes	Yes	Yes
202T	Diploid	Yes	NT	NT
203T	Aneuploid	Yes	NT	NT
335T	Diploid	Yes	NT	NT
336T	Questionable	Yes	NT	NT
343T	Aneuploid	NT	Yes	Yes
407T	Aneuploid	Yes	Yes	Yes
469T	Questionable	Yes	Yes	Yes

NT = not tested

necessary therefore to explain why the aneuploid cells are preferentially lost from cultures of primary carcinomas. Aneuploid cells appear to be lost during the initial tissue digestion, since we have found that the cells isolated from an aneuploid tumor were diploid prior to subsequent culturing (Fig 1). It is possible that

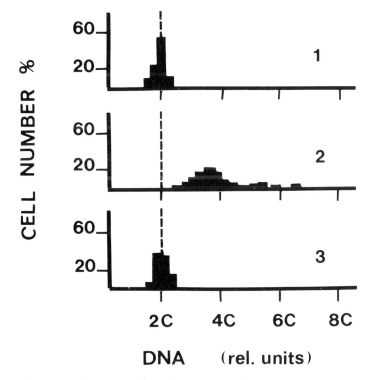

FREQUENCY HISTOGRAMS OF NUCLEAR DNA CONTENT
(Feulgen positive material stained as in ref. 46)
1. Normal diploid mammary cells (control)
2. Paraffin section of original tumor (specimen 343T)
3. Cells isolated from tumor specimen 343T by enzymatic digestion is described in ref. 8. Briefly, the minced specimen was digested overnight with collagenase and hyaluronidase. Tumor clumps, separated from single cells by filtration, were cryopreserved in 10% DMSO (dimethyl sulfoxide). Subsequently, the clumps were thawed, removed from DMSO, fixed in formalin, paraffin embedded, and sectioned.

the aneuploid cells within primary tumors are viable in vivo but are relatively fragile and therefore preferentially lost during isolation. Those tumor populations which can be mechanically dissociated to single cells are enriched for both aneuploid and nonviable cells when compared to populations isolated from the same tumors by enzymatic digestion (11,12). Possibly the shear forces necessary to generate single cells from the tightly apposed tumor cell clumps are lethal. However, we have found that tumor cell clumps gently "spilled" from the tissue sometimes are also largely nonviable. We suggest an alternative explanation for the absence of aneuploid cells in the isolates from primary carcinomas. We hypothesize that many of the aneuploid cells are nonviable even in vivo. It is known from kinetic studies that most of the cells in primary carcinomas are lost from the proliferative compartment (44). We suggest here that many of these cells are permanently rather than reversibly nonproliferating. Small subpopulations of viable aneuploid cells present within primary carcinomas may be responsible for proliferation and metastasis. We suggest that metastasizing subpopulations can be generated from diploid, invasive cells by a process of genetic instability similar to that originally proposed by Nowell (56). Most of the aneuploid cells generated by this process are probably nonviable; however, an occasional cell could retain viability while gaining the capacity for metastatic growth. Although a close relationship between aneuploidy and tumor progression seems clear, whichever alternative proves correct, a fundamental point which has been illustrated is that diploid cells within breast cancers are capable of invasive growth. We suggest that such cells may be more informative than tumor cell lines with grossly aberrant karyotypes for investigating early somatic genetic changes as well as other alterations involved in the acquisition of malignant characteristics.

ACKNOWLEDGEMENTS

This work was supported in part by Grants CA34192 and CA38739 to Helene S. Smith, Ph.D. from the National Cancer Institute of the United States.

REFERENCES

1. Talmadge, J., Wolman, S., Fidler, I. (1982) Science 217:361-363.
2. Wolman, S.R., Leff. S., Smith, H.S., Hackett, A.J. (1985) Cancer Genetics & Cytogenetics, In Press (abstract).
3. Smith, H.S., Wolman, S.R., Hancock,M.C., Lippman, M.E., Hackett, A.J. (1985) In Vitro, In Press (abstract).
4. Gazdar, A.F., Carney, D.N., Minna, J.D. (1983) Seminars in Oncology 10:3-19.
5. Weber, M., Sekeley, L. In Vitro Models for Human Cancers CRC Press, In Press 1985.
6. Stampfer, M.R., Hallowes, R.C., Hackett, A.J. (1980) In Vitro, 16:415-425.
7. Smith, H.S., Hackett, A.J., Lan, S., Stampfer, M.R. (1981) Cancer Chemo. and Pharm., 6:237-244.
8. Smith, H.S., Lan, S., Ceriani, R., Hackett, A.J., Stampfer, M.R. (1981) Cancer Res., 41:4637-4643.
9. Stampfer, M.R. (1982) In Vitro, 18:531:537.
10. Smith, H.S., Stampfer, M.R., Hancock, M.C., and Hackett, A.J. (1983) in (T. Pretlow ed.) Cell Separation: Methods and Selected Applications II Acad. Press pp. 183-202.
11. Chassevent, A., Daver, A., Bertrand, G., Coic, H., Geslin, J., Bidabe, M-Cl., George, P., Larra, F. (1984) Cytometry 5:263-267.
12. Frankfurt, O.S., Slocum, H.K., Rustum, Y.M., Arbuck, S.G., Pavelic, Z.P., Petrelli, N., Huben, R.P., Pontes, E.J., Greco, W.R. (1984) Cytometry 5:71-80.
13. Easty, G.C., Easty, D.M., Monoghan, P., Ormerod,M.G., Neville, A.M. (1980) Int'l J. Cancer, 26:577-584.
14. Stoker, M.G.P., Pigott, D., Taylor-Papadimitriou, J. (1976) Nature, 264:764-767.
15. Taylor-Papadimitriou, J., Purkiss, P., and Fentimen, I.S. (1979) J. Cell. Physiol., 102:317-321.
16. Kirklan, W.L., Yang, H., Jorgensen, T., Langley, C., Furmanski, P. (1979) JNCI 63:29-42.
17. Taylor-Papadimitriou, J., Fentiman, I.S., Burchell, J. (1980) in Problems and Directions in Cell Biology of Breast Cancer (eds. McGrath, C., Brennan, M.J., Rich, M.A.) Academic Press, pp. 347-362.
18. Yang, J., Richards, J., Guzman, R., Imagawa, W. and Nandi, S. (1980) PNAS, USA, 77:2088-2092.
19. Hammond, S.L., Ham, R.G., Stampfer, M.R. (1985) Proc. Nat'l Acad. Sci. 81:5435-5439.
20. Taylor-Papadimitriou, Shearer, M., Tilly, R. (1977) JNCI, 58:1563-1571.
21. Stampfer, M.R., Hackett, A.J., Hancock, M.C., Leung, J.P., Edgington, T.S., Smith, H.S. (1982) Cold Springs Harbor Symposium on Cell Proliferation, 9:819-829.
22. Biran, S., Horowitz, A.T., Fuks, Z., Vlodavsky, I. (1983) Int. J. Cancer, 31:557-566.
23. Wolman, S.R., Smith, H.S., Stampfer, M.R., Hackett, A.J. (1985) Cancer Genetics & Cytogenetics, 16:49-64.
24. Stampfer, M.R., Vlodavsky, I., Smith, H.S., Ford, R., Becker, F.F., Riggs, J. (1981) JNCI, 67:253-261.
25. Taylor-Papadimitriou, J., Burchell, J., Hurst, J. (1981) Cancer Res., 41:2491-2500.

26. Taylor-Papadimitriou, J., Peterson, J.A., Arklie, J., Burchell, J., Ceriani, R.L., Bodmer, W.F., (1981) Int. J. Cancer, 28:17-21.

27. Hallowes, R.C., Millis, R., Pigott, D., Shearer, M., Stoker, M.G.P., and Taylor-Papadimitriou, J. (1977) Clin. Oncol., 3:81-90.

28. Asaga, T., Suzuki, K., Takemiya, S., Okamoto, T., Tamura, N. and Umeda, M. (1983) Gann, 74:95-99.

29. Medina, D., Osborn, C.J., Ash, B.B. (1980) Cancer Res., 40:329-333.

30. Ceriani, R.L., Peterson, J.A., Blank, E.W. (1984) Cancer Res. 44:3033-3039.

31. Leung, J.P., Plow, E.F., Nakamura, R.M., Edgington, T.S. (1978) J. Immunol., 121:1287-1296.

32. Leung, J.P., Borden, G.M., Nakamura, R.M., DeHeer, D.H., Edgington, T.S. (1979) Cancer Res., 39:2057-2061.

33. Smith, H.S., Liotta, L.A., Hancock, M.C., Wolman, S.R., Hackett, A.J. (1985) Proc. Natl. Acad., USA, 82:1805-1809.

34. Russo, R.G., Thorglirsson, W., and Liotta, L.A. (1982) (eds. L.A. Liotta and I.R. Hart) The Hague, Boston and London: Martimes and Nijhoff Pub., 173-187.

35. Russo, R.G., Foltz, C.M., Liotta, L.A. (1983) Clin. Expl. Metastasis, 1:115-127.

36. Smith, H.S., Acton, E.M., Hackett, A.J. (1983) in Rational Basis for Chemotherapy, Vol. 4, A.R. Liss, Inc., NY, pp 119-136.

37. Smith, H.S., Lippman, M.E., Hiller, A.J., Stampfer, M.R., Hackett, A.J. (1985) J. Nat'l Cancer Inst. 74:341-347.

38. Lasfargues, E.Y., Coritinho, W.G. (1981) in New Frontiers in Mammary Pathology (eds. K.H. Hollman, J. de Brux, J.M. Verley) Plenum Press, London, pp. 117-143.

39. Smith, H.S., and Dollbaum, C.M. (1982) in Handbook of Experimental Pharmacology: Tissue Growth Factors. ed. Renato Barserga, Vol. 57, pp. 451-478.

40. Engel, L.W., Young, N.A. (1978) Cancer Res., 38:4327-4339.

41. Cailleau, R., Olive, M., Cruciger, Q.V.J. (1978) In Vitro, 14:911-915.

42. Hackett, A.J., Smith, H.S. (1985) in In Vitro Models for Human Cancer (ed. Weber and Sekeley), CRC Press, FL., In Press.

43. Smith, H.S., Wolman, S.R., Hackett, A.J. (1984) Biochem & Biophysica Acta 738:103-123.

44. Meyer, J.S., McDivitt, R.W., Stone, K.R., Prey, M.U., Bauer, W.C. (1984) Breast Cancer Res. and Treat. 4, 79-88

45. Auer, G.U., Caspersson, T.O., Wallgren, A.S. (1980) Anal. Quant. Cytol., 2:161-165.

46. Auer, G., Erikson, E., Azavido, E., Caspersson, T.O., Wallgren, A.S. (1984) Cancer Res. 44:394-396.

47. Fossa, S.D., Marton, P.F., Knudson, O.S., Kaalhus, O., Bormer, O., Vaage, S. (1982) Human Pathology, 13:626-630.

48. Fossa, S.D., Thorud, E., Vaage, S., Shoaib, M.C. (1983) Acta. Path. Microbiol. Immunol. Scand., Section A, 91:235-243.

49. Kute, T.E., Muss, H.B., Anderson, D., Crumb, K., Miller, B., Burnes, D., Dube, L.A. (1981) Cancer Res., 41:3524-3529.

50. Lazzari, G., Vineis, C. (1980) Ann. Osp. Maria Vittoria Torino, 23:112-125.

51. Sandberg, A.A.(1983) Cancer Genet. and Cytogenet., 8:277-285.

52. Wolman, S.R., (1983) Cancer Metastasis Reviews, 2:257-293.
53. Rodgers, C.S., Hill, S.M., Hulten, M.A. (1984) Cancer Genetics & Cytogenetics 13:95-119.
54. Gebhart, E., Bruderlein, S., Tuluson, A.H., Maillot, K.V. Birkmann (1984) Int. J. Cancer 34:369-373.
55. Auer, G., Ono, J., Caspersson, T.O. (1983) Anal. and Quant. Cytol 5:5-8.
56. Nowell, P.C. (1976) The Clonal Evolution of Tumor Cell Populations. Science, 194:23-28.

8

WORKSHOP ON IN VITRO CULTURE SYSTEMS

R. HALLOWES and M. STAMPFER

Imperial Cancer Research Fund, London WC2A 3PX, England, and Lawrence
Berkeley Laboratory, Berkeley, California, USA 94720.

In vitro cell culture allows for experimental evaluation of cell
properties with greater control of external conditions than whole animal
studies. For studies of human cellular biology, where "in vivo"
experimentation is not an option, the availability of well characterized
culture systems is essential for scientific research. Much progress has
been made in recent years in the development of a variety of mammary
epithelial culture systems that permit active cell growth, utilize
serum-free conditions, and/or provide potentially useful clinical
correlates, such as sensitivity to chemotherapeutic drugs. At the same
time, there have been rapid advances in markers for identification and
characterization of mammary cells (see reference 1 for the status report of
in vitro culture at the previous workshop in 1983). The current workshop
addressed some of the outstanding unresolved issues in mammary cell
culture, including (a) the effects of culture conditions on both
maintenance of survival of specific cell types and regulation of specific
cell functions; (b) how can malignant cells be identified in culture; (c)
what possible role may fibroblast cells be playing in development of breast
pathology.

Dr. Martha Stampfer (University of California) introduced the meeting
and described some effects of culture medium upon the expression of
differentiated function. Human mammary epithelium from reduction
mammoplasties was grown on plastic dishes in two different media: MM (2)
which contains conditioned medium, growth factors, and foetal calf serum,
and MCDB 170 (3) a chemically defined medium containing one undefined
growth factor, bovine pituitary extract. Four differentiated properties
were examined, (a) Metabolism of glucose: Emerman et al. (4) had shown that
glucose metabolites of virgin-derived and pregnancy-derived mouse mammary
cells were different. The present study showed that the metabolic pattern
of cells maintained in MM was similar to that of pregnant mice, high in

glycogen and lactate, whereas in MCBD 170 it resembled that of the virgin. These differences were maintained whilst the cells were passaged in the same medium. However when cells that had been passaged 8 times in MCBD 170 were transferred to MM, the glucose metabolites rapidly changed to that characteristic of MM. The reverse was also true. (b) Milk fat globulin antigen expression: some expression was found in MM, increasing from 2nd to the 5th passage, whereas little or none was seen in MCBD 170. (c) 35 S incorporation into proteins secreted into the medium probed with whey protein antibodies: In MM, several bands were detected by Western blots that reacted with the antibodies, whereas only one was seen in MCBD 170. (d) Benzo(a)pyrene metabolism: increasing passage of cells in MCBD 170 resulted in lower levels of water soluble metabolites but the general pattern and quantity of organosolubles was little changed. This presentation clearly demonstrated the profound effects that the choice of medium may have on the metabolic pathways expressed by mammary epithelial cells in culture and underlined the importance of comparing the effects of different media where investigating cell function in culture.

Dr. O.W. Petersen (University of Copenhagen) demonstrated the importance of cell identification when wishing to study human breast cancer cells in culture before attempting to define media specifically for their growth. Primary tumours contain a heterogeneous epithelial cell population. Ideally all of these populations should be present in the initial primary cultures if these are to be representative of the situation in vivo. A histochemical method for detecting glucose 6-phosphogluconate de-hydrogenase (G6-PDH) activity may be suitable for distinguishing among normal, dysplastic, and cancer cells. Cryosections were cut from reduction mammoplasties (RM) and from caricnomas. G6-PDH was present in the epithelium from both but by raising the oxygen (O_2) tension during the histochemical incubation it was possible to totally inhibit G6-PDH in the normal epithelium whilst retaining high activity in more than 50% of the cancers. Cryosections from benign dysplasias incubated under these conditions showed G6-PDH activity that overlapped the lowest range from carcinomas. Three patterns of G6-PDH localization were seen on epithelial islands grown from breast tissues. (a) The central explant and its surrounding island of cells were strongly positive; this pattern was seen in cultures from 1^0 and 2^0 cancer. (b) The explant was weakly positive as was the peripheral ring of island cells; found in many 1^0 but no 2^0 cancers, and in benign tissues. (c) all positive; found in some benign tissues and the only pattern seen from RM tissue. Recently dihydro-nicotinamide adenine dinucleotide diaphorase (NADPH) is being evaluated, and examination of cryosections has shown that raised O_2 tension resulted in both normal and dysplastic epithelium being negative whilst cancer remained positive. Two chemically defined media, CCDM 1 & 2 were evaluated for their ability to maintain survival of cancer cells in culture. CCDM1 selectively encouraged growth of non-malignant epithelium (NADPH negative cells) whereas CCDM2 was less selective. However the NADPH negative cells soon overgrew the positive cells. In was concluded that a simple histochemical test enables non-malignant and malignant epithelium to be identified and this could be used for designing media to their specific requirements.

Dr. J.C. Heuson (Institut Jules Bordet, Brussels) described his studies applying his human tumour cloning systen (HTCS) to primary breast cancers. The system was first tested with MCF-7 cells; the cloning efficiency fell from 20% to 4% during a 2 to 3 wk exposure to 4-hydroxy Tamoxifan (OHT) at concentrations of 10^{-8} M to 10^{-6} M. This inhibition was reversed by the addition of equimolar amounts of estradiol (E_2). Nineteen breast cancer tumor tissues were then assayed. Epithelial clusters from the enzyma-tically dissociated tumour tissue were cultured from 1-2 wks before place-ment in agar with OHT. The E_2 receptor (E_2R) level obtained from the original tumour showed no correlation with response to OHT in the HTCS. Additionally, the E_2R level was measured in the cultured cells from 6 patients just prior to the cells being suspended in agar. Each sample was negative whereas in the 1^0 tumours E_2R levels ranged from 19-262 fmoles/mg protein. Dr. Heuson concluded that although the method may work for a cell line, it does not for patient-derived cells. He suggested some possible explanations: that the clonogenic assay may be irrelevant to the clinical course of the disease, the clonogenic cells may not be tumour cells, the clonogenic cells may represent progenitor cells devoid of E_2 dependance or that the HTCS technique used requires modification.

Dr. G. Calaf (Acadmia de Ciencia Pedegogicas de Santiago, Chile) described her work done in Dr. J. Russo's laboratory, Detroit, using organ culture and autoradiography to study cell kinetics of epithelium in explants from RM's. The tissues were reduced to $1mm^3$ explants and maintained in serum-free M199. Insulin (I, 5 ug/ml), hydrocortisone (HC, 1 ug/ml), estradiol (E_2 0.05 ug/ml) and progesterone (Pg 1 ug/ml) were added as appropriate. DNA labelling index (LI) was measured using a 1 hr pulse of ^{3}H-thymidine, length of S phase (Ts) using ^{3}H- and 14 C- labelled thymidine and 2-layered autoradiography, and growth fraction (GF) using a 5 day continuous exposure to ^{3}H-thymidine. A comparison was made between large ducts, intralobular ducts, and alveoli after 5 days in culture. The LI (1%) was greater in explants from younger women (mean age 26 yr) than in older women (0.42%) (mean age 49 yr). Ts was similar in both age groups. GF was higher in intralobular ducts vs. large ducts or alveoli, and in younger women vs. older. The length of the cell cycle (TC) was 40 hrs in younger women compared with 260 hrs in older, F1 was shorter too in the younger group. The addition of I + HC increased the LI compared with control and this was further increased by adding E_2 but not by Pg. However the mitotic index was similar in all hormonal additions. All the hormones increased the GF, but E_2 specifically reduced the length of the cell cycle (TC). It was concluded that kinetic data and how it may be modulated by hormonal additions can be determined using short term organ culture.

Dr. N.H. Sarkar (Memorial Sloan-Kettering Cancer Center, N.Y.) used organ culture techniques to demonstrate factors that operate in the induction and maintenance of hyperplastic mammary alveolar lesions (MAL) which develop due to MMTV infection in the mouse. Whole mammary glands from 7 month old mice were maintained for 8 days on Dacron rafts in NB7/52 type 1 medium that contained additional insulin, aldosterone, hydrocortisone and prolactin (lactogenic medium). The organ culture was then continued in medium plus insulin only, to which were added, as modulators, either a retinoic acid analogue (hydroxyphenylretinamide, HPR) or the fatty acids arachadonic or stearic, or the prostaglandin synthesis inhibitor, indomethacin. Twenty four days later the number of MAL/gland was counted, the medium content of prostaglandin PGE_2 determined, the tissue core fatty acids and ^{3}H-thymidine incorporation into DNA measured. The results showed that both lobules and MALs were well maintained in the lactogenic medium during this time, but the lobules degenerated when subsequently placed in insulin-containing medium, while the MALs were unaffected. The number of MALs present in each mammary gland remained constant for 24 days, but addition of HPR for only 14 days reduced the number 30%. HPR also reduced MAL/mammary gland 50% where the glands were not maintained initially in lactogenic medium. Stearic acid had a similar effect. Exposure to arachadonic acid increased 3H thymidine labelling and PGE_2 synthesis whereas indomethacin decreased both parameters. Virus expression was also modulated by those factors. It was concluded that some of the factors which regulate growth and survival of pre-neoplastic mammary lesions may readily be studied by using this simple organ culture method.

Dr. S. Schor (Paterson Laboratories, Manchester) introduced fibroblasts into the workshop with the study of fibroblast migration into 3-dimensional (3-D) type I collagen gels. Cell density markedly affects the migratory response (5) and this affect was different in foetal vs. adult human skin fibroblasts and in normal (WI 38) vs. transformed (SV WI38) cells. Increasing cell density from 10^3 to 10^6 cells/cm^2 decreased the percentage of infiltrating normal cells whereas it increased that of transformed cells. The cell density migration index (CDMI), defined as

$$\frac{\% \text{ of cells in gel at low cell density}}{\% \text{ of cell in gel at high cell density}} \times \log^{10}$$

was used to compare the dynamic infiltrating capacity of cells. The CDMIs of foreskin and adult fibroblast lines gave positive indices similar to WI38, subsequently called "N range". 15 transformed lines give negative indices similar to SV WI38, subsequently called "T range". 24 lines of foetal mesenchymal cells gave indices intermediate between N & T, subsequently called "FN" or "TF range". Normal adult fibroblasts, foetal fibroblasts and transformed fibroblasts were tested for CDMI during 75 population doublings or 1 years growth. Whereas the adult cells maintained CDMI in the N range, and transformed cells in the T range, at passage 25 foetal cells changed from the FN to the N range, and remained there till senescence. Thus the foetal cells undergo a transition at some point in their life in culture to an adult like state. The CDMI of fibroblasts from within breast cancers was then compared with that of the patient's skin fibroblasts. A CDMI in the FN/TF range was found in 13 out of 27 patients. Other tumours, (retinoblastoma, soft tissue sarcoma, Wilms tumour, familiar polyposis coli) also showed both skin and tumour fibroblasts with CDMI in the FN range. A comparison was then made of skin fibroblast CDMI between controls (n=24) with no breast pathology, patients with benign disease, with breast cancer (n=37), and patients with both abnormal breast pathology and a family history of breast disease (n=11). Ninety percent of controls, 50% of benigns with no family history, and 50% of breast cancer with no family history were N range, whereas 100% of breast cancer with a family history were FN. Some of those cells also formed colonies in soft agar, grew in both serum-containing and platelet-poor-plasma- containing medium, produced a PDGF type growth factor and secreted a foetal type fibronectin. The importance of epithelial mesenchymal interactions in the regulation of epithelial cell biology is well documented and the present study shows the isoformic transition of foetal cells to a normal adult phenotype. It was postulated that this transition may not occur in certain individuals, thereby altering control mechanisms and increasing the risk of certain cancers developing in these individuals.

Dr. F. Feuilhade (Creteil, France) presented the final paper which described studies on the estrogen receptor (E_2R) and progesterone receptor (PgR) levels in cultured fibroblasts obtained from breast cancer tissue. Part of the tissue from 11 patients was homogenized to determine E_2R and PgR levels and the remainder was digested with collagenase. The resulting cells were grown in medium F12 plus 10% foetal calf serum (FCS) for 6 days, then treated with trypsin EDTA to selectively release fibroblasts, which were then grown in F12 plus steroid-stripped FCS. Similar procedures were performed upon 19 soft tissue sarcomas. E_2R and PgR levels in the cultured fibroblasts were determined as for the parent tissue. The results showed that cultured breast fibroblasts had higher E_2R levels but lower PgR levels than the parent tissue; 1381 ± 406 f mols/mg protein versus 55.1 ± 38 for E_2R and 12.9 ± 8 versus 103 ± 50 for PgR. The fibroblasts grown from the soft tissue sarcomas were negative for E_2R and PgR, the parent tissues having absent or very low levels themselves. It was concluded that cultured fibroblasts from breast cancer tissue contain receptors for both E_2 and Pg but that these did not correlate with either parent tissue level, age, or hormonal status of patient. Such receptors are absent from the transformed fibroblasts tested.

SUMMARY

Numerous techniques now exist for mammary cell culture; current efforts are being directed towards improving these in vitro systems by identifying specific cell types and developing culture conditions that may shed light on the normal and aberrant processes that occur in vivo. The results reported here illustrate advances in these directions. For example, methods to distinguish among normal, dysplastic, and malignant mammary epithelial cells, as well as serum-free medium that encourages growth of malignant cells, are important tools for understanding the nature of the malignant breast epithelial cell. Similarly, a recognition that abnormalities in mesenchymal cells could influence epithelial cell pathology may broaden the persepctive of breast cancer etiology. Furthermore, the examination of how different factors may regulate cell behavior in vitro underlines the realization that culture systems are only approximations of the in vivo situation. Therefore, it is of great importance to carefully explore the variables influencing these different culture systems (e.g. organ, monolayer, agar), to determine the effect of the culture environment, and how to create in vitro systems that will most accurately reflect the in vivo situation.

REFERENCES

1. Furmanski, P. In: Understanding Breast Cancer (eds. M.A. Rich, J.C. Hager and P. Furmanski), Marcel Dekker Inc., New York, 1983, pp. 371-375.
2. Stampfer, M.R., Hallowes, R.C., and Hackett, A.J. In Vitro 16: 415-425, 1980.
3. Hammond, S.L., Ham, R.G., and Stampfer, M.R. Proc. Natl. Acad. Sci. USA 81: 5435-5439, 1984.
4. Emerman, J.T., Bartley, J.C., and Bissell, M.J. Exp. Cell Res. 134: 241-250, 1981.
5. Schor, S.L., Schor, A.M., Winn, B., and Rushton, G. Int. J. Cancer 29: 57-62, 1982.

9

NEW APPROACHES TO THE PATHOLOGY OF BREAST CANCER;
CAN IMMUNOHISTOCHEMISTRY ADD NEW INFORMATION?

PH. HAGEMAN and J.L. PETERSE

Division of Clinical Oncology and Department of Pathology,
Netherlands Cancer Institute, Amsterdam, The Netherlands

INTRODUCTION

If we want to evaluate the contribution of immunohistochemistry to
the understanding of breast disease, we must first consider the role of
histopathology. The aims of histopathological studies are:
1. differentiation between benign and malignant lesions.
2. classification and grading of malignancy (relevant for prognosis).
3. staging and extent of disease (relevant for prognosis).
4. in case of metastasis of occult primary tumor: differential diagnosis
   of possible primary tumor.
5. giving insight in histogenesis and tumor biology.
Especially in the last decade a large number of polyclonal and monoclonal antibodies and fluorescein- or enzymeconjugated lectins has been
developed to define more precisely the composition and functional characteristics of the mammary gland. Some recent developments which may contribute to histopathological studies will be reviewed, without the pre-
tention to be complete. Emphasis will be given to markers that can be
applied to routinely fixed, paraffin-embedded material.

METHODS

Immunohistochemical reactions are most commonly visualized by an
immunoperoxidase test using either a peroxidase-labeled second antibody,
a peroxidase-antiperoxidase complex (the unlabeled antibody method of
Sternberger) or one of the variations of the avidin-biotin method. Evaluations of these methods are given by Naritoku and Taylor (1) and
De Jong et al. (2).

PRECAUTIONS

Heyderman (3) gave an excellent description of immunohistochemical methods in pathology and the controls that have to be included in such tests. A few of the problems that are encountered by the evaluation of immunohistochemical methods applied to human pathology are reviewed by Erlandson (4). A main difficulty can be caused by the lack of specifity of polyclonal but also of monoclonal antibodies. This is demonstrated in the literature concerning immunohistochemical detection of carcinoembryonic antigen in breast tumors. Carcinoembryonic antigen (CEA) is a glycoprotein that shares many epitopes with cross-reacting antigens of which the Nonspecific Cross-reacting Antigen I and II and biliary protein are well known (for a review see Von Kleist, 5). Nearly all polyclonal antisera against CEA show these cross-reactions, but also many monoclonal antibodies are directed against epitopes that are not unique to CEA. Walker (6) and Nap et al. (7) have paid much attention to these cross-reactions and they published absorption methods to obtain monospecific polyclonal antisera against CEA. One should be aware of the fact that complete disappearance of the activity of an antibody after absorption with pure CEA does not prove the specifity for CEA of this antibody because the cross-reacting epitopes are part of the CEA molecule. Work on the presence of casein is another example of difficult interpretable results due to unwanted crossreactivity. Bussolati et al. (8) reported that some antisera against casein contain antibodies to epithelial membrane antigens of the breast. Monoclonal antibodies have their own specificity problem: they are specific for a certain epitope that can be present on several molecules. An example are the antibodies to epithelial membrane antigens that react with an epitope that is shared by different molecules present in epithelial cells and lymphoid cells (9).

Variations in the frequency of occurrence of an antigen as mentioned by different authors may be caused by differences in technique, in strength of reaction or by sampling errors. The expression of antigens in a tumor is often heterogeneous and small samples might lead to false negative results.

Pretreatment with trypsin or pronase may enhance the sensitivity of immunohistochemical tests but Foster and Neville (10) observed a reduction in the binding of peanut agglutinin.

SURVEY OF MARKERS

Epithelial markers.

A vast number of the recently developed monoclonal and polyclonal antibodies are directed against differentiation antigens of the mammary gland. Different keratins can be used as markers for epithelial breast cells, though they are also found in myoepithelial cells (11).

The presence of the oncofetal protein CEA is considered to be of significance for the determination of the malignancy of epithelial mammary tumor cells.

Probes directed against the sugarmoiety of glycoproteins can be of importance, especially as indicators of misprocessing of sugars, a phenomenon that seems to occur frequently on the surface of transformed mammary cells (10, 12). In addition, fluorescein- or peroxidase-labeled lectins have been used to visualize sugar determinants of antigens.

Myoepithelial markers: actin and myosin.

Basement membrane markers: laminin, type IV collagen (Gusterson et al., 13)

Hormone receptors:

In addition to already existing probes for hormone receptors, recently monoclonal antibodies to estrogen receptors became available (14) and have been succesfully applied to frozen and to paraffin sections of human breast tumors (15, 16).

Special products of the mammary gland:(lactalbumin, casein) related to its secretional function identify mammary cells and indicate the functional state of the cells.

Stromal markers: vimentin.

Miscellaneous markers have been used for special histological problems, for instance neuron specific enolase to identify an endocrine variant of ductal carcinoma in situ (17).

ANTIBODIES PREPARED AGAINST MAMMARY (TUMOR) CELLS

Numerous markers have been used as tools in breast pathology, but monoclonal and polyclonal antibodies that have been raised against membranes of mammary tumor cells or human milkfat globule membranes deserve special attention. A selection of these antibodies is shown in table I, II and III. A number of antibodies of different sources has a comparable reaction pattern: apical staining of cells of normal ducts, benign lesions or differentiated areas in mammary carcinomas and cytoplasmic or focal

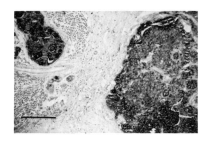 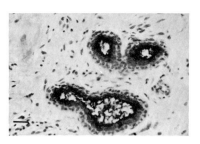

Fig. 1. Cytoplasmic reaction of antibody 115-D8 on mammary tumor

Fig. 2. Apical staining of normal mammary duct with 115-D8. Bar: 100 µ

staining in the cells of poorly differentiated tumors (Fig. 1 and 2). This comparable reaction pattern does not indicate that the corresponding antigens are identical: some antigens are expressed on nearly all mammary carcinomas, others on a limited number. Heterogeneous expression of the antigens is a generally observed phenomenon. Edwards and Brooks (48) used an ingenious dissection technique to demonstrate that antibodies

Table 1. Antibodies against human milkfat globule membranes

antibody	antigen	references
*rabbit α-HME	large glycoprotein	Ceriani (18)
mouse Mc5	400 kD glycoprotein	Ceriani (19)
*rabbit α-EMA	large glycoprotein	Heyderman (20), Sloane (21), Ormerod (22)
mouse HMFG-1	large glycoprotein	Arklie (23)
mouse HMFG-2	large glycoprotein	Taylor-Papadimitriou (24)
mouse 115-D8	large glycoprotein	Hilkens (25)
mouse M8	large glycoprotein	Foster (26, 27)
mouse M18	glycoprotein (I/Ma-epitope)	
mouse M24	39-59 kD glycoprotein	
*rabbit αgp70	70 kD glycoprotein	Imam (28)
*rabbit	antigen binds with PNA correlation with steroid hormone receptor	Klein (29)

*polyclonal

M8, M18 and M24 (26, 27) reacted with different cell types in the normal ducts. The heterogeneity in the tumor would be a reflection of the heterogeneity in the normal tissue. The heterogeneity of antigen expression was not related to the mitotic cell cycle, but as several of the antibodies are directed against a glycoprotein, it is possible that the heterogeneity partly is caused by variations in carbohydrate structures on otherwise identical molecules (for review see 49 and 50). An increased heterogeneity in breast carcinomas compared to normal and hyperplastic human breast was also reported of binding sites of wheat germ agglutinin that detects acetyl-D-glucosamine endgroups (51, 52).

Peterson et al. (53) and Ceriani et al. (54) observed a heterogeneous expression of a cell surface glycoprotein with molecular weight 400 kD recognized by their antibody Mc5 both on normal and malignant

Table 2. Mouse monoclonal antibodies against human mammary tumor cell lines

antibody	antigen	references
MBr1	large glycolipid	Mènard (30), Canevari (31) Mariani-Costantini (32)
H59	glycoprotein in estrogen receptor pos. tumors	Yuan (33), Hendler (34)
F36/22	glycoprotein	Papsidero (35), Croghan (36)
24-17.2	100 kD molecule	Thompson (37)

Table 3. Antibodies against human mammary tumor cells

antibody	antigen	references
mouse B 72.3	220-400 kD glycoprotein	Colcher (38), Nuti (39)
mouse NCRC-11	large glycoprotein	Ellis (40)
mouse DF3	290 kD antigen	Kufe (41)
human MBE6	cytoplasmic antigen	Schlom (42) Teramoto (43)
human CF 29/34	antigen preferently on poorly differentiated tumors	Imam (44)
*rabbit	mammary tumor associated antigen	Yu (45)
*rabbit MTGP	53 kD glycoprotein	Leung (46, 47)

*polyclonal

breast tissue. Malignant cells exhibited a higher rate of genotypic variability, cells from tumor tissue gave more frequently rise to mixed
clones in respect to their antigen expression than cells from normal or
benign breast tissue. Study of this phenomenon may give information about
the lability of the cells and the grade of malignancy of a tumor.

APPLICATIONS OF THE MARKERS TO HISTOLOGICAL PROBLEMS
Malignancy

The differential diagnosis of malignant versus benign breast tissue
is one of the main problems of breast pathology and one of the objectives
for the development of monoclonal antibodies is to improve the characterization of the malignant cell.

Though a number of the monoclonal antibodies raised against human
milkfat globule membranes or mammary tumor cell membranes shows a different
pattern of reaction on normal and on malignant breast tissue (apical
staining and cytoplasmic staining respectively), this is complicated by
the reaction in well-differentiated tumors that show apical staining in
areas that exhibit tubule formation. The human monoclonal antibody MBE6
(42, 43) and CF29/34 (44) and the antisera against Mammary Tumor Glyco-
Protein (46, 47) and mammary tumor associated antigen (45) seem to have
a strong preference for binding to malignant mammary cells.

Cal antibody was specially selected to recognize malignant cells
in different tissues (55). An extensive study of Simpson et al. (56)
showed that at least for breast tissue this marker has no specificity
for malignancy as the antibody reacted with 20 out of 20 normal breast
tissues and with nearly all fibroadenomas tested.

Peanut agglutinin (PNA) reacts with molecules carrying the dissacha-
ride β-D-Gal(1$\rightarrow$3)D-GalNac as a terminal group. This configuration is the
antigenic determinant of the Thomsen-Friedenreich antigen, a precursor
of the blood group antigens MN. Thomsen-Friedenreich antigen is supposed
to be present on human mammary tumors in a free state and to be absent
or masked by sialic acid in normal breast tissue (Springer et al., 12;
Howard, 58). Several authors (59, 60, 61, 62) found binding of PNA both
on normal and malignant breast tissue. Howard et al. (63) and Newman et
al. (64) observed a staining with peanut agglutinin in the apical region
of the cells in normal breast tissue and well-differentiated carcinomas,
in poorly differentiated tumors the reaction was cytoplasmic or absent.

This secretion-associated binding pattern in tumors was related with presence of estrogen and progestrone receptors in the tumors (Klein et al., 65). In a recent publication Springer et al. (66) indicate that the Tn antigen, a precursor of the Thomsen-Friedenreich antigen lacking the β-galactose terminal group could be a promising marker for the detection of malignancy in the breast though they detected also some Tn activity on a limited number of cells in normal ducts.

Cytoplasmic staining of cells with monospecific polyclonal antisera or well-defined monoclonal antibodies against CEA can be considered as a marker for malignant mammary cells (Papotti et al., 67; Nap et al., 68) though only 50% of the carcinomas is positive for this marker.

Antibodies against epithelial markers (keratin), myoepithelial cells (actin, myosin) and markers of the basement membrane (laminin, collagen IV) are promising tools for the differential diagnosis of proliferative and neoplastic lesions. Reactions with these markers may provide insight in the histogenesis of breast cancer. In benign proliferative lesions (adenosis, epitheliosis, intraductal adenosis, papillomas) the proliferations consist of myoepithelial and epithelial cells, often arranged in bilayers as in normal breast tissue. In ductal carcinoma in situ and papillary carcinoma, lesions microscopically often mimicking benign lesions, the proliferation consists of epithelial cells only (Busolatti, 8, 69; Gusterson, 13, 70; Papotti, 67). Papotti (71) found in cases of multiple ductal papillomas areas lacking myoepithelium, with CEA-positive cells, microscopically arranged as ductal carcinoma in situ. He considered this as indication of transformation of a proliferative lesion into malignancy, a phenomenon against which many pathologists oppose (Azzopardi, 72).

The absence of myoepithelial cells is one of the main characteristics of tubular carcinoma, distinguishing it from adenosis.

Destruction of basement membrane, revealed by staining with antibodies against laminin and type IV collagen and absence of myoepithelial cells may be helpful in distinguishing in situ and infiltrating carcinoma. In highly differentiated infiltraing carcinoma basement membrane protein can be formed, however (70).

Prognosis

One of the aims of tumor classification is to identify groups of tumors that are different in respect to prognosis. Shousa and Lyssiotis

(73) found a correlation between the presence of carcinoembryonic antigen in tissue sections and presence of lymph node metastases. They concluded (74) that immunohistochemically detectable carcinoembryonic antigen was a useful prognostic indicator, especially since patients with CEA negative tumors had significantly higher survival rates. Unfortunately these authors used a polyclonal antiserum that probably contained antibodies against cross-reacting antigens. Other groups (Walker, 6; Rolf-Smit et al., 75; Nap, 68) could not confirm the relationship between CEA content of the primary tumor with poor prognosis.

Wilkinson et al. (76) described a relationship between the reaction pattern of mammary tumor sections with the antibodies HMFG-1 and HMFG-2 and prognosis. Unfortunately Berry et al. (77) using the same antibodies but a slightly different staining technique and different method of grading of the results of the immunoperoxidase test could not confirm the association of the reaction with these antibodies and prognosis.

The presence of immunohistochemically detectable pregnancy-associated β1-glycoprotein was considered to be related to poor prognosis (78), at least in small infiltrating ductal carcinomas (79). Barry et al. (80) studied immunohistochemically the markers: casein, human placental lactogen, alpha-lactalbumin, pregnancy specific β1-glycoprotein, secretory component, CEA and receptor for peanut agglutinin and could not find any difference in reaction pattern between patients who had recurrent cancer compared to those who remained at least five years disease-free.

Keydar et al. (81) suggested that presence of an antigen related to gp52, a 52 000 dalton major glycoprotein of mouse mammary tumor virus was related to poor prognosis. Moreover, the incidence of this antigen seems to be higher in tumors of patients with a family history (Mesa-Tejada et al., 82). The relationship did not hold for a group of Tunesian women studied by Levine (83). Though in this group a high incidence of gp52-related antigen was found, no correlation with aggressiveness of the tumor or survival time was observed. As many sera against mouse mammary tumor virus do not show this cross-reaction with human mammary tumors, we will have to wait for monoclonal antibodies directed against the cross-reacting epitope. This is even more interesting because the epitope seems to be restricted to malignant tissue and to breast tumors only (81, 82, 84). As often many tumor cells in a positive reacting mammary tumor are negative,it seems unlikely that this marker can be generally used as a marker for malignancy in breast tissue.

Origin of a primary tumor and detection of metastases

Several of the monoclonal and polyclonal antibodies raised against
milkfat globule membranes or mammary tumor cells are currently used to
recognize mammary tumor cells in pathological specimens. The antigens detected by these antibodies are not tissue-specific, in addition to their
reaction with mammary tumors reactions are reported with a large selection of other epithelial tumors such as carcinomas of ovary, lung and
gastrointestinal tract. No evaluation should be made on the basis of a
single antibody reaction (85) but the antibodies should be used as part
of a panel (9). Gatter and Mason (86) describe such a panel of antibodies
including HMFG-1 and HMFG-2 (24) for the diagnosis of cancer of unknown
primary site, and Henzen-Logmans et al. (87) included 115-D8 (25) in
their panel for the diagnosis of large cell tumors. The panels help to
discriminate adenocarcinomas from lymphoma, melanoma, sarcoma or tumors
of the nervous system. Several of these antibodies that were originally
raised against mammary tissue are easier to apply on formalin-fixed and
paraffin-embedded tissue than most antikeratins, that do not react on
fixed material or require a preincubation of the tissue with trypsin or
pronase.

As the majority of the above-mentioned antibodies is directed against
differentiation antigens of the breast one would expect that their contribution in the recognition of the origin of a tumor would be small.
When cells and tissues are well-differentiated they likely express differentiation antigens, but then the microscopical diagnosis of the tumor

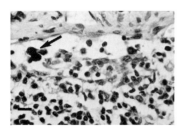

Fig. 3 Micrometastases of mammary
tumor in lymph node positive with
115-D8 (arrow). Bar: 100 μ.

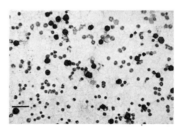

Fig. 4 Metastatic tumor cells in
ascitis fluid positive with 115-D8
Bar: 100 μ

is usually easy and the immunohistochemical reaction only confirms the diagnosis that was already made with conventional light microscopy. Because some of the monoclonal antibodies as anti epithelial membrane antigen and 115-D8 (25) react positively on nearly all mammary tumors the corresponding antigens are probably not limited to a very restricted differentiation stage of the cell. Such antibodies that stain nearly all mammary tumors and a large percentage of the cells in a tumor can well be applied to detect metastatic tumor cells in lymph nodes, bone marrow and effusion fluids (31, 37, 40, 88, 89, 90, 91). Fig. 3 shows mammary tumor cells in a lymph node and Fig. 4 tumor cells in ascites fluid detected with antibody 115-D8.

Redding et al. (92) using antibody against epithelial membrane antigen demonstrated that in a surprisingly high percentage ($\pm$ 30%) of breast cancer patients micrometastases could be detected in bone marrow. A complication in these tests might be a cross-reaction with plasma cells that is reported for epithelial membrane antigen (9, 85, 93, 94), for antibody NCRC-11 (40) and that we also occasionally observe with antibody 115-D8 (25). For the detection of mammary tumor cells in effusion fluids only those antibodies are suitable that do not react with mesothelium (for instance MBr1, tested by Mariani-Costantini et al., 32).

When searching for the tissue origin of a tumor one should not overlook antibodies against other milk proteins. Especially alphalactalbumin is reported to be a suitable marker. 60% of mammary tumors and their metastases was positive for this marker (95, 96) and of the other tumors tested only those originating from salivary glands or skin appendages contained alphalactalbumin.

Histogenesis

Apart from the work on the epithelial and myoepithelial markers that we already described the stromal marker vimentin can be used in combination with epithelial markers to study the structure and histogenesis of carcinosarcoma, a tumor containing malignant cells of both epithelial and mesenchymal appearance. The carcinomatous elements in carcinosarcoma can be easily detected by antibody 115-D8, (Fig. 5), the mesenchymal cells by antivimentin. Some authors suggest that the two components of carcinosarcoma are derived from distinct cell types (97) but they probably overestimate the specificity of vimentin as a marker for cells of mesenchymal origin.

Amongst cases of ductal carcinoma in situ a subgroup of tumors can be distinguished containing argyrophilic cells. This endocrine variant of ductal carcinoma in situ can be recognized by a
strong positivity for neuron specific enolase and is negative for
α-lactalbunin (17).

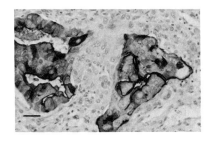

Fig. 5 Carcinosarcoma of the breast:
115-D8 stains epithelial elements.
Bar: 100μ.

FUTURE OUTLOOK

Despite many efforts an absolute marker for the differential diagnosis between proliferative lesions of the breast and neoplasia has not
been found yet. Studies related to the structure and histogenesis of the
tumor have yielded the most satisfactory results. The protein products
of onc genes form the most exciting group of tentative markers for malignancy and progression. Hand et al. (98) were able to detect expression
of the ras gene product p21 in the majority of a series of mammary carcinomas and not in normal breast cells. The presence of the ras gene product in such a high percentage of tumors was remarkable because Kraus et
al. (99) could detect a transforming ras gene only in one out of 21 human
mammary carcinomas. Hand mentions the possibility that enhanced expression of normal c-ras gene might occur in mammary tumors.

Though the recently developed markers have not revolutionized breast
pathology to a degree that some of us expected, immunohistochemical markers have become indispensable for the pathologist. Especially promising
are the studies on myoepithelial markers and on onc gene products whereas the possibilities of monoclonal antibodies directed against tumor cell
constituents have not been fully explored yet.

REFERENCES

1. Naritoku, W.U. and Taylor, C.R. J. Histochem. Cytochem. 30: 253-260,
    1982.
2. De Jong, A.S.H., Van Kessel-van Vark, M. and Raap, A.K. Histochem. J.
    (submitted for publication).
3. Heyderman, E. J. Clin. Pathol. 312: 971-978, 1979.
4. Erlandson, R.A. Am. J. Surg. Path. 8: 615-624, 1984.
5. Von Kleist, S. In: Carcinoembryonic proteins, Vol. 1 (Ed. F.G. Lehman),
    Elsevier, pp. 35-39, 1979.

6. Walker, R.A. J. Clin. Pathol. 33: 356-360, 1980.
7. Nap, M., Ter Hoor, K.A. and Fleuren, G.J. Am. J. Clin. Pathol. 79: 25-31, 1983.
8. Bussolati, G., Gugliotta,P. and Papotti, M. In: New Frontiers in mamma pathology, Vol. 2 (Eds. K.M. Hollmann, J.M. Verley), Plenum Press, New York, pp. 249-264, 1983.
9. Taylor-Papadimitriou, J., Burchell, J. Lancet i: 458-459, 1985.
10. Foster, C.S. and Neville, A.M. Human Pathol. 15: 502-513, 1984.
11. Altmannsberger, M., Osborn, M., Hölscher, A., Schauer, A. and Weber, K. Virchows Arch. B (Cell Pathol.)37: 277-284, 1981.
12. Springer, G.F., Desai, P.R. and Banatwala, I. J. Natl. Cancer Inst. 54: 335-339, 1975.
13. Gusterson, B.A., Warburton, M.J., Monaghan, T., Foster, C., Edwards, P., Kraft, N., Smith, C., Mitchell, D., Rudland, P.S., Neville, A.M. and Hancock, W. Behring Inst. Mitt. 74: 39-48, 1984.
14. King, W.J., Greene, G.L. Nature 307: 745-747, 1984.
15. King, W.J., De Sombre, E.R., Jensen, E.V. and Greene, G.L. Cancer Res. 45: 293-304, 1985.
16. Skovgaard Poulsen, H., Ozzello, L., King, W.J. and Greene, G.L. J. Histochem. Cytochem. 33: 87-92, 1985.
17. Cross, A.S., Azzopardi, J.G., Krausz, T., Van Noorden, S. and Polak, J.M. Histopathology 9: 21-37, 1985.
18. Ceriani, R.L., Thompson, K., Peterson, J.A. and Abraham, S. Proc. Natl. Acad. Sci. 74: 582-586, 1977.
19. Ceriani, R.L., Peterson, J.A., Lee, J.Y., Moncada, R. and Blank, E.W. Somat. Cell Genet. 9: 415-427, 1983.
20. Heyderman, E., Steele, K. and Ormerod, M.G. J. Clin. Pathol. 32: 35-39, 1979.
21. Sloane, J.P. and Ormerod, M.G. Cancer 47: 1786-1795, 1981.
22. Ormerod, M.G., Steele, K., Westwood, J.H. and Mazzini, M.N. Br. J. Cancer 48: 533-541, 1983.
23. Arklie, J., Taylor-Papadimitriou, J., Bodmer W., Egan, M. and Millis, R. Int. J. Cancer 28: 23-30, 1981.
24. Taylor-Papadimitriou, J., Peterson, J.A., Arklie, J., Burchell, J. Ceriani, R.L. and Bodmer, W.F. Int. J. Cancer 28: 17-21, 1981.
25. Hilkens, J., Buys, F., Hilgers, J., Hageman, Ph., Calafat, J. Sonnenberg, A. and van der Valk, M. Int. J. Cancer 34: 197-206, 1984.
26. Foster, C.S., Edwards, P.A.W., Dinsdale,E.A. and Neville, A.M. Virchows Archiv A 394: 279-293, 1982.
27. Foster, C.S., Dinsdale, E.A., Edwards, P.A.W. and Neville, A.M. Virchows Archiv A 394: 295-305, 1982.
28. Imam A., Taylor, C.R. and Tökes, Z.A. Cancer Res. 44: 2016-2022, 1984.
29. Klein, P.J., Vierbuchen, M., Schulz, K.D., Farrar, G., Fischer, J. Uhlenbruck G. and Fischer, R. Cancer Det. Prev. 6: 199-206, 1983.
30. Ménard, S., Tagliabue, E., Canevari , S., Fossati, G. and Colnaghi,M.I. Cancer Res. 43: 1295-1300, 1983.
31. Canevari, S., Fossati, G., Balsari, A., Sonnino, S. and Colnaghi, M.I. Cancer Res. 43: 1301-1305, 1983.
32. Mariani-Costantini, R., Colnaghi, M.I., Leoni, F., Ménard, S., Cerasoli, S. and Rilke, F. Virchows Arch. (Pathol. Anat.) 402: 389-404, 1984.
33. Yuan, D., Hendler, F.J. and Vitetta, E.S. J. Natl. Cancer Inst. 68: 719-728, 1982.
34. Hendler, F.J. and Yuan, D. Cancer Res. 45: 421-429, 1985.

35. Papsidero, L.D., Croghan, G.A., O'Connell,M.J., Valenzuela, L.D. Nemoto, T. and Ming Chu, T. Cancer Res. 43: 1741-1747, 1983.
36. Croghan, G.A., Papsidero, L.D., Valenzuela, L.A., Nemoto, T., Penetrante, R. and Ming Chu, T. Cancer Res. 43: 4980-4988, 1983.
37. Thompson, C.H., Jones, S.L., Whitehead, R.M. and Mckenzie, I.F.C. J. Natl. Cancer Inst. 70: 409-420, 1983.
38. Colcher, D., Hand, P.H., Nuti, M. and Schlom, J. Proc. Natl. Acad. Sci. 78: 3199-3203, 1981.
39. Nuti, M., Teramoto, Y.A., Mariani-Costantini, R., Horan Hand, P., Colcher, D., Schlom, J. Int. J. Cancer 29: 539-545, 1982.
40. Ellis, I.O., Robbins, R.A., Elston, C.W., Blamey, R.W., Ferry, B. and Baldwin, R.W. Histopathology 8: 501-516, 1984.
41. Kufe, D., Inghirami, G., Abe, M., Hayes, A., Justi-Wheeler, H. and Schlom, J. Hybridoma 3: 223-232, 1984.
42. Schlom, J., Wunderlich, D. and Teramoto, Y.A. Proc. Natl. Acad. Sci. 77: 6841-6845, 1980.
43. Teramoto, Y.A., Mariani, R., Wunderlich, D., Schlom, J. Cancer 50: 2411249, 1982.
44. Imam A., Drushella, M.M., Taylor, C.R. and Tökes, Z.A. Cancer Res. 45: 263-271, 1985.
45. Yu, G.S.M., Kadish, A.S., Johnson, A.B., Marcus, D.M. Am. J. Clin. Path. 74: 453-457, 1980.
46. Leung, J.P., Plow, E.F., Nakamura, R.M. and Edgington, T. S. J. Immunol. 121: 1287-1296, 1978.
47. Leung, J.P., Edgington, T.S. Cancer Res. 40: 662-666, 1980.
48. Edwards, P.A. and Brooks, I.M. J. Histochem. Cytochem. 32: 531-537, 1984.
49. Edwards, P.A.W. Br. J. Cancer 51: 149-160, 1985.
50. Feizi, T. Nature 314: 53-57, 1985.
51. Walker, R.A. J. Pathol. 142: 279-291, 1984.
52. Walker, R.A. J. Pathol. 144: 101-108, 1984.
53. Peterson, J.A., Ceriani, R.L., Blank, E.W. and Osvaldo, L. Cancer Res 43: 4291-4296, 1983.
54. Ceriani, R.L., Peterson, J.A. and Blank, E.W. Cancer Res. 44: 3033-3039, 1984.
55. Ashall, F., Bramwell, M.E. and Harris, H. Lancet ii, 1-6, 1982.
56. Simpson, H.W., Candlish, W., Liddle, C., McGregor, M., Mutch, F. and Tinkler, B. Histopathology 8: 481-499, 1984.
57. Springer, G.F., Desai, P.R., Murthy, M.S., Yang, H.J. and Scanlon, E.F. Transfusion 19: 233-249, 1979.
58. Howard, D.R. and Taylor, C.R. Cancer Res. 43: 2279-2287, 1979.
59. Klein, P.J., Newman, R.A., Müller, P., Uhlenbruck, G., Citoler, P., Schäfer, H.E., Lennartz, K.J. and Fischer, R.F. J. Cancer Res. Clin. Oncol. 93: 205-214, 1979.
60. Stegner, H.E., Fischer, K. and Poschmann, A. Tumor Diagnostik 3: 127-130, 1981.
61. Hageman, Ph., Bobrow, L., Van der Valk, M.A., Misdorp, W., and Hilkens, J. In: The lectins, Vol. 3 (Eds. T.C. Bøg-Hanssen, G.A. Spengler) W. de Gruyter, Berlin, pp. 105-118, 1983.
62. Franklin, W.A. Cancer 51: 295-300, 1983.
63. Howard, D.R., Ferguson, P. and Batsakis, J.G. Cancer 47: 2872-2877, 1981.
64. Newman, R.A., Klein, P.J. and Rudland, P.S. J. Natl. Cancer Inst. 63: 1339-1346, 1979.
65. Klein, P.J., Vierbuchen,M., Wurtz, H., Schulz, K.D. and Newman, R.A.

Br.J.Cancer 44: 746-748, 1981

66. Springer, G.F., Taylor, C.R., Howard, D.R., Tegtmeyer,H., Desai,P.R.,
    Murthy, S.M., Felder, B. and Scanlon, E.F. Cancer 55: 561-569, 1985.
67. Papotti, M., Gugliotta, P., Eusebi, V. and Bussolati,G. Am.J.Surg.
    Pathol. 7: 457-461, 1983.
68. Nap, M.,Keuning, H., Burtin, P.,Oosterhuis, J.W. and Fleuren, G.J.
    Am.J.Clin.Pathol. 82: 526-534, 1984.
69. Bussolati, G., Botta, G. and Gugliotta, P. Virchows Archiv B 34: 251-
    259, 1980.
70. Gusterson, B.A., Warburton, M.J., Mitchell, D., Ellison, M.L.,
    Neville, A.M., Rudland, P.S. Cancer Res. 42: 4763-4770, 1982.
71. Papotti, M., Gugliotta, P., Ghiringhello, B. and Bussolati, G.
    Histopathology 8: 963-975, 1984.
72. Azzopardi, J.G. Problems in breast pathology. W.B.Saunders, London, 1979
73. Shousha, S. and Lyssiotis, T. Histopathology 2: 433-447, 1978.
74. Shousha, S., Lyssiotis, T., Godfrey, V.M. and Scheuer, P.J. Br.Med.
    J. 1: 777-779, 1979.
75. Rolf Smith, S., Howell, A., Minawa, A. and Morrison, J.M. Br. J.
    Cancer 46: 757-764, 1982.
76. Wilkinson, M.J.S., Howell, A., Harris, M., Taylor-Papadimitriou, J.,
    Swindell, R., and Sellwood, R.A. Int.J.Cancer 33: 299-304, 1984.
77. Berry, N., Jones, D.B., Smallwood, J., Taylor, I., Kirkham, N.,
    Taylor-Papadimitriou, J. Br.J.Cancer 51: 179-186, 1985.
78. Horne, C.W., Reid, I.N. and Milne, G.D. Lancet ii:279-282, 1976.
79. Kuhajda, F.P., Bohn, H. and Mendelsohn, G. Cancer 54: 1392-1396, 1984.
80. Barry, J.D., Koch, T.J., Cohen, C., Brigati, D.J. and Sharkey, F.E.
    Am.J.Clin.Pathol. 82: 582-585, 1984.
81. Keydar, I., Selzer, G., Chaitili, S., Hareuveni, M., Karbi, S. and Hizi, A
    Eur.J.Cancer Clin.Oncol. 18: 1321-1328, 1982.
82. Mesa-Tejada, R., Keydar, I., Ramanarayanan, M., Ohno, T., Fenoglio, C. and
    Spiegelman, S. AACR Proc. 20: 276, 1979.
83. Levine, P.H., Mesa-Tejada, R., Keydar, I. and Tabbane, F. Int.J.
    Cancer 33: 305-308, 1984.
84. Mesa-Tejada, R., Keydar, I., Ramanarayanan, M., Ohno, T., Fenoglio, C. and
    Spiegelman, S. Proc.Natl. Acad. Sci. 75: 1529-1533, 1978.
85. Heyderman, E. and Macartney, J.C. Lancet i: 109, 1985.
86. Gatter, K.C. and Mason, D.Y. Seminars in Oncology 9: 517-525, 1982.
87. Henzen-Logmans, S.C., Mullink, H., Vennegoor, C., Hilgers, J. and Meyer,
    C.J.L.M. Am.J.Clin.Pathol. submitted for publication.
88. Sloane, J.P., Ormerod, M.G., Imrie, S. and Coombes, R.C. Br.J.Cancer 42:
    392-398, 1980.
89. Dearnaley, D.P., Sloane, J.P., Ormerod, M.G., Steele, K., Coombes, R.C.,
    Clink, H., Powles, T.J., Ford, H.T., Gazet, J.C. and Neville, A.M.
    Br.J.Cancer 44: 85-90, 1981.
90. Gugliotta, P., Botta, G. and Bussolati, G. Histochem.J.13: 953-959, 1981.
91. Wells, C.A., Heryet, A., Brochier, J., Gatter, K.C. and Mason, D.Y.
    Br.J.Cancer 50: 193-197, 1984.
92. Redding, W.H., Monaghan, P., Imrie, S.F., Ormerod, M.G., Gazet, J.C.,
    Coombes, R.C., Clink, H.M., Dearnaly, D.P., Sloane, J.P., Powles, T.J. and
    Neville, A.M. Lancet ii: 1271-1274, 1983.
93. Delsol, G., Gatter, K.C., Stein, H., Erber, W.N., Pulford, K.A.F.,
    Zinne, K. and Mason, D.V. Lancet ii: 1124-1129, 1984.
94. Sloane, J.P., Dearnaley, D.P. and Ormerod, M.G. Lancet i: 109-110, 1985.
95. Clayton, F., Nelson, G.O. and Hanssen, G.M. Arch.Pathol.106: 268-270,198
96. Lee, A.K., Delellis, R.A. and Rosen, R.P. Am.J.Surg.Pathol. 8:93-100, 198

97. Huszar, M., Herczeg, E., Lieberman, Y. and Geiger, B. Hum.Pathol. 15: 532-538, 1984.
98. Horan-Hand, P., Thor, A., Wunderlich, D., Muraro, R., Caruso, A. and Schlom, J. Proc.Natl. Acad.Sci. 81: 5227-5231, 1984.
99. Kraus, M.H., Yuasa, Y. and Aaronson, S.A. Proc.Natl.Acad.Sci. 81: 5348-5388, 1984.

10

NEW DEVELOPMENTS IN BREAST CANCER IMMUNOLOGY

DIANA M. LOPEZ

Department of Microbiology and Immunology, University of Miami School
of Medicine and the Comprehensive Cancer Center for the State of Florida,
P.O. Box 016960, Miami, Florida 33101

INTRODUCTION

During the past five years a great number of investigators have
applied immunological methods in their quest against breast cancer. A
great proportion of the studies have been dedicated to the application
of the hybridoma technology to obtain monoclonal antibodies to define
breast tumor markers that could help in the diagnosis of primary and metastatic lesions. The ultimate goal is to direct chemotherapeutic agents
with great efficiency to the tumor mass sparing the surrounding normal
tissues. Another area that has received considerable attention is the
assessment of host immune reactions in relationship to mammary tumor development. In this connection several investigators have studied the humoral
immune factors and their modulating effects on the lymphoreticular cells.
Realizing that the activities detected in peripheral lymphoid organs may
not be as relevant as those of tumor infiltrating cells, many researchers
have analyzed the in situ immune responses and the cells mediating them.
In recent years molecular biologic data has been generated that indicates
a possible association between mouse mammary tumor virus (MMTV) and human
breast carcinoma. Various immunological studies have been published that
also establish a relationship between the murine agent and the human tumors.
In the following sections the various reports are discussed and analyzed
in order to obtain new perspectives as we evaluate the progress made up to
date and formulate future plans aimed at the eventual control of breast cancer.

DEVELOPMENT OF MONOCLONAL ANTIBODIES RELATED TO MAMMARY TUMORS.

The first reports about the generation of monoclonal antibodies against human breast epithelial cells date only since 1980. At present there are quite a number of such reagents available that are being used in research projects and that appear to have potential use for diagnosis and therapy. To generate the monoclonal antibody producing hybridoma, mice of various strains have been immunized with different types of breast tumors as well as human milk or breast tissue derived products. Spleen lymphocytes from these sensitized animals have been subsequently fused with mouse myeloma cell lines. Among the antigens used for the immunizations are human breast carcinoma cell lines, primary and metastatic human breast tumor materials, normal breast tissues or subcellular fractions, human breast cystic fluid, human milk fat globule membrane and purified estrogen receptors and estrogen regulated proteins. A possible limitation to the eventual clinical application of these monoclonal reagents is their murine origin. Therefore, hybridizations of human lymphocytes and mouse myelomas have been performed to obtain monoclonal antibodies of human origin that should pose less of an immunological problem upon administration in vivo. The main source of these lymphocytes are axillary lymph nodes or peripheral blood of breast cancer patients.

The hybridoma technology is characterized by the production of numerous antibodies specific for different antigens and even different epitopes within one given antigen. The specificity of a given monoclonal antibody may not be easily determined in all cases and the potential biological relevance of the antigens recognized might not be fully understood. Therefore, it is necessary to screen carefully the obtained products and choose those reagents that are capable of distinguishing qualitatively or at least quantitatively between normal and tumor tissues. Various monoclonal

reagents generated by different researchers have now been characterized at
least in part, and in some cases a great deal of information about such
immunoglobulins is available. For example, monoclonal antibodies raised
to epithelium specific components of the delipidated human milk fat globule
membrane (1, 2) appear to have not only diagnostic but prognostic significance
when used as detectors of surface antigens in primary human breast carcinomas
(3, 4). Soule et al (5) have reported on a hybridoma antibody designated
10-3D2 that binds to all tested breast carcinoma cell lines as well as to
a number of other human carcinomas. This antibody does not bind to normal
mammary epithelium and other normal tissues but recognizes a membrane
126-Kd protein which is indistinguishable in different tumor cells, suggesting
that it may represent a tumor associated antigen present in mammary tumors
and other human neoplasms. Colcher et al (6) generated a spectrum of
mouse monoclonal antibodies non-reactive with normal cells of several types
of human tissues but with an apparent "pancarcinoma" reactivity. Papsidero
et al (7) and White et al (8) have also described the selective reactivities
of murine monoclonal antibodies generated by their respective laboratories
to human breast cancer cells. The antigen(s) recognized by these reagents
have not been characterized. However, Horan-Hand et al (9,10) have recent
evidence that one of their monoclonal antibodies (B72.3) reacts with a
tumor-associated glycoprotein complex of high molecular weight present in
50% of primary breast tumors and 85% of colon carcinomas. This antigen
termed TAG-72 is not present in tumor cell lines of comparable origin and
it appears to be modulated by the spatial configuration of the cells (10).
An attempt to characterize the tumor associated antigens responsible for
induction of autologous immune responses was undertaken by Imam et al (11).
These investigators fused lymphocytes from lymph nodes of metastatic breast
cancer patients with a nonsecretory variant of murine myeloma cells. A

screen of the products obtained indicated that 15 of 81 human immunoglobulin-producing clones showed preferential binding to breast carcinoma cells. Other monoclonal antibodies that appear to be of potential use in the diagnosis of breast cancer are those directed against estrogen regulated proteins studied by Brabon et al (12) and Garcia et al (13). The relative expression of HLA antigens (14, 15) and carcinoembryonic antigen (16) in breast carcinoma cells may serve under controlled conditions as a suitable tumor marker that could be detected by immunological methods. In a recent international workshop held in California (17), data were presented about the detection of cytokeratins by monoclonal antibodies, as well as glyco-sphingolipids and the human ras antigenic determinant in breast cancer cells.

In vivo use of the monoclonal reagents has been limited up to now. However, localization of human mammary tumors implanted in athymic mice (18) and of metastatic human carcinomas in patients (19) by radiolabelled monoclonal antibodies have been reported. Recently, there have been attempts to utilize the hybridoma products in immunotherapeutic protocols. Capone et al (20) have established a relationship between the antigen density and the immunotherapeutic response elicited by monoclonal antibodies against solid tumors indicating that it may be necessary to use a mixture of these antibodies to obtain a significant effect. Very limited studies in the area of breast cancer have dealt with the use of immunotoxins, i.e. antibodies covalently linked to a toxin moiety. Krolick et al (21) conjugated ricin toxin A-chain to a murine monoclonal antibody specific for a subset of estrogen receptor-positive human breast tumors and this conjugate was cytotoxic to a human breast tumor cell line. Bjorn et al (22) using an extensive panel of breast tumor selective monoclonal antibodies found that many of these immunotoxins were cytotoxic for the breast tumor cells, but not to control fibroblast cell lines. A preliminary report by Nepo et al (23) indicates that daunorubicin-conjugated monoclonal antibody which recognizes an antigen found on the surface and cytoplasm of T47D human breast carcinoma cells, retained its ability to find the relevant antigen and be taken up by cells in suspension. These results underline the considerable potential of immunotoxic conjugates for the eventual therapy of human breast cancer.

ASSESSMENT OF HOST IMMUNE REACTIONS IN RELATIONSHIP TO MAMMARY TUMOR DEVELOPMENT

Humoral factors and their modulating effects

In the search for a suitable marker for breast tumors, several investigators have analyzed the various humoral factors in the circulation of patients at different stages of disease. The results of various laboratories indicate that in the sera of breast cancer patients it is possible to detect antigens, antibodies and immune complexes which are either absent or at differential levels in the sera of normal subjects. In addition, the levels of acute phase reactants may be of possible monitoring significance.

Among the antigens that have been described in circulation are human mammary epithelial antigens. Thus, Ceriani et al (24) were able to detect high levels of such antigens, which are normally present in the human milk fat globule membrane and breast epithelial cells, in the sera of patients with disseminated cancer of the breast. Patients with disseminated non-breast cancer, as well as normal female controls, do not possess those antigens in circulation. Furthermore, these authors were able to extract and characterize these antigens, and with the help of monoclonal antibodies defined a 46,000 dalton antigen that may prove to be valuable in breast cancer diagnosis. Several studies have analyzed the possibility of using the levels of carcinoembryonic antigen in the management of metastatic disease (25, 26), while other investigators have performed serial analyses of plasma gross cystic disease fluid protein (27) to predict therapeutic outcome.

Humoral immune responses to tumor associated antigens are demonstrable in patients with mammary carcinomas. Thus, in the sera of breast cancer patients, Crawford et al (28) were able to detect antibodies against the cellular protein p53 associated with transformed cells, and Tomana et al (29) described antibodies to MMTV related proteins. By far the majority of the tumor related antibodies generated by the cancer patients appeared to be tied up in the form of immune complexes which have been shown in animal models and in humans to play an important role in the pathogenesis of tumors and in the down-regulation of immune responses that might be beneficial to tumor bearing hosts. The clinical value of circulating immune complexes as an aid to prognosis however, does not appear to be very high (30). Acute phase reactants have been shown to reach high levels in the serum of cancer patients and as such, represent markers of tumor burden. Advanced breast cancer patients are immunologically compromised and some of their cell mediated immune functions appeared highly depressed. As an example, in Table 1, we present data from our laboratories indicating the progressive

Table 1. Concanavalin A-induced blastogenic responses of breast cancer patients at different stages of disease.

Lymphocyte donors	^{3}H-thymidine incorporation
Normal subjects	$57,014 \pm 4,272$
Non-metastatic patients	$54,083 \pm 3,592$
Untreated patients with metastases	$33,987 \pm 4,612$
Metastatic patients treated with chemotherapy	$21,520 \pm 2,378$

Results are expressed in mean cpm $\pm$ S.E. of Con A stimulated cultures minus the cpm of unstimulated control cultures.

decline of the blastogenic response of patients with advancing tumor status.

We have investigated the possibility that the inhibition of the blastogenesis

responses may be due to a modulatory effect of an acute phase protein such

as α_1-acid glycoprotein (orosomucoid), which might be interacting with

lymphocyte membranes and altering their capacity to be stimulated by mitogen

(31). In Table 2 evidence is presented of a positive correlation between

the levels of α_1-acid glycoprotein in the sera of breast cancer patients

and the potential of such sera to abrogate the blastogenic responses of

Table 2. Blastogenic responses of lymphoid cells from normal subjects
incubated in normal or breast cancer sera and levels of
α_1-acid glycoprotein in these sera.

Serum source	[a]Blastogenic responses induced by		Mean serum levels of α_1-acid glycoprotein
Normal subjects	[b]PHA Con A PWM	38,271 + 1,542 50,346 + 5,157 17,956 + 912	0.77 mg/ml [c] (n = 28)
Breast cancer patients	PHA Con A PWM	27,120 + 1,789 37,345 + 2,734 13,033 + 733	1.47 mg/ml (n = 25)

[a] Results expressed in mean cpm + S.E.
[b] PHA: phytohemagglutinin P; Con A: concanavalin A; PWM: pokeweed mitogen.
[c] n: number of individuals tested.

peripheral blood lymphocytes from normal subjects when exposed to three

different mitogenic stimuli. These results underline the complexity of

the interplay between humoral factors and the effector cells of the

immune system during tumorigenesis. Although our knowledge in these areas

is still far from complete, the purification and characterization of these

factors and cells will give insight about the mechanisms involved in these

interactions.

Cellular immune responses in peripheral organs

Cell mediated immunity has been studied by several kinds of techniques in breast cancer. Some of the assays used are general assessments of immunocompetence, while other investigations have analyzed the specific cellular responsiveness of hosts to tumor associated antigens. The majority of these studies appear to indicate that breast cancer patients are generally immunosuppressed as indicated by one or more parameters of in vivo and in vitro cell mediated immune correlates. A concomitant increase in suppressor cell activity has been reported in animal models and in humans,paralleling tumor development and metastasis. Decreased blastogenic responses to phytohemagglutinin (32), to concanavalin A (33) and diminished dermal hypersensitivity to recall antigens (32) appear to be indicative of poor prognosis. It should be noted that when a comparison is made between lymph nodes and systemic reactivity (34), patients with small primary tumors possess lymph node lymphocytes that react in blastogenic assays to a much greater extent than peripheral blood lymphocytes (PBL). However, in patients with very large tumors, the nodal reactivity is much lower than the corresponding PBL.

Although early studies utilized the leukocyte migration inhibition assay, many investigators have instead employed the leukocyte adherence inhibition (LAI) test as a diagnostic procedure of breast cancer patients. There is a great discrepancy about the usefulness of this technique. Thus, Kotlar and Sanner (35) in a blind study of sera collected from patients with breast cancer 0.5 to 2 years before indirect LAI measurements, found that 83% of the patients had a positive response when KCl extracts from breast carcinomas were used as antigens. In contrast, Fritze et al (36) contend that breast-tissue specific rather than tumor-specific responses can be detected by LAI testing. In this connection, Tsang et al (37) have found that T lymphocytes of patients with breast cancer exhibit breast cancer extract-specific LAI responses, B lymphocytes do not respond, and monocytes from these patients show a nonspecific LAI response to several unrelated tumor extracts. Cytophilic antibodies can be found in the sera from breast cancer patients that are capable of arming guinea pig peritoneal macrophages in a modification of a LAI assay. This test, named serum-armed macrophage adherence inhibition by Harris et al (38), appears to have potential as a diagnostic means of early breast cancer.

Various types of cytotoxicity reactions have been analyzed in connection with mammary tumor progression. Cunningham-Rundles et al (39) studied the natural cytotoxicity of PBL and regional lymph node cells of women with breast cancer. Their results confirm previous reports of an association of reduced natural killer (NK) activity and malignant disease in general, but also suggest that host defenses against mammary tumors may be associated with the appearance of NK activity in the regional node. Recently, Fulton et al (40) reported a negative correlation between NK levels and maximum tumor diameter in patients with primary human breast cancer. The mean NK activity determined at approximately 6 months postoperative was significantly lower than the subsequest tests. At around 12 months postsurgery, there is a recovery of NK activity to preoperative levels. These results are in accordance with those of Uchida et al (41) who reported on the detection of suppressor cells for NK activity in the peripheral blood of patients with breast carcinoma of stages I or II after surgery. These suppressor cells appeared to be of the monocytic line and did not exert any regulatory activity to the mitogenic potential of normal lymphocytes. Other types of cytotoxic reactions have been studied in connection with mammary tumors. Thus, antibody-dependent-cellular-cytotoxicity (ADCC) against cultured breast cancer cells mediated by human effector cells using monoclonal and polyclonal antibodies have been reported by Gore et al (42). Although the

exact role of the various cytotoxic cells is not fully known, they have
been implicated as potential effectors for tumor cell destruction.
Furthermore, some of these cells have been shown to be modulated by various
lymphokines (43), supporting the rationale for adopting regimens that include
addition of such soluble factors as part of the therapy of neoplastic breast
disease.

In situ immune responses

In many reports concerning the role of the immune system in the emergence and progression of neoplasms, there is a disparity between the observed
in vitro reactivity in peripheral lymphoid organs and the development of
the tumor in vivo. In order to better understand the inability of the immune
system to check neoplastic development, investigators have turned to the
study of the immune cells which actively infiltrate the tumor mass.

According to Vaage and Pepin (44) the accumulation of a large number
of lymphoid cells in the stroma around implants of syngeneic mammary
carcinomas in C3H/He mice, is a constant feature of the early primary host
response. Dvorak et al (45) have observed fibrin deposits in the stroma
of all human infiltrating breast carcinomas studied, particularly at their
growing edge, but the lymphocytes penetrated the fibrous tumor stroma
poorly. Similar results were obtained by Vaage and Pepin (46) in a more
recent study where they report that in the developing phase of concomitant
immunity to primary subcutaneous implants of mammary tumors, B and T cell
subsets show little tendency to infiltrate among the cells of the implants,
while macrophages are closely associated with the formation of a fibrous
cellular capsule. In more advanced stages of tumor development these
authors observed greater tendency of these macrophages to infiltrate the
tumor cells. Furthermore, there are reports of a differential distribution
of macrophages invading metastatic and nonmetastatic tumors (47). There

appears to be a general consensus that of the tumor infiltrating lymphocytes, the majority appears to be of the T cell lineage (48, 49). More
of these lymphocytes are of the suppressor/cytotoxic subset than the
helper/inducer subset, as characterized with monoclonal antibodies against
mouse (50) and human (51) leukocyte antigens. Lymphoreticular cells
possessing surface markers characteristic of granulocytes and natural killer
cells were virtually absent from malignant tissue (49).

The functional reactivities of mammary tumor infiltrating lymphoreticular cells has been the subject of several reports. Blastogenic
responsiveness to mitogens and tumor associated antigens can not be detected
using lymphocytes infiltrating large mammary tumors (50). In regressing
tumor models, phagocytosis of seemingly intact mammary tumor cells, is
common and appears to account for much of the loss in tumor cell numbers
(52). Macrophage mediated cytotoxicity and cytostasis have been detected
by several investigators and according to Loveless and Heppner (53) there
is a significant association between a tumor's ability to metastasize
spontaneously to the lung and the tumoricidal activity of that tumor's
infiltrating macrophages. Lymphocytes infiltrating human primary mammary
carcinomas lack ADCC and show very low levels of natural cytotoxicity (54).
It should be pointed out that although NK activity has not been correlated
with control of primary tumors, there is recent direct evidence using a
rat mammary adenocarcinoma model system (55), that the large granular
lymphocytes play a role in the inhibition of tumor metastases. The depression
of the various types of cell mediated immune reactions within the micro-
environment of mammary tumors appears to be a result of a down-regulation
by suppressor cells (56). Table 3 presents a summary of the known
morphological and functional characteristics of the cells that infiltrate
mammary tumors. As our knowledge about in situ cells and their functions

is enhanced, it would be theoretically possible to manipulate the altered

mechanisms to overcome the adverse effects on the immune system brought

about by the process of tumorigenesis.

Table 3.   Nature and functional characterization of mammary tumor
           infiltrating lymphoreticular cells.

General characteristics of the leukocyte infiltrates	Functional reactivity of in situ lymphocytes
Increase in total number of lympho-reticular infiltrating cells	Diminished blastogenic responses to mitogens and antigens
Leukocyte more numerous in malignant than in benign tumors	Active phagocytosis
	Limited macrophage mediated ADCC
Monocytes/macrophage mainly around the capsules	Detectable macrophage mediated cytotoxicity and cytostasis
Few cells with NK markers	Absence of NK activity
Majority of the in situ lymphocytes of the T cell lineage	High levels of suppressor cell activity
Increase in the levels of cytotoxic/ suppressor T cells in comparison to helper/inducer T cells	a) Macrophage mediated b) Lymphocyte mediated

IMMUNOLOGICAL ASSOCIATION OF MMTV AND HUMAN MAMMARY TUMORS

Evidence for an immunological relationship between mouse mammary

tumor virus and human carcinoma of the breast has been available for over

a decade since Black et al (57) presented their original observations that

leukocytes of patients with breast cancer react with MMTV in leukocyte

migration assays. These studies have been substantiated by subsequent

reports by Mesa Tejada et al (58) and Dion et al (59) who reported on the

presence of an antigen related to the major envelope glycoprotein of MMTV

in human mammary tumors. This human antigen has been considered as a

possible marker in the diagnosis (60) and prognosis (61) of breast cancer,

and it appears to be expressed in both male (62) and female (61) human
mammary carcinomas. An increased incidence of the MMTV-related antigen
has been detected in Tunisian patients suffering of a rapidly progressive
form of breast cancer initially designated as poussee evolutive (63).
This antigen is also expressed in metastatic lesions of human mammary
tumors, as well as in human breast carcinoma cell lines. Clonal derivatives
of such lines have been shown to release soluble proteins and particles
that have the biochemical characteristics of a retrovirus and these possess
antigens cross reactive with gp52, the major external protein of MMTV (64).
A recent study by Segev et al (65) provides evidence that the human cross-
reacting antigens are located on polypeptides with molecular weights of
about 68,000 and 60,000. Both appear to be glycosylated and the larger
one is present in the viral particles whereas both are found in the soluble
fraction. Therefore, the MMTV gp52 and the immunologically related human
proteins share a restricted similarity.

Antibodies reactive with murine mammary tumor virus have been detected
by several investigators in the sera of american women with breast cancer
(29, 66). Such antibodies can also be detected, albeit at lower percentages,
in healthy women and in some patients with benign breast disease. Strik-
ingly, less than 5.0% of women from mainland China with breast cancer had
MMTV-reactive antibodies in their sera (66). Although the inhibition of
direct and indirect leukocyte migration inhibition assays to MMTV is well
documented (57), more recent studies have indicated that these tests may
not be very valuable in breast cancer diagnosis. Instead, they may help
to identify a group of benign breast disease patients, whose breast
pathology is thought to be associated with a high risk for developing
breast cancer (67). The specificity of these reactions to MMTV antigens
and not to contaminating components of the host cells from which the virus

is derived, is the subject of a recent report by McCoy et al (68). Another parameter of cell mediated immunity, lymphoblastogenesis to MMTV, appears to be elevated in breast cancer patients (69). Data from our laboratory summarized in Table 4, indicate that while women with breast metastatic disease have diminished responsiveness to mitogens, their T lymphocytes appear to have immunologic hyperactivity to selected antigenic stimuli, such as MMTV. These results may be a reflection of altered proportions of T cell subsets in the peripheral blood of the stage IV breast cancer patients.

The possible association between the mouse retrovirus and the putative human mammary tumor virus is strengthened by the presence of retrovirus like particles with reverse transcriptase activity in human milk samples (70) and by the detection of sequences related to the MMTV genome in the DNA of human mammary tumors (71, 72). We have explored the possibility that such genetic information may be expressed in non transformed cells of human origin. In this connection, we have presented recent evidence (73) that in the surface of peripheral blood lymphocytes of both male and female normal subjects, it is possible to detect antigenic determinants cross reactive with two monoclonal antibodies against different epitopes of the MMTV gp52. Similar findings have been obtained by Tax and Manson (74) who have detected the gp52 related antigen in 60% of human tonsil cells and in 5 to 10% of peripheral blood cells. Based on the presence on their surfaces of an MMTV related antigen, a subset of B lymphocytes can be likewise defined in the spleens of Balb/c mice, which are devoid of exogenous MMTV (75). This protein is not expressed in normal or chemically-induced neoplastic Balb/c mammary cells nor in thymus derived lymphocytes. Molecular biological studies (73) have shown that in T cell enriched Balb/c spleen cells, MMTV-RNA expression is absent. In contrast, B cell enriched

Table 4. Lymphoproliferative responses to mitogens and MMTV in unseparated and E-rosette separated peripheral blood lymphocytes from metastatic breast cancer patients.

Blood donors	Stimulant	Unseparated mononuclear cells	E-rosetting lymphocytes	Non E-rosetting lymphocytes
Normal subjects	PHA	62,234 ± 4,173	65,379 ± 7,018	4,976 ± 228
	Con A	54,172 ± 5,998	58,333 ± 4,973	4,124 ± 629
	Sp A	76,883 ± 6,002	10,431 ± 983	22,837 ± 2,946
	MMTV	895 ± 482	3,965 ± 1,389	743 ± 523
Patients with metastatic breast cancer	PHA	41,397 ± 3,893	37,275 ± 4,283	3,004 ± 137
	Con A	32,116 ± 2,439	29,996 ± 3,500	1,931 ± 88
	Sp A	44,272 ± 2,910	6,413 ± 892	12,294 ± 983
	MMTV	4,782 ± 594	13,633 ± 3,366	443 ± 57

Results expressed in mean cpm ± S.E. of stimulated cultures with 10% bovine serum supplement in the growth medium, minus cpm of unstimulated control cultures.
PHA: phytohemagglutin; Con A: concanavalin A: Sp A: Staphylococcus aureus lysate.

preparations from the same sources have significant elevated expressions

of MMTV RNA, as compared to the levels observed in the liver, thymus,

retired breeder mammary glands and carcinogen-induced mammary tumors of

Balb/c mice. Although similar studies of molecular biology have not been

as yet performed using human lymphocytes, it is tempting to speculate that

the expression of an antigen from a retrovirus not known to actively

replicate in lymphoid cells, may play a role in the growth and/or

differentiation of cells of the bone marrow derived lymphoid lineage.

ACKNOWLEDGEMENT

The work from this laboratory cited here, was supported by Public
Health Service Grant CA-25583 awarded by the National Cancer Institute,
DHHS.

REFERENCES

1. Taylor-Papadimitriou, J., Peterson, J.A., Arklie, J., Burchell, J. and Ceriani, R.L. Int. J. Cancer 28: 7-21, 1981.
2. Hilkens, J., Bujis, I., Hilgers, J., Hageman, Ph, Sonnenberg, A., Koldovsky, U., Karande, K., van Hooven, R.P., Feltkamp, C. and van de Rijn, J.M. Proct. Biol. Fluids 29: 813-816, 1981.
3. Wilkinson, M.J.S., Howell, A., Harris, M., Taylor-Papadimitriou, J., Swindell, R. and Sellwood, R.A. Int. J. Cancer 33: 299-304, 1984.
4. Rasmussen, B.B., Pedersen, B.V., Thorpe, S.M., Hilkens, J., Hilgers, J. and Rose, C. Cancer Res. 45: 1424-1427, 1985.
5. Soule, H.R., Linden, E. and Edgington, T.S. Proc. Natl. Acad. Sci. U.S.A. 80: 1332-1336, 1983.
6. Colcher, D., Horan-Hand, P., Nuti, M. and Schlom, J. Proc. Natl. Acad. Sci. U.S.A. 78: 3199-3203, 1981.
7. Papsidero, L.D., Croghan, G.A., O'Connell, M.J., Valenzuela, L.A., Nemoto, T. and Cho, T.M. Cancer Res. 43: 1741-1747, 1983.
8. White, C.A., Dulbecco, R., Allen, R., Bowman, M. and Armstrong, B. Cancer Res. 45: 1337-1343, 1985.
9. Horan-Hand, P., Colcher, D., Wunderlich, D., Nuti, M., Teramoto, Y.A., Kufe, D. and Schlom, J. In: Rational Basis for Chemotherapy, UCLA Symposia on Molecular and Cellular Biology (Ed. B.A. Chabner), N.Y. Alan R. Liss Inc., Vol. 1, 1982, pp. 315-318.
10. Horan-Hand, P., Colcher, D., Salmon, D., Ridge, J., Noguchi, P. and Schlom, J. Cancer Res. 45: 833-840, 1985.
11. Imam, A., Drushella, M.M., Taylor, C.R. and Tokes, Z.A. Cancer Res. 45: 263-271, 1985.
12. Brabon, A.C., Williams, J.F. and Cardiff, R.D. Cancer Res. 44: 2704-2710, 1984.

13. Garcia, M., Capony, F., Derocq, D., Simon, D., Pav, B. and Rochefort, H. Cancer Res. 45: 709-716, 1985.
14. Natali, P.G., Giacomini, P., Bigotti, A., Imai, K., Nicotra, M.R., Ng, A.K. and Ferrone, S. Cancer Res. 43: 660-668, 1983.
15. Bernard, D.J., Maurizis, J.C., Chassagne, J., Chollet, P. and Plagne, R. Cancer Res. 45: 1152-1158, 1985.
16. Colcher, D., Horan-Hand, P., Nuti, M. and Schlom, J. Cancer Investigation 1: 127-138, 1983.
17. Peterson, J.A. and Ceriani, R.L. Breast Cancer Res. and Treat. 1985 (In press).
18. Colcher, D., Zalutsky, M., Kaplan, W., Kufe, D., Austin, F. and Schlom, J. Cancer Res. 43: 736-742, 1983.
19. Smedley, H.M., Finan, P., Lennox, E.S., Ritson, A., Takei, F., Wraight, P. and Sikora, K. Br. J. Cancer 47: 253-159, 1983.
20. Capone, P.M., Papsidero, L.D. and Cho, T.M. J. Natl. Cancer Inst. 72: 673-677, 1981.
21. Krolick, K.A., Yuan, D. and Vitetta, E.S. Cancer Immunol. Immunother. 12 39-41, 1981.
22. Bjorn, M.J., Ring, D. and Frankel, A. Cancer Res. 45: 1214-1221, 1985.
23. Nepo, A.G., Greaton, C.J., Taub, R.N. and Mesa-Tejada, R. Proc. Biennial Int. Breast Cancer Res. Conf. p. 197, 1985.
24. Ceriani, R.L., Sasaki, M., Sussman, H., Waka, W.M. and Blank, E.W. Proc. Natl. Acad. Sci. U.S.A. 79: 5420-5424, 1982.
25. Falkson, H.C., Falkson, G., Portugal, M.A., Van Der Watt, J.J. and Schoeman, H.S. Cancer 49: 1859-1865, 1982.
26. Lee, Y.T. Am. J. Clin. Oncol. 6: 287-293, 1983.
27. Silva, J.S., Leight, G.S., Haagensen, D.E., Tallos, P.B., Cox, E.B., Dilley, W.G. and Wells, S.A. Cancer 49: 1236-1242, 1982.
28. Crawford, L.V., Pim, D.C. and Bulbrook, R.D. Int. J. Cancer 30: 403-408, 1982.
29. Tomana, M., Kajdos, A.H., Niedermeier, W., Durkin, W.J. and Mestecky, J. Cancer 47: 2696-2703, 1981.
30. Krieger, G., Hehl, A., Wander, H.E., Salo, A.M. Rauschecker, and Nagel, G.A. Int. J. Cancer 31: 207-211, 1983.
31. Cheresh, D.A., Distasio, J.A., Vogel, C.L. and Lopez, D.M. J. Natl. Cancer Inst. 68: 779-783, 1982.
32. Mandeville, R., Lamoureux, G., Legault-Poisson, S. and Poisson, R. Cancer 50: 1280-1288, 1982.
33. Distasio, J.A., Cheresh, D.A., Schilder, R.J., Vogel, C.L., Silverman, M.A. and Lopez, D.M. J. Natl. Cancer Inst. 68: 69-74, 1982.
34. Reiss, C.K., Volence, F.J., Humphrey, M., Singla, O. and Humphrey, L.J. J. Surg. Onc. 22: 249-253, 1983.
35. Kotlar, H.K., and Sanner, T. J. Natl. Cancer Inst. 66: 265-271, 1981.
36. Fritze, D., Fedra, G. and Kaufmann, M. Int. J. Cancer 29: 261-264, 1982.
37. Tsang, P.H., Holland, J.F. and Bekesi, J.G. J. Clin. Lab Immunol. 9: 151-157, 1982.
38. Harris, L.F., Miller, L.L. and Hickok, D.F. Cancer Res. 42: 4985-4990, 1982.
39. Cunningham-Rundles, S., Filippa, D.A., Braun, Jr., D.W., Antonelli, P. and Ashikari, H. J. Natl. Cancer Inst. 67: 585-590, 1981.
40. Fulton, A., Heppner, G., Roi, L., Howard, L., Russo, J. and Brennan, M. Breast Cancer Res. and Treat. 4: 109-116, 1984.

41. Uchida, A., Kolb, R. and Micksche, M. J. Natl. Cancer Inst. 68: 735-741, 1982.
42. Gore, M.E., Skilton, R.A. and Coombes, R.C. Br. J. Cancer 48: 877-879, 1983.
43. Merluzzi, V.J., Savage, D.M., Souza, L., Boone, T., Mertelsmann, R., Welte, K. and Last-Barney, K. Cancer Res. 45: 203-206, 1985.
44. Vaage, J. and Pepin, K. J. Natl. Cancer Inst. 71: 147-154, 1983.
45. Dvorak, H.F., Dickersin, G.R., Dvorak, A.M., Manseau, E.J. and Pyne, K. J. Natl. Cancer Inst. 67: 335-340, 1981.
46. Vaage, J. and Pepin, K. Cancer Res. 45: 659-666, 1985.
47. Mahoney, K.H., Fulton, A.M. and Heppner, G.H. J. Immunol. 131: 2079-2085, 1983.
48. Rios, A.M., Miller, F.R. and Heppner, G.H. Cancer Immunol. Immunother. 15: 87-91, 1983.
49. Whitwell, H.L., Hughes, H.P.A., Moore, M. and Ahmed, A. Br. J. Cancer 49: 161-172, 1984.
50. Buessow, S.C., Paul, R.D. and Lopez, D.M. J. Natl. Cancer Inst. 73: 249-255, 1984.
51. Rowe, D.J. and Beverley, P.C.L. Br. J. Cancer 49: 149-159, 1984.
52. Key, M. and Haskill, J.S. Int. J. Cancer 28: 225-236, 1981.
53. Loveless, S.E. and Heppner, G.H. J. Immunol. 131: 2074-2078, 1983.
54. Eremin, O., Coombs, R.A. and Ashley, J. Br. J. Cancer 44: 166-176, 1981.
55. Barlozzari, T., Leonhardt, J., Wiltrout, R.H., Herberman, R.B. and Reynolds, C.W. J. Immunol. 134: 2783-2789, 1985.
56. Buessow, S.C., Paul, R.D., Miller, A.M. and Lopez, D.M. Int. J. Cancer 33: 79-85, 1984.
57. Black, M.M., Moore, D.H., Shore, B., Zachrau, R.E. and Leis, Jr. H.P. Cancer Res. 34: 1054-1060, 1974.
58. Mesa-Tejada, R., Keydar, I., Ramanarayanan, M., Ohno, T., Fenoglio, C. and Spiegelman, S. Proc. Natl. Acad. Sci. U.S.A. 75: 1529-1533, 1978.
59. Dion, A.S., Farwell, D.C., Pomenti, A.A. and Girardi, A.J. Proc. Natl. Acad. Sci. U.S.A. 77: 1301-1305, 1980.
60. Mesa-Tejada, R., Oster, M.W., Fenoglio, C.M., Magidson, J. and Spiegelman, S. Cancer 49: 261-268, 1982.
61. Keydar, I., Selzer, G., Chaitchik, S., Hareuveni, M., Karby, S. and Hizi, A. Eur. J. Clin. Oncol. 18: 1321-1328, 1982.
62. Lloyd, R.V., Rosen, P.P., Sarkar, N.H., Jimenez, D., Kinne, D.W., Menendez-Botet, C. and Schwartz, M.K. Cancer 51: 654-661, 1983.
63. Levine, P.H., Mesa-Tejada, R., Keydar, I., Tabbane, F., Spiegelman, S. and Mourali, N. Int. J. Cancer 33: 305-308, 1984.
64. Keydar, I., Ohno, T., Nayak, R., Sweet, R., Simoni, F., Weiss, F., Karby, S., Mesa-Tejada, R. and Spiegelman, S. Proc. Natl. Acad. Sci. U.S.A. 81: 4188-4192, 1984.
65. Segev, N., Hizi, A., Kirenberg, F. and Keydar, I. Proc. Natl. Acad. Sci. U.S.A. 82: 1531-1535, 1985.
66. Day, N.K., Witkin, S.S., Sarkar, N.H., Kinne, D., Jussawala, D.J., Levin, A., Hsia, C.C., Geller, N. and Good, R.A. Proc. Natl. Acad. Sci. U.S.A. 78: 2483-2487, 1981.
67. Cannon, G.B., Barsky, S.H., Alford, T.C., Jerome, L.F., Tinley, V., McCoy, J.L. and Dean, J.H. J. Natl. Cancer Inst. 68: 935-943, 1982.
68. McCoy, J.L., Tagliabue, A., Ames, R.E., Teramoto, Y.A., Cannon, G.B., Alford, C., Herberman, R.B. and Schlom, J. J. Natl. Cancer Inst. 72: 569-576, 1984.

69. Lopez, D.M., Parks, W.P. Silverman, M.A. and Distasio, J.A. J. Natl. Cancer Inst. 67: 353-358, 1981.
70. Keydar, I., Mesa-Tejada, R., Ramanarayanan, M., Ohno, T., Hu, R., and Spiegelman, S. Proc. Natl. Acad. Sci. U.S.A. 75: 1524-1528, 1978.
71. Callahan, R., Drohan, W., Tronick, S. and Schlom, J. Proc. Natl. Acad. Sci. U.S.A. 79: 5503-5507, 1982.
72. May, F.E., Westley, B.R., Rockefort, H., Buetti, E. and Diggelman, H. Nucleic Acid Res. 11: 4127-4139, 1983.
73. Lopez, D.M., Pauley, R.J. and Paul, R.D. In: Viruses, Immunity and Immunodeficiency (Eds. H. Friedman and S. Specter). Plenum Press, (In press).
74. Tax, A. and Manson, L.A. Proc. Biennial Int. Breast Cancer Res. Conf. p. 169, 1985.
75. Lopez, D.M., Charyulu, V. and Paul, R.D. J. Immunol. 134: 603-607, 1985.

11

MOLECULAR MARKERS AND THE MANIFESTATION OF METASTASIS

ZOLTÁN A. TÖKÉS

Department of Biochemistry, Comprehensive Cancer Center, University of Southern California, School of Medicine, Los Angeles, CA 90033, USA

INTRODUCTION

There are two ways to conceptualize tumor invasion and metastasis, which are the major causes of treatment failure for patients with malignancy. In one approach, the researcher classifies molecular or histological markers as manifestations of favorable factors. Such a conceptualization realizes that either the high expression of one set of parameters or the diminished presence of another set would suggest a low incidence of metastasis and good prognosis. The low efficiency of metastatic events would also be stressed. For example, an intravenous or subcutaneous injection of fifty-thousand mammary carcinoma cells into a Fisher rat (as in the case of experimental or spontaneous models for metastases) can result in fifty to a hundred colonies of lung metastasis. The experiment would be perceived as evidence for the rather low efficiency of metastatic success.

The former approach offers an anomaly to the one more commonly taken, in which the researcher interprets the same manifestations as unfavorable. In fact, an approximate ratio of forty to one publications describe what one might term as "bad news" markers, resulting in abundant reports describing two types of molecular markers whose increased or decreased expression signify poor prognosis. Regardless of how the complex cascade of events is conceptualized, however, almost all investigators share the conviction that early identification of primary malignancies with a high metastatic potential will allow the application of appropriate treatment modalities and thus result in an increased number of disease-free survivals. Furthermore, it is also believed that better understanding of the molecular events pertinent to invasion will prevent the emergence of highly metastatic phenotypes.

This summary explores ramifications of recent investigations and highlights some of the most promising parameters, with the understanding that a comprehensive review is not within the scope of this chapter. Each increased expression of a parameter signifying poor prognosis will have a reciprocal relationship, and its diminished expression can be interpreted as an indication of "good news". Conversely, when the low expression of a marker indicates higher risk of invasion, its elevated expression signifies favorable prognosis. Examples of parameters which may signify increased metastatic potential are given in Table 1.

Table 1. Examples of molecular and cellular parameters whose increased expressions may signify enhanced metastatic potential

> Aneuploidity and increased rate of diversification
> Peritumoral vessel invasion
> Plasminogen activator, 55 kd
> Tissue-matrix degrading enzymes
> > Collagenases
> > Cathepsin B
> > Endoglycoglycosidases
> Laminin and laminin receptors
> Cell-surface glycoproteins
> > gp 580, gp 52, Con-A binding sites
> Carcinoembryonic antigen, CEA
> Homotypic aggregation
> Autocrine growth factors

During the last few years, more than ten reasonable molecular parameters representing poor prognosis have been described. Since, in surgical pathology, one or two such parameters would already represent significant improvement, the gradual application of some of these markers within the next two years to evaluate invasive potentials in newly diagnosed surgical specimens is clearly foreseeable. Outstanding reviews exist on the topics of tumor invasion and metastasis, on the genesis and regulation of cellular heterogeneity in metastatic tumors (1-6) and on breast cancer markers (7). Consequently, only some of the most recent observations will be reviewed here. This research area progresses with such agility, that a blink may result in missing an important development. For this reason, I have included a few exceptionally promising references to recently presented abstracts, recognizing that such a practice is seldom desirable and anticipating that the quoted authors' work will have been published in detail by the time this volume is published. Since the focus will be on parameters associated with intact cells or detected in tissue specimens, diagnostic markers present in sera of breast cancer patients will receive no emphasis here.

MOLECULAR AND CELLULAR PARAMETERS

Aneuploidy and the rate of generating genetic or epigenetic diversity.

Aneuploidy and the rate of generating genetic or epigenetic diversity appear to be the central issue for the appearance of metastatic capabilities (3). The question remains as to the extent to which the metastatic potential is related to an increased diversification of the genetic information. There is increasing evidence to suggest a correlating relationship. For example, in a recent study of prognostic indicators including DNA histogram type, receptor content and staging related to human breast cancer, survival was evaluated in 74 patients (9). Among the 24 patients who died during the 36-month follow-up, 92% were classified as aneuploid. After 36 months, the lowest survival rates occurred in patients over 67 years of age who had aneuploid tumors, compared with 100% survival in patients over 67 years of age who had diploid tumors. However, it is not completely resolved whether there is an essential prerequisite for a diversified genome or for an aneuploid state before the appearance of metastatic phenotype (10).

Of fundamental significance are the number of genes necessary to express an invasive or metastatic phenotype. The most recent observations made with murine RAW 117 large cell lymphoma and fibrosarcoma models indicate that only a few genes are differentially expressed in the highly metastatic as compared with the low metastatic cells (11,12). Hybridization of cDNA with RNA were used in the studies cited. Their conclusions showed that a difference of less than 5% was detectable between the two RNA populations of the high and low metastatic clones despite the significant phenotypic differences between them (12). If these observations continue to elicit support, it will become apparent that only minute changes (genetic or epigenetic) in the genome will suffice to result in the metastatic phenotype. However, it remains to be seen how many different sets of such minor changes in gene expression could be utilized to result in a metastatic cascade.

Tumor progression in evolving neoplasia need not occur only by genetic alterations. DNA hypomethylation or remethylation is one epigenetic mechanism which could cause transient changes in gene expression and, therefore, in the expression of the metastatic phenotype (8,13). Experimental evidence for the relevance of this mechanism was obtained with 5-azacytidine-treated Lewis lung carcinoma cells. Such treatment interferes with DNA methylation and results in a change of tumorigenic (T+) but not metastatic (M-) cell lines to become metastatic (M+). Conversely, stable T+/M+ cell lines could lose their metastatic phenotype by similar treatments. Analogous experimental approaches with metastatic mammary carcinoma would be of considerable interest. However, cautious interpretation of relevant data is warranted here since hypomethylation is an alteration in the DNA that precedes malignancy, as was recently demonstrated in human benign and malignant colon tumors (14). The level of methylation of only a few pertinent genes or gene-segments may be relevant to the whole process of metastasis.

Contributions from the host toward the induction of mammary tumor variants deserve special attention. The demonstration that mammary tumor-associated macrophages or human neutrophils are mutagenic due to the generation of superoxide moieties indicates their possible role in accelerating the diversification process within a tumor cell population (15,16). It would therefore be of interest to demonstrate the conversion of a T+/M- clone to the T+/M+ phenotype, since this is one process where the application of oxygen scavengers, such as superoxide dismutases, may have an immediate and beneficial result.

The contribution of chemotherapy to tumor diversification also requires further attention, in particular with regard to the mutagenic anthracyclines (doxorubicin for example). In an experimental model of osteosarcoma in Wistar-Lewis rats treated with doxorubicin, metastasis to the long-bone increased frequently (17). It follows that a detailed evaluation of the rates and sites of metastatic appearances should be made in patients receiving chemotherapy involving mutagenic drugs or drugs capable of inducing mutagenic superoxides.

Different growth patterns were reported with varying aneuploidy in a new human breast carcinoma cell line (PMC 42) with stem cell characteristics (18). Thus floating cord cells were hypodiploid (mode 39), whereas the monolayer cultures were subtriploid (mode 66). In addition, cultures were bimodal when cords of cells have attached and where cells grew out as monolayers. Ten to 20% of the attached cells became progressively pseudotetraploid with a mode of 77. These experiments demonstrate that there may be a relationship between ploidity and growth patterns.

The fact that cellular DNA content influences the disease-free survival of Stage II breast cancer patients points to the possible clinical relevance of aneuploidy (19). Using a novel flow cytometric method to analyze paraffin-embedded archival material, it was found that 44% of patients with aneuploid tumors had relapsed compared with 23% of patients with diploid tumors. This correlation was even more pronounced in the premenopausal patients, further suggesting that aneuploid tumors have either a different natural history or a higher probability of developing drug resistance (19). Similar observations have been made in other solid tumors as well, for example in human prostate cancer. In this system, 80% of aneuploid tumors and only 7.1% of diploid tumors formed metastases (18). It will be of interest to investigate in greater detail these so-called "metastatic diploid cells", since the applied flow cytometry and DNA histograms might not detect minor variations in DNA content which would suffice to express a metastatic capability. These issues and relevant questions to ploidy and invasiveness are further summarized by H.S. Smith and collaborators in this volume.

Peritumoral vessel invasion

The prognostic significance of peritumoral vessel invasion has been recognized, and its significance was further emphasized in a recent study involving adjuvant treated breast cancer patients with axillary lymph node metastasis (21,22). Vessel invasion was recently evaluated histologically by the Ludwig Breast Cancer Group using data on 1510 women who were entered into trials for the evaluation of adjuvant therapy on operable breast cancer with axillary nodal metastasis. Vessel invasion was identified with routine light microscopy and, more recently, with improved immuno-cytochemistry (23). Depending on the subpopulations, patients with vessel invasion had a 41-54% greater risk of treatment failure than those without invasion. They also had a 29-64% greater risk of death. A higher percentage of treatment failures at distant sites was observed for women with invasion compared to those without vessel invasion (27% vs. 18%, p = 0.003). Thus histological recognition of vascular invasion may become one of the most significant parameters. The application of this prognostic factor would be relevant to patients who are lymph-node negative. In these cases, the invasive phenotype would be detected in the vicinity of primary tumor sites prior to invasion of lymph nodes. The significance of vascular invasion may be comparable to the identification of micrometastasis in bone marrow.

Plasminogen activators

Plasminogen activators, PA, a family of proteases which are active blood coagulants, may be important in the expression of certain phenotypes associated, but not exclusively, with malignancy. Tissue invasion by endothelial cells, macrophages or regenerating nerve growth-cones are usually associated with elevated PA activity. Plasmin generated from plasminogen by a tumor-cell-associated plasminogen activator may be crucial for matrix hydrolysis at low cell densities, as demonstrated with human rhabdomyosarcoma and fibrosarcoma cells, and with mouse melanoma cells (24). Rhabdomyosarcoma cells continued to degrade matrix glycoproteins in the presence of plasminogen at higher cell densities as well, but the human fibrosarcoma cells continued the digestion even in the absence of zymogen (24). A true idea of the complexity of possible correlations between metastasis and PA activity is beginning to emerge from such studies. Relevant to this complexity are the multiple forms of PA and their variations found in tumors, plasma and in lymph nodes containing the metastasis (25). The pattern of isoelectric molecular forms of PA, active at pH 8, showed two groups of several isotypes: in plasma from breast cancer-bearing patients and controls, these isotypes were in the pI ranges of 6.6 to 6.8 and 8.0 to 8.5. In mammary adenocarcinoma tissue, the ranges were 6.8 to 7.9 and 9.0 to 9.4. PA activity in tumor-bearing patients was very high in malignant tissue and considerably decreased in plasma. The latter decrease correlated with the presence of metastasis in the axillary lymph nodes (25). These results suggested that the high PA activity in the tumor tissue might participate in the destruction of the peritumoral tissue, thus allowing its invasion by tumor cells. The low activity of PA in the plasma might increase plasma fibrin, reflecting an early disorder in blood coagulation which would increase the likelihood of the formation of metastasis (25).

Recurrence of breast cancer within two years after surgical removal of the primary cancer and the presence of PA in the primary lesion have been investigated (26). No recurrence was found when the tissue had undetectable amounts of PA. These investigators distinguished two major types of PA, the 100 kd or 73 kd tissue activator and the 55 kd activator. When only the tissue activator was detectable, the recurrence rate was 7%. This rate increased to 36% when both the 73 kd and 55 kd were detectable, and to 46% when only the 55 kd PA was present. Such correlations with poor prognosis clearly establish the 55 kd PA as one of the most important molecular parameters to be considered for evaluation by the surgical pathologist. Either the application of PA-specific monoclonal antibodies or fluorescent substrates capable of binding to the active site of this enzyme may be useful for evaluating their prognostic significance in tissue sections.

The expression of PA in clones with high metastatic potential may be regulated by epigenetic mechanisms. High PA presence could be temporary and relate to the cell's capacity to migrate. The location of PA in the cells is also significant. The existence of plasminogen independent novel receptor for the catalytic site of PA was recently suggested (27). The number of these receptors on the cell surface decreased in virally transformed mouse fibroblasts. Cells in general fail to bind the 33 kd breakdown-product of PA, further suggesting the role of membrane receptors (28). Cell lines with more invasive characteristics appear to have increased membrane-associated PA activity. In addition to the expression of PA by the tumor cells, the contribution of the host's environment needs further study. The integrity of the matrix itself may influence the levels and types of PA isozyme activities of mammary epithelial cells (29). It is also conceivable that tumor-activated macrophages containing significantly elevated PA participate in the matrix degradation at the vicinity of the tumor (30). Alternatively, endothelial cells during the process of angiogenesis could contribute significant quantities of this factor.

Tissue-matrix degrading enzymes

Light- or electron-microscopic examination of tissue sections from malignant specimens gives an impression of disappearance of normal basal membrane structures and destruction of surrounding tissue matrix. Most investigators assumed that the tumor cell is the primary cause of destruction. However, increased recognition is given to numerous other intricate mechanisms, whereby host factors may only temporarily influence the tumor cells or the tumor cells may stimulate host cells such as fibroblasts, endothelial cells and leukocytes to degrade the tissue matrix. The multitude of such intricate signal-processes can overwhelming, especially since virtually every degrading enzyme has its own endogenous inhibitor which could in turn be regulated by yet another set of signals. Nevertheless, some of the enzymes show promising correlations with invasive capabilities, examples of which will be high-lighted here. In addition, it needs to be acknowledged that some of the crucial enzymes involved in the metastatic cascade may not yet have been discovered.

Collagenases

Collagen is considered an essential component of the matrix and constitutes the structural scaffolding upon which several other components are assembled. Tumor-derived collagenases have been implicated in the destruction of interstitial collagen Types I,II, and III and of Type IV located in basal membranes. The relevance of these enzymes to invasion and metastasis has been reviewed (4,31). These enzymes are calcium and zinc-dependent enzymes, active at neutral pH and capable of producing single cleavages in the collagen molecule. There are increasing numbers of studies demonstrating that the amount of tumor collagenase can be correlated with the aggressive behavior of the tumor. This relationship has been particularly well demonstrated for bladder cancer (32). Although the capacity of some invasive tumor cells to degrade basement membranes is known, a convincing argument for a relationship between Type IV collagenase and metastasis in human breast cancer is just beginning to emerge (33). On the basis of experimental findings with murine and rat mammary adenocarcinomas and the support obtained with human surgical specimens, one anticipates that of Type IV collagenase will become one of the useful molecular markers (4,34,35,36). Use of monoclonal antibodies or fluorescent labeled specific substrates should permit the evaluation of the presence of Type IV collagenase in a tissue section within the settings available for surgical pathologists (33).

Increased amounts of collagenases can result from tumor host-interaction, as has been demonstrated with the rabbit V2 carcinoma (37). Co-cultures of intraperitoneally grown tumor and normal subcutaneous tissue of the rabbit resulted in significantly higher production of cysteine proteinases and collagenase, compared with the sum of the activities of the separate tissues. Similarly, did explants of subcutaneous tissue of tumor-bearing rabbits secreted significantly more cysteine proteinases and collagenase than explants from normal animals. Normal subcutaneous tissue explants stimulated with tumor-conditioned culture medium secreted both enzymes in higher amounts than controls. It was suggested that diffusible factors derived from the tumor or from immigrated cells promote an increased synthesis and secretion of collagenase and cysteine proteinase in the host. These enzymes may play a cooperative role during invasion (37).

Similar observations are emerging with rat 13762 NF adenocarcinoma cells (38). Tumor cells released soluble factors which stimulated fibroblasts to release collagenolytic activity (39). Similar findings have been noted with endothelial cells (40). It is of interest that endothelial cells have been reported to produce inhibitors to enzymes which are involved in degrading cell-free extracellular matrices (41).

It remains to be seen how wide the correlations between Type IV collagenase activity and tumor metastasis will prove to be. Exceptions, using highly metastatic and nonmetastatic clones of Lewis lung carcinoma and T10 sarcoma, have been reported, where no correlation was detected between degradation activity and metastatic capacity (42).

Cathepsin B-like enzymes

More than ten years ago cathepsin-B, a cysteine proteinase, was detected in elevated quantities in malignant breast cancer specimens when compared with benign fibroadenomas or noninvasive hyperplasias (43). Continuous support for this finding emerges not only in mammary carcinoma but in other tumor models as well. The activity of cathepsin B-like proteinases was determined both in nonmetastatic and highly metastatic variants of spontaneous BDX rat sarcoma (44). The metastatic clones manifest exceedingly high intracellular cathepsin B-like activity compared with the nonmetastatic variant. In this model, other proteinases such as elastase-like and collagenase-like enzymes and plasminogen activators showed low and essentially comparable activity patterns.

Cathepsin B-like enzyme was six to 20 times greater in homogenates of human melanoma, fibrosarcoma, and mammary, lung and colon adenocarcinoma when compared with liver homogenates (45). The enzyme was purified to homogeneity from each of these tissues. These enzyme preparations had similar physical, chemical and kinetic properties, similar substrate specificities and pH optima. However, differences were demonstrated in isoenzyme patterns and the tumor-derived enzyme exhibited greater stability above pH 7 compared with the preparation from normal tissue. Mouse mammary tissue secretes cathepsin B-like enzyme, which has a larger molecular weight (46). This component is immunologically related to the one produced by the spleen and may represent an abnormally secreted precursor form of the lysosomal enzyme. Secretion studies using various mammary gland explants suggest the presence of a subpopulation of cells in the mammary gland, cells that are capable of secreting elevated amounts of cathepsin B-precursor. The corresponding cell population appears to be more abundant in glands of mice with high incidence of spontaneous tumors and thus might indicate the presence of pre-neoplastic lesions. Visualization of this proteinase using novel fluorescent transition-state analog probes would be of interest and may lead to the establishment of a parameter of prognostic significance (47).

General comments on proteinases

The development, maintenance and dynamic rearrangement of the well defined glandular architecture in breast tissue present a particularly challenging problem to molecular biology. Mechanisms not yet fully understood exist to create the characteristic three-dimensional glandular architecture and to expand it for the special demands of pregnancy and lactation. Well controlled processes are triggered for the involution of this tissue after lactation is terminated. Proteinases play a vital role in structuring and restructuring the tissue. However, their role in this task is vastly different from the ordinary enzyme - substrate type of reactions which may take place in a solution. In a three-dimensional tissue structure, the enzyme's position and relationship to well defined topographic and microenvironmental factors must be taken into consideration (48). Untimely degradation and gradual disorganization of tissue architecture are characteristics of neoplastic growth. Such processes may not be entirely due to increased levels of degrading enzymes, but could be explained by positional effects as well. It is therefore conceivable, for example, that aberrant release of minute quantities of enzymes to lateral-lateral or to basement membrane domains could gradually disrupt the tissue and induce cell migration. Such minute deviations may not be detectable when enzyme levels are measured in tissue homogenates or in homogenates of monolayers of cells maintained under cell-culture conditions. Preliminary results have been reported indicating that preferential localization of plasminogen activator activity and cathepsin B to the plasma membrane and to the cell surface increases the metastatic potential of rat mammary adenocarcinoma and murine melanoma cells (49,50).

More attention needs to be focused on the possibility that the proteinases most relevant for invasion and metastasis, or for growth control, have not yet been discovered. The role of a novel proteinase was, for example, suggested recently from studies on cloning and sequence analysis of a cDNA for rat transforming growth factor, TGF-alpha (51). This cDNA hybridizes to a 4.5-kilobase messenger RNA that is 30 times larger than necessary to code for a 50-amino acid polypeptide; it is present not only in retrovirus-transformed rat cell but also at lower levels in normal rat tissues. The nucleotide sequence of the cDNA predicts that TGF-alpha is synthesized as a larger product and that the larger form may exist as a transmembrane protein. However, unlike many polypeptide hormones, including EGF, the cleavage of the 50-amino acid TGF-alpha from the larger form does not occur at paired basic residues, but rather between alanine and valine residues, suggesting the influence of a novel protease (51).

Proteinase inhibitors

There are three major mechanisms by which a given cell can control the availability of proteinases: the synthesis of corresponding messenger RNA, conversion of inactive zymogen forms to active enzymes, and regulation by specific inhibitors. This latter mechanism has not yet received adequate attention, although the significance of such inhibitors may be equal to the availability of tissue-degrading proteases.

The major glycoproteins synthesized and released by human breast epithelial cells have been characterized (52-54). Gp 68 is one of the five major families of glycoproteins observed both in organ-culture supernatants from surgical specimens and in established breast carcinoma cell lines. This glyprotein is identical to serum alpha-1-antichymotrypsin (Achy) as determined by two-dimensional gel electrophoresis and by immunological techniques. Gp 68 was detected in organ-culture supernatants from uninvolved breast surgical specimens, fibroadenomas and infiltrating ductal carcinomas. Quantitative immunoprecipitation did not show significant variations among the three different types of cultures. The same protein is a prominent component of the supernatants from primary cultures of normal epithelial cells, MCF-7 and MDA-MB-231 cells, but it is present only in trace quantities in

ZR-75-1 cells (54). Immunohistochemical studies demonstrated the expression of Achy on normal and malignant breast epithelial cells and on their lymph node metastases. The inhibitor from MCF-7 cells can form an irreversible complex with chymotrypsin indicating that it is functionally active.

The name alpha-1-antichymotrypsin is a misnomer because it is actually a more potent inhibitor of cathepsin G than of chymotrypsin. Cathepsin G is a matrix-degrading enzyme released by leukocytes and mast cells. Thus, the fact that an active Achy is synthesized by human breast epithelial cells suggests that the function of this inhibitor may be to protect the integrity of glandular tissue structures from degrading enzymes released by invading leukocytes (54).

In addition to the de novo synthesized inhibitor, another component is adsorbed from fetal bovine serum by the MCF-7 cells and subsequently released into serum-free media. This component also forms an irreversible, 88,000-dalton complex with chymotrypsin. The biological role of this component is not clear, but the observation suggests that host-factors may likewise be relevant in the stabilization of cell surface components and that they could also be involved in the protection of extracellular matrices from untimely degradation (53).

These studies were extended to clones of rat mammary adenocarcinoma cells, MTLn2 and MTLn3, representing low and high spontaneous metastatic potentials respectively (55). The experiments have shown that both cell lines express active proteinase inhibitors, which form stable enzyme-inhibitor complexes of 70,-80,000 daltons. The inhibitors for these complexes are derived from fetal bovine serum. MTLn2 (low metastatic potential) cells exhibited five times more proteinase inhibitory activity than MTLn3 cells under identical conditions. Only MTLn2 cells have expressed molecules which formed 40,-50,000-dalton complexes with chymotrypsin when the cells were maintained in media containing only proteinase inhibitor-free bovine serum albumin and no other serum component. These findings further point to the possible involvement of tumor-cell-produced and serum-derived proteinase inhibitors in metastasis (55).

Endoglycosidases

Glycosaminoglycans are prominent components of vascular endothelial basal lamina. Heparan sulfate, heparin, chondroitin 6-sulfate, chondroitin 4-sulfate, dermatan sulfate, keratan sulfate and hyaluronic acid were all tested as potential substrates for endoglycosidases produced by highly metastatic clones of mouse B16 melanoma. Of all these matrix components only heparan sulfate (HS) was extensively degraded (56-59). The HS degrading enzyme was purified and characterized as an endoglucuronidase capable of cleaving at intrachain sites. It is inhibited by heparin and the inhibitory activity requires the -N-sulfate groups. Tissues from human malignant melanoma metastases also showed high heparanase activity (58). Of particular interest is the binding of HS to Type IV collagen and the inhibiting of its degradation by the Type IV specific collagenase. Since all cell clones of metastatic rat 13762 NF mammary adenocarcinoma exhibited uninhibited Type IV collagenolytic activity, it would seem to indicate that HS was not available or that HS must be degraded prior to the effective destruction of basal lamina (60). Insufficient deposits of HS may make Type IV collagen more prone to degradation. This latter interpretation appears more likely since most of the rat mammary tumor clones failed to cleave HS extracted from bovine lung.

Beta-N-acetylglucosaminidase, together with cathepsin B were observed in association with plasma membranes in highly metastatic melanoma cells (49). None of the other lysosomal hydrolases showed such an association, further indicating that hydrolytic enzymes bound to the cell surface may be important factors for extravasation of tumor cells during the metastatic cascade.

Cell motility and response to chemoattractants

Motility is an essential component of the invasive process. Investigation has been carried out on differential cell migration into synthetic membranes with stromal protein impregnated and the effects on migration of various tumor extracts (61,82). Autocrine chemoattractants produced by malignant cells may promote metastasis both by stimulating motility of tumor cells invading secondary targets and, later, by recruiting cells from circulation. Materials originating from local necrotic regions of tumors also appear to affect the rates at which dissemination patterns develop. However, as of today, the chemoattractant factors for mammary adenocarcinoma cells have not been identified. Certain tumor models, such as the M5076 reticulum sarcoma cells known to be highly invasive in vivo, respond to the synthetic chemoattractant peptide N-formylmethionyl-leucyl-phenylalanine (FMLP). Human amnion membrane denuded of its epithelium was penetrated 600% more effectively by reticulum sarcoma cells when 10^{-7}M FMLP was introduced (62). The chemoattractant-induced invasion did not result in increased collagenase activity. Five-fold decrease of invasion was obtained, however, when inhibitors of both serine and metalloproteinases from bovine cartilage extract were introduced. Collagenase treatment appears to increase motility in four murine tumor models (63). Active cell movement was observed with Walker rat carcinoma but not with 13762 cells in lymph node metastasis (64), further demonstrating that generalizations regarding the role of cell motility and invasion are not yet appropriate. At this time, it is seems unlikely that a routine assay measuring cell motility will become applicable for prognostic evaluations. Nevertheless, the penetration of human amnion membrane serves as a powerful tool for investigating the mechanisms involved in invasion and for screening potential chemoattractants.

Laminin and laminin receptors

Laminin is a glycoprotein associated with the basement membrane and promotes the binding of cells to Type IV collagen. Mammary carcinoma cells have receptors for laminin on their surfaces which may be involved in the initial interaction of tumor cells with the vascular basement membrane to facilitate invasion and subsequent promotion of metastasis (65). The relevant molecular events have been reviewed recently (4).

A variety of biological phenomena related to cell attachment, migration, growth and morphology may be regulated by laminin. This glycoprotein has a multidomain structure and a cross-shaped configuration, with three short arms and one long arm. Globular end regions are located at the end of each four arms. A protease insensitive intersection forms the central portion of the molecule. This is the section that binds to a specific cell surface receptor on the cell. The globular end regions are the apparent binding sites for Type IV collagen and the long arm of laminin contains the heparin-binding site. Breast carcinoma tissue contains a higher number of unoccupied laminin receptors than does the benign tissue. The existence of exposed receptors might be caused by the incomplete basement membrane found in the vicinity of invading cells. The availability of laminin receptors appear to play a role in blood-borne metastases. Ten times more metastases were observed in experimental models after intravenous injection of tumor cells selected for their ability to attach to basement membrane via laminin. When the receptors on these cells are blocked with fragments of laminin, devoid of collagen binding domains, a marked reduction in pulmonary metastases is observed. Such experiments indicate the possibility that a quantitation of laminin receptors may have prognostic significance. Furthermore, they represent the beginning of experimental designs for therapeutic or preventive approaches whereby metastasis might be retarded by nontoxic substances (4,66).

Cell surface glycoproteins

Extensive reviews are available on cancer-associated glycoproteins, on the cell surface carbohydrates, including sialic acid, and on the heterogeneous expression of cell surface antigens in normal epithelia and their tumors as revealed by monoclonal antibodies (67-69). Only selected examples will be used here to illustrate some of the most recent developments.

The availability of rat 13762 NF mammary adenocarcinoma clones with varying metastatic potentials made it possible to systematically investigate lectin binding sites and glycoproteins at the cell surface and to study their possible relationship with metastasis (70,71). After neuraminidase treatment, the highly metastatic MTLn3 cells express approximately twice the quantity of peanut agglutinin (PNA) binding sites than do clones of lower metastatic potential. Concanavalin A (Con-A)-binding sites were similar, and the number of wheat germ agglutinin (WGA)-binding sites decreased slightly as the metastatic potential of the clones increased. The major PNA binding protein was subsequently identified as a 580,000-dalton protein, expressing terminal galactose residues on the oligosaccharide side-chains, gp 580. The expression of this galactoprotein appears to correlate with the metastatic potential of various cell clones (70). Monoclonal antibodies to rat gp 580 react with tissue sections of human breast cancer, indicating the possibility that a similar molecule may have prognostic significance and application in surgical pathology. Another major sialoglycoprotein, gp 80, identified by similar techniques, showed consistent decrease on the increasingly metastatic clones.

The prognostic value of Con-A reactivity with primary human breast cancer cells has been investigated in detail (72). Patients whose tumors were highly reactive with Con-A were at significantly greater risk of developing early recurrence than patients with low-reactivity tumors. These findings are in apparent contradiction to what was observed in rat mammary carcinoma models (70). However, it must be kept in mind that the techniques for evaluating Con-A binding activity were also different. In the study of human specimens, no correlation was found between Con-A reactivity and the age of the patients, their menopausal status, the number of axillary lymph nodes infiltrated with tumor, the estrogen receptor content of the tumor, or the clinical stage of the disease (72). The study thus shows that the Con-A reactivity is an independent discriminator for identifying patients at high risk of developing early recurrent disease.

Examination of glycoprotein synthesis by human surgical specimens of uninvolved and malignant breast tissues offers a unique opportunity to identify molecules synthesized while the cells are maintained in their undisrupted tissue environment (68,73,74). These isotope-labeled gps have been characterized by two-dimensional gel electrophoresis and fluorography. The labeled gps from monolayer cultures of normal epithelial cells and of two established malignant cell lines, MCF-7 and ZR-75-1 have been investigated by similar techniques. In the molecular weight range of 20,000 to 200,000 daltons, twenty families of gps were detected, and their apparent pIs and molecular weights have been described. The types of gps recognized in the supernatants of the organ cultures were similar to the gps detected in the supernatants of monolayer cultures, although there were significant variations from specimen to specimen (73,74).

Two types of variations were observed when a comparison was made between gp patterns of uninvolved and malignant surgical specimens. A marked increase in three families of gps with apparent molecular weights of 55, 39-42 and 38-39 kd was observed from specimens of infiltrating ductal carcinomas. Conversely, two families of gps with molecular weights of 117 and 130 kd are released in greater quantities from the uninvolved specimens. Comparison of the gp patterns released by monolayers of normal epithelial cells and the malignant MCF-7 and ZR-75-1 cells in cultures confirmed the variations observed with organ cultures. Although the variations among specimens were extensive, no novel transformation-specific gp family emerged, suggesting that the differences in gps caused by transformation are more quantitative than qualitative. A comparison of glycoprotein patterns from highly invasive cells and from cells already metastasized to the lymph nodes or to other distant sites, using organ cultures, would be of interest, for it may lead to the direct identification of molecules whose expression may be indicative of increased metastatic potentials.

An estrogen-regulated glycoprotein of 52,000 molecular weight, gp 52, appears to be released by metastatic human breast cancer cells in culture (75,76). Frozen sections of human breast cancer samples were stained by the peroxidase anti-peroxidase method using monoclonal antibodies raised specifically to gp 52. In 20 of 25 cancer specimens, cytoplasmic staining was observed with six monoclonal antibodies specific for gp 52. The five samples that were not stained contained no detectable estrogen receptor. All the six normal mammary gland specimens were negative. It would be of interest to extend these studies to the process of tissue invasion and to find out whether cancer cells in lymph nodes produce elevated levels of gp 52. The prognostic significance of high, medium and low expression of this glycoprotein should become available shortly.

Carcinoembryonic antigen, CEA

At this time, the measurement of CEA in serum is considered a useful procedure to monitor the progress of breast carcinoma (7,79). Rising plasma levels can be detected in about 50% of patients with a lead time of 3-6 months. Generally, it is associated with either greater tumor burden or with a more aggressive tumor type. Such an association, however, represents a paradox, for even normal epithelial cells, when placed in primary cultures, express CEA as demonstrated by fluorescent-labeled antibodies to CEA. Since normal tissue sections do not stain for this glycoprotein, it would seem that the disruption of tissue architecture alone is sufficient for its induction. The staining is cell-surface associated, which is consistent with a location in or near the plasma membrane. CEA is released by malignant cells into the culture supernatant. It would be of interest to see whether more aggressive or invasive tumor types release CEA faster and whether the rate is related to the availability of proteolytic enzymes.

Another aspect of the CEA-paradox is that the prognostic parameters obtained from immunohistological studies are different from those obtained from the determination of serum levels (80). Based on a study of 167 breast cancer cases, the overall expression of CEA was 65%. There was no significant correlation in expression and survival in either regional or localized breast cancer cases, and there was no association with number of lymph node involved, size of tumor, parity or menopausal status. There were, however, a statistically significant number of short survivors whose primary tumor was negative for CEA but whose metastatic tumor expressed the marker (80). If this finding is substantiated in further studies, CEA expression in histological sections of primary breast cancer may signify favorable prognosis.

Homotypic aggregation factors

An intriguing set of experiments were performed recently with murine melanoma cells in which aggregation was induced with various concentrations of asialofetuin. Variant cell lines were selected which had reduced tendency to undergo such homotypic aggregation in the presence of syngeneic serum (77). The non-aggregating cells spread on solid substrate more than the parental cell lines, formed more focal contacts, and proliferated more slowly. A variety of tumor cells have also been identified with the capacity to produce galactose-specific agglutinating lectins (78). Monoclonal antibodies raised against such lectins inhibited colony formation in soft agar without any detectable cytotoxic effects. Colony formation in semisolid medium and the development of experimental metastasis in the lungs of syngeneic mice are markedly reduced in cells with low honotypic aggregation. Thus, the ability to undergo aggregation in the presence of glycoproteins with exposed terminal galactose residues is a property of malignant cells capable of influencing anchorage-independent growth and the formation of metastases. The extension of these findings to models of mammary carcinoma is eagerly awaited.

Autocrine growth factors

Mechanisms exist by which autonomous cells in a mammary carcinoma can replace the steroid requirement for growth promotion (81,83). The process is accomplished by the secretion of factors which not only stimulate their own proliferation but might also stimulate adjacent dependent or responsive cells. Proteins expressing such activity have been purified and shown to be resistant to low pH and elevated temperatures. Proteolytic degradation by cathepsin D results in active peptides with molecular weight range of 2,100-5,200 dalton. These peptide mimic the action of mitogens, participate in stimulating autonomous mammary tumor growth and represent an escape mechanism from estrogen dependence.

Indirect evidence for the in vivo relevance of these growth factors comes from studies on clonal heterogeneity in two mammary carcinomas which metastasize spontaneously in mice (84). When clonal interactions were studied by the simultaneous injection of different clones, injected at different subcutaneous sites, it was found that a slow growing line failed to modify the growth rate of a rapidly growing line, but did accelerate the growth of a second slow growing line injected simultaneously on the contralateral side. This enhancement of tumor growth was radioresistant. Interclonal growth regulation can be invoked to explain these findings, further emphasizing the possible role of autocrine growth factors in assisting the metastatic process by promoting growth which is independent of factors released by the host. Quantitation of these factors in a given surgical specimen could result in the identification of significant prognostic indicators.

EXAMPLES OF PARAMETERS WHOSE DIMINISHED EXPRESSION MAY SIGNIFY INCREASED METASTATIC POTENTIAL

The loss of molecular markers associated with well differentiated phenotypes lead to conclusions which suggest poor prognosis. Although such evaluations are made adequate by using light microscopy and morphological criteria, the addition of refined cytological and molecular parameters may improve such evaluations. For example, the loss of basement membrane can be better visualized with immunohistological techniques using specific antibodies to Type IV collagen (85). In fibroadenoma of the breast, the Type IV collagen was present in basement membranes as a continuous sheet, but in invasive, well differentiated ductal carcinoma, it was present only as thin irregular filaments surrounding some epitheliomatous clusters. Minor sites of disruption Type IV collagen deposits were visible in intraductal carcinoma of the breast. Since studies of more invasive tumors showed Type IV collagen diminished or became absent, the application of immunostaining techniques for this component could be of value.

Loss of myoepithelial cell characteristics were observed recently in metastasizing rat mammary tumors relative to their nonmetastasizing counterparts (86,87). In these studies, cell lines were isolated from the metastasizing rat mammary tumor cell strain by single-cell cloning. Incidence of metastasis was determined by injection of cells into the mammary fat pads and by assessing the dissemination to the lungs and to axillary and paraaortic lymph nodes. Antisera to keratin, actin, laminin and fibronectin, which normally stain myoepithelial cells and basement membranes, failed to stain the metastatic cell lines. The study suggests that the metastatic epithelial-derived cell lines lack the ability to express features of myoepithelial cells, in contrast to cell lines isolated previously from nonmetastasizing rat mammary tumors (87).

Analysis of tumor antigen profiles in combination with established surface markers may provide important information relevant to prognosis and to differentiation status (88-90). A study of the expression of beta 2-microglobulin, HLA, CEA, and two breast tumor-associated antigens (TAAs) as detected by B 6.2 and B 72.3 monoclonal antibodies demonstrated that poorly differentiated tumors lose surface antigens selectively. Beta 2-microglobulin and HLA expression correlated with differentiated tumor types. The detection of TAAs, however, was not related to differentiation (88), as observed in the tissue sections of primary tumors. The levels of ABO(H) cell surface antigens diminished in carcinoma as compared with benign lesions (89). On the basis of immunoabsorption studies using sera from primary breast cancer patients and tumor specimens from distant metastasis, it was possible to demonstrate the decreased capacity of metastatic cells to bind to circulating antibodies (90). Two types of interpretations are raised. The first would associate the shift of antigens normally expressed on the cell surface to the cytoplasmic domains with the decreasing efficiency of antibody binding. The second would argue that antigenically silent clones emerge with tumor progression. There is evidence for both types of reasoning, which underlines one of the limitations of extracting information on prognostic factors from examining primary tumor cell populations. Since these cells will shed some of their molecular markers as tumor progression proceeds, it would seem that the rate of antigen-shedding events would be significant rather than their evaluation at the time of initial diagnosis.

The successful cloning of human lymphocytes capable of producing antibodies against the surface antigens of malignant breast epithelial cells has opened up opportunities to study changes in TAA expressions (91,92). Human monoclonal antibodies, MAb, have been identified with preferential binding to malignant cells. The majority of such antibodies are not breast-specific, and indeed one wonders whether there are any such molecules characterized so far. Antigenic heterogeneity among the primary tumor cells are readily demonstrated by human MAb. Clones exist which produce antibodies that recognize only a minor population, 5-10%, of transformed epithelial cells. Other clones bind to the majority of malignant cells both at the primary and metastatic sites. As of today, there appears to be no convincing correlation between prognosis and the expression of antigens recognized by these antibodies. Nevertheless, the probability of finding one is favorable mainly because of the ever increasing number of hybridoma clones being generated and being screened for this property.

Human MAb's show diffuse staining of cytoplasmic components and evidence for cell-surface expression is rare. This shift from the surface to the cytoplasmic compartment is puzzling, for it may signify an altered intracellular processing of membrane components (91). It may also explain the emergence of antigenically silent clones during tumor invasion and metastasis (91).

A similar shift from the membrane to cytoplasmic domains has also been observed with epithelial membrane antigens EMA and with glycoproteins derived from the milk-fat-globule membranes, MFGM (93-95). Milk-fat-globule membrane contains more than 35 proteins, as detected by 2D-gel electrophoresis (93). Some of these have been purified to homogeneity, for example MFGM gp 70 and gp 155; specific polyclonal antibodies have been raised against them (93,96). Antisera to both of these components stained the luminal apical portion of epithelial cells using immunohistochemistry. Antibodies to gp 155 preferentially bind to the luminal epithelial cells of the lobules and show promise for distinguishing lobular from ductal carcinomas (96). Both sets of antibodies almost exclusively stained the apical surface of normal and well differentiated malignant cells. Poorly differentiated ductal adenocarcinoma cells had diminished staining with anti-MFGM gp 70 which was predominantly in the cytoplasm. Antibodies against MFGM gp 155 stained lobular carcinoma better than ductal carcinoma cells over the cytoplasmic region. Although a diminished staining was observed on specimens from distant metastatis, their quantitation needs further investigation. One can, however, now raise the precise question as to the prognostic significance, if any, of a diminished expression of these differentiation-controlled membrane glycoproteins.

SUMMATION AND PERSPECTIVE

It seems evident that the last few years have witnessed an information explosion in the area of metastasis. Diversified models have become available and the rationale for experimental designs have become better defined. As a result, the metastatic cascade becomes increasingly organized into events that can be better scrutinized: i.e. matrix degradation, attachment to vascular endothelia, invasion of basal lamina, escape from immune-lysis by blood-borne tumor cells and organ specific homing. Understanding each of these events at the molecular level paves the way for our comprehension of the whole metastatic process.

Caution must be applied in the following aspects of investigation. The first is the extent to which it is possible to extrapolate from one tumor model to another, for example, whether the parameters relevant to the metastatic potential of B 16 melanoma are equally relevant to mammary adenocarcinoma. Tabulation of organ-related distinguishing features may help investigators avoid over-extrapolations from one set of experiments to another. Quite clearly, there are molecular parameters such as the laminin receptor, plasminogen activator or Type IV collagenase whose elevated expressions are shared by many invasive tumor types. The distinguishing parameters for the malignancies of a given organ will likewise need to be carefully delineated.

Particular caution is also suggested when extrapolation is made from a single event to the whole metastatic cascade. Excellent correlations are emerging between vessel invasion and distant micrometastasis, and between degradation of basal lamina and tumor spread. On the other hand, models with a pausity of correlation offer opportunity for new considerations, for example, the possible contributions by the host to the degradation of the basal lamina, or the participation of the host's lymphatic system in carring away the tumor cells as "passive passengers".

The impact of molecular biology, the capability of gene cloning and the selection of clone-specific gene products will certainly change our concept of the events involved in metastasis. Of particular interest will be the more precise definition of histological cell-types. Certain histological types of malignancies originating from different subsets of stem cells appear to have unique metastatic routes. For example, infiltrating lobular carcinomas, ILC, have a different pattern of metastasis compared with the infiltrating ductal carcinomas, IDC (97,98). At post mortem, diffuse retroperitoneal involvement was found in 92% of ILC patients and in only 9% of IDC patients. Similarly, diffuse involvement of the stomach was seen in 38% of ILC patients and 3% of IDC patients. In short, the recognition of membrane glycoproteins which are preferentially expressed by ILC could significantly aid the histological classification of the malignant tissue and help predict the most likely metastatic pattern expected.

Our understanding of these events at the molecular level will undoubtedly be refined by experiments using transfection of noninvasive, nonmetastatic clones of cells with unique copies of genes whose products may be involved in the invasive processes. Conversely, transfection with genes to inhibit these processes may lead to a better understanding of metastasis control.

MuMTV virus may serve as a tool in these types of experimental designs. Infection of murine epithelial cells with viral genomes which have been constructed to yield more aggressive or less invasive phenotypes of adenocarcinoma cells may further our understanding of possible genetic mechanisms essential for metastasis. Experiments are in progress along this line and mammary cells transformed by MuMTV variants have been obtained with different and apparently stable metastasizing capability (99).

RNA translation profiles have been obtained recently from highly metastatic sublines of already metastatic M2 melanoma cells. Six specific mRNAs were recognized from the most invasive cell lines whose translation was quantitatively increased when compared with the RNA from the parental subline (100). Such approaches will be dominant in metastasis research and may lead to the characterization of "metastatic-specific" gene products and gene probes of cDNA. The results, however, will rely ostensibly on the validity of the cellular models chosen for the characterization of the so-called specific gene products.

To reiterate a point made in the introduction of this paper, just a few reliable molecular markers are all that are needed to make significant contributions to the correct diagnosis, assessment of prognosis and treatment of breast cancer. And yet, while the rationality of experimental approaches are debated and scrutinized, one has the unsettling notion that the fascinating drama will play itself out with the appearance of undefined monoclonal antibodies which might provide correlations with prognosis. While thoughtful experiments and innovation continue, so does the laborious task of screening for relevant monoclonal antibodies. The offspring of this latter effort might just be antibodies whose binding will provide a more reliable marker for metastatic prognosis than those parameters based on sound theoretical judgment. Regardless of what the markers turn out to be a large number of investigators and surgical pathologists are ready to apply them to improve the management of cancer patients.

ACKNOWLEDGEMENT

The author thanks Diana Irons and Jean Hilbert for the preparation of this manuscript. Helpful editorial comments of Dorcas Vanian-Tokes" ' and Dr. Mary Test are greatfully acknowledged. The work quoted from the author's laboratory was supported by grant-CA 24645 from the National Cancer Institute.

REFERENCES

1. Nicolson, G.L., Poste, G. Int. Rev. Exp. Pathol. 25: 77-181, 1983.
2. Nicolson, G.L. Exp. Cell. Res. 150: 3-22, 1984.
3. Poste, G. and Greig, R. Invasion Metastasis 2: 137-176, 1982.
4. Liotta, L.A. Am. J. Path. 117: 339-348, 1984.
5. Nicolson, G.L. and Poste, G. Curr. Probl. Cancer 7: 1-42, 1983.
6. Fidler, I.J. and Hart, I.R. Science 217: 998-1003, 1982.
7. Edgington, T.S. and Nakamura, R.M. In: Human Cancer Markers (Eds. S. Sell and B. Wahren), Humana Press, Clifton, New Jersey, 1982, pp. 191-232.
8. Kerbel, R.S., Frost, P., Liteplo, R.G. and Fidler, I.J. Proc. Am. Assoc. Cancer Res. 26: 394-395, 1985.
9. Coulson, P.B., Thornthwaite, J.T., Wooley, T.W., Sugarbaker, E.V., Seckinger, D. Canc. Res. 44: 4187-4196, 1984.
10. Nicolson, G.L. Cancer Metastasis Rev. 3: 25-42, 1984.
11. Sanchez, J., Varani, J., Wicha, M. and Miller, D. Proc. Am. Ass. Canc. Res. 26: 59 (233) 1985.
12. LaBiche, R.A., Frazier, M.L., Brock, W.A. and Nicolson, G.L. Proc. Am. Assoc. Canc. Res. 26: 48 (191) 1985.
13. Olsson, L. and Forchhammer, J. Proc. Natl. Acad. Sci. USA, 81: 3389-3393, 1984.
14. Goelz, S.E., Vogelstein, B., Hamilton, S.R. and Feinberg, A.P. Science 228: 187-190, 1985.
15. Yamashina, K. and Heppner, G.H. Proc. Am. Assoc. Canc. Res. 26: 43 (169) 1985.
16. Weitzman, S.A., Weitberg, A.B., Clark, E.P. and Stossel, T.P. Science 227: 1231-1233, 1985.
17. Kempf, R.A., Cebul, R.D. and Mitchell, M.S. J. Immunopharmacology 2: 509-525, 1980.
18. Whitehead, R.H., Monaghan, P., Webber, L.M., Bertoncello, I. and Vitali, A. J. Natl. Canc. Inst. 71: 1193-1203, 1983.
19. Hedley, D.W., Rugg, C.A., Ng, A.B.P. and Taylor, I.W. Canc. Res. 44: 5395-5398, 1984.
20. Frankfurt, O.S., Chin, J.L., Englander, L.S., Greco, W.R., Pontes, J.E. and Rustum, Y.M. Canc. Res. 45: 1418-1423, 1985.
21. Bettelheim, R., Penman, H.G., Thornton-Jones, H. and Neville, A.M. Br. J. Cancer 50: 771-777, 1984.
22. Davis, B.W., Gelber, R., Goldhirsch, A., Hartmann, W.H., Hollaway, L., Russell, I. and Rudenstam, C.M. Annual Report for the Ludwig Breast Cancer Study Group, Bern, 1985.
23. Bettelheim, R., Mitchell, D. and Gusterson, B.A. J. Clin. Path. 37: 364-366, 1984.
24. Bogenman, E. and Jones, P.A. J. Natl. Canc. Inst. 71: 1177-1182, 1983.
25. Colombi, M., Barlati, S., Magdelenat, H. and Fiszer-Szafarz, B. Canc. Res. 44: 2971-2975, 1984.

26. Furmanski, P. Intern. Workshop on Monoclonal Antibodies and Breast Cancer, San Francisco, USA, 1984.
27. Del Rosso, M., Dini, G. and Fibbi, G. Canc. Res. 45: 630-636, 1985.
28. Vassalli, J.D., Baccino, D. and Belin, D. J. Cell Biol. 100: 86-92, 1985.
29. Yang, N.S., Park, C., Longley, C. and Furmanski, P. Mol. Cell. Biol. 3: 982-990, 1983.
30. Eisenbach, L., Segal, S. and Feldman, M. J. Natl. Canc. Inst. 74: 77-85, 1985.
31. Liotta, L.A., Thorglirsson, U.P., Garbisa, S. Canc. Metas. Rev. 1: 277-297, 1982.
32. Wirl, G. and Frick, J. Urol. Res. 7: 103, 1979.
33. Barsky, S.H., Siegal, G., Jannotta, F. and Liotta, L.A. Lab. Invest. 49: 140-148, 1983.
34. Fessler, L., Duncan, K., Fessler, J., Salo, T. and Tryggvason, K. J. Biol. Chem. (In press) 1985.
35. Starkey, J.R., Hosick, H.L., Stanford, D.R. and Liggitt, H.D. Canc. Res. 44: 1585-1594, 1984.
36. Nakajima, M., Custead, S.E., Welch, D.R. and Nicolson, G.L. Proc. Am. Assoc. Canc. Res. 244: 162, 1984.
37. Baici, A., Gyger-Marazzi, M. and Strauli, P. Invasion Metastasis 4: 13-27, 1984.
38. Dabbous, M.Kn., Haney, L., Carter, L., Brinkley, Sr., Nakajima, M. and Nicolson, G.L. Fed. Proc. 44(5): 1430 (5958), 1985.
39. Biswas, C. Fed. Proc. 44(4): 1337 (5419), 1985.
40. Rifkin, D. and Moscatelli, D. Proc. Fed. Am. Soc. Exp. Biol. p. 587 (1765), 1984.
41. Heisel, M., Laug, W.E. and Jones, P.A. J. Natl. Canc. Inst. 71: 1183-1187, 1983.
42. Eisenbach, L., Segal, S. and Feldman, M. J. Natl. Canc. Inst. 74: 83-93, 1985.
43. Bosmann, H.B. and Hall, T.C. Proc. Natl. Acad. Sci. USA 71: 1833-1837, 1974.
44. Koppel, P., Baici, A., Keist, R., Matzku, S. and Keller, R. Exp. Cell Biol. 52: 293-299, 1984.
45. Sloane, B.F., Bajkowski, A.S., Day, N.A., Honn, K.V. and Gissman, J.D. Proc. Am. Assoc. Cancer Res. 25: 4, 1984.
46. Recklies, A.D., White, C. and Poole, A.R. Proc. Fed. Am. Soc. Exp. Biol. 87a:(327), 1984.
47. Kozlowski, K.A., Wezeman, F.H. and Schultz, R.M. Proc. Natl. Acad. Sci. USA 81: 1135-1139, 1984.
48. Unemori, E.N. and Werb, Z. Proc. Fed. Am. Soc. Exp. Biol. 86a:(322), 1984.
49. Ng, R. and Keller, J.A. Proc. Am. Assoc. Canc. Res. 25: 53 (208), 1984.
50. Rozhin, J., Crissman, J.D., Honn, K.V. and Sloane, B.F. Proc. Am. Assoc. Canc. Res. 26: 57 (226), 1985.
51. Lee, D.C., Rose, T.M., Webb, N.R. and Todaro, G.J. Nature 313: 489-491, 1985.
52. Tökés, Z.A., Gendler, S.J. and Dermer, G.B. J. Supramol. Struct. Cell. Biochem. 17: 69-77, 1981.
53. Gendler, S.J., Dermer, G.B., Silverman, L.M. and Tökés, Z.A. Canc. Res. 42: 4567-4573, 1982.
54. Gendler, S.J. and Tökés, Z.A. J. Cell. Biochem. 26: 157-167, 1984.
55. Neri, A. and Tökés, Z.A. Proc. Am. Assoc. Canc. Res. 26: 51 (203), 1985.
56. Nakajima, M., Irimura, T., Di Ferrante, D., Di Ferrante, N. and Nicolson, G.L. Science 220: 611-613, 1983.
57. Nakajima, M., Irimura, T., Di Ferrante, N. and Nicolson, G.L. J. Biol. Chem. 259: 2283-2290, 1984.
58. Nakajima, M., Irimura, T. and Nicolson, G.L. Proc. Am. Assoc. Canc. Res. 26: 49 (192), 1984.
59. Kramer, R.H., and Vogel, K.G. J. Natl. Canc. Inst. 72: 889-899, 1984.
60. Nakajima, M., Custead, S.E., Welch, D.R. and Nicolson, G.L. Proc. Am. Assoc. Canc. Res. 25: 62 (244), 1984.

154

61. Turner, G.A. and Weiss, L. Invasion Metastasis 2: 361-368, 1982.
62. Thorgeirsson, U.P., Liotta, L.A., Kalebic, T., Margulies, I.M., Thomas, K., Rios-Candelore, M. and Russo, R.G. J. Natl. Canc. Inst. 69: 1049-1054, 1982.
63. Maslow, D.E. Proc. Am. Assoc. Canc. Res. 26: 51 (201), 1985.
64. Carr, I., Levy, M. and Orr, K. Fed. Proc. 44(4): 913 (2937), 1985.
65. Terranova, V.P., Rao, C.N., Kalebic, T., Margulies, I.M. and Liotta, L.A. Proc. Natl. Acad. Sci. USA 80: 444-448, 1983.
66. Basara, M.L., McCarthy, J.B., Palm, S.L. and Furcht, L.T. Fed. Proc. 44(4): 5418, 1985.
67. Schirrmacher, V., Altevogt, P., Fogel, M., Dennis, J., Waller, C.A., Barz, D., Schwartz, R., Cheingsong-Popov, R., Springer, G., Robinson, P.J., Nebe, T., Brossmer, W., Vlodavsky, I., Parveletz, N., Zimmermann, H.P. and Uhlenbruck, G. Invasion Metastasis 2: 313-360, 1982.
68. Tökés, Z.A., Gendler, S.J., Imam, A., Pullano, T.G. and Ross, K.L. In Cellular Oncology, New Approaches in Biology, Diagnosis and Treatment (Ed. P.J. Moley and G.L. Nicolson) Praeger Press, New York, pp. 28-62, 1982.
69. Edwards, P.A.W. Br. J. Cancer 51: 149-160, 1985.
70. Steck, P.A. and Nicolson, G.L. Exp. Cell Res. 147: 255-267, 1983.
71. Steck, P.A. and Nicolson, G.L. Transplant Proc. 16: 355-360, 1984.
72. Furmanski, P., Kirkland, W.L., Gargola, T., Rich, M.A., and the Breast Cancer Prognostic Study Clinical Associates. Canc. Res. 41: 4087-4092, 1981.
73. Gendler, S.J. and Tökés, Z.A. Breast Canc. Res. and Treat. 4: 353 (75), 1984.
74. Gendler, S.J. and Tökés, Z.A. Cancer Res. (manuscript submitted), 1985.
75. Garcia, M., Salazar-Retana, G., Richer, G., Domerque, J., Capony, F., Pujol, H., Laffarque, F., Pau, B. and Rochefort, H. J. Clin. Endocrinol. Metab. 59: 564-566, 1984.
76. Garcia, M., Capony, F., Derocq, D., Simon, D., Pau, B. and Rochefort, H. Canc. Res. 45: 709-716, 1985.
77. Lotan, R. and Raz, A. Canc. Res. 43: 2088-2093, 1983.
78. Lotan, R., Lotan, D. and Raz, A. Proc. Am. Assoc. Canc. Res. 26: 53 (208), 1985.
79. Neville, D.M. Invasion Metastasis 2: 2-11, 1982.
80. Halter, S.A., Fraker, L.D., Parmenter, M., Dupont, W.D. Oncology 41: 297-302, 1984.
81. Sirbasku, D.A. and Danielpour, D. Proc. Am. Assoc. Canc. Res. 26: 393-394, 1985.
82. Mandler, R., Katz, D., Murano, G., Liotta, L. and Schiffman, E. Fed. Proc. 44 (4): 1337 (5420), 1985.
83. Sporn, M.B. and Todaro, G.J. New Eng. J. Med. 303: 878-880, 1980.
84. Brodt, P., Parhar, R., Sankar, P. and Lala, P.K. Int. J. Canc. 35: 265-273, 1985.
85. Cam, Y., Bellon, G., Poulin, G., Caron, Y. and Birembout, P. Invasion Metastasis 4: 61-72, 1984.
86. Dunnington, D.J., Kim, U., Hughes, C.M., Monagham, P., Ormerod, E.J. and Rudland, P.S. J. Natl. Canc. Ins. 72: 455-466, 1984.
87. Dunnington, D.J., Kim, U., Hughes, C.M., Monagham, P. and Rudland, P.S. Canc. Res. 44: 5338-5346, 1984.
88. Sawtelle, N.M., DiPersio, L., Michael, J.G., Pesce, A.J. and Weiss, M.A. Lab. Invest. 51: 225-232, 1984.
89. Shull, J.H., Javadpour, N., Soares, T. and DeMoss, E.V. J. Surg. Onc. 18: 193-196, 1981.
90. Sheikh, K.M.A., Quismario, F.A., Friou, G.J. and Lee, Y. Cancer 44: 2083-2089, 1979.
91. Imam, A., Drushella, M.M., Taylor, C.R. and Tökés, Z.A. Canc. Res. 45: 263-271, 1985.
92. Schlom, J., Wunderlich, D. and Teramoto, Y. Proc. Natl. Acad. Sci. USA, 77: 6841-6845, 1980.

93. Imam, A., Taylor, C.R. and Tökes, Z.A. Canc. Res. 44: 2016-2022, 1984.
94. Ceriani, R.L., Thompson, K., Peterson, J.A. and Abraham, S. Proc. Natl. Acad. Sci. USA, 74: 582-586, 1977.
95. Chang, S.E. and Taylor-Papadimitriou, J. Cell Differentiation 12: 143-154, 1983.
96. Imam, A., Taylor, C.R. and Tökes, Z.A. Proc. Am. Assoc. Canc. Res. 25: 251 (995), 1984.
97. Harris, A. Br. J. Canc. 50: 23-30, 1984.
98. Harris, A., Harris, M., Chrissohoou, M., Hudson, M., Swindell, R. and Sellwood, R.A. Int. Workshop on Monoclonal Antibodies and Breast Cancer, San Francisco, p. 139, 1984.
99. Basolo, F., Toniolo, A. and Squartini, F. Biennial Int. Breast Cancer Res. Conf. London, 6-06, 1985.
100. Steeg, P., Kalebic, T., Claysmith, A., Liotta, L. and Sobel, M. Fed. Proc. 44 (4): 1336 (5413), 1985.

12

MuMTV GENOTYPE, PROTONEOPLASIA, AND TUMOR PROGRESSION

R.D. CARDIFF, D.W. MORRIS, L.J.T. YOUNG and R. STRANGE

Department of Pathology, University of California Medical School, Davis, California, 95616

If we are to understand cancer, we must understand its origins and its evolution. The current concept, that cancer results from somatic cell mutation, means that the molecular origin and evolution of the disease must also be understood. At present, most of our information about the molecular biology of neoplastic progression comes from either lymphoid cells or fibroblasts in tissue culture (1-3). Unfortunately, breast cancer is a solid tumor of epithelial origin. In fact, most cancers develop in solid organs and, with rare exception, we know very little about the origin and evolution of such neoplasms.

Recently, the mouse mammary tumor model, a classical system for the study of neoplastic progression, has provided insight into the molecular origin and evolution of solid tumors (4-5). The mouse mammary epithelium has markers which permit the tracking of cell populations through various stages of tumor progression. These markers include the mouse mammary tumor virus and several host integration sites. Studies of these markers in normal, hyperplastic and neoplastic tissues from the mouse mammary gland have provided the first information concerning neoplastic progression in solid tumors at a molecular level (5).

The Mouse Mammary Tumor Virus (MuMTV)

The mouse mammary tumor virus appears as two forms of proviral DNA: exogenous and endogenous. The endogenous proviruses are generally silent. The exogenous virus is the infectious agent and is transmitted primarily through the milk (6). Once in a new host, the virus infects the mammary epithelium. At this point the viral genomic RNA is converted to double stranded DNA utilizing the enzyme reverse transcriptase and this newly produced double stranded exogenous viral DNA integrates into the host genome (7). MuMTV does not have a viral oncogene in its genome, so it is generally proposed that host genome/virus genome interactions at the site of integration lead to transformation (4).

Several aspects of the integration event merit our consideration. First, the proviral DNA integrates randomly into the host DNA (8). Each integration creates an insertional mutation by the introduction of 10 kbp of proviral DNA which permanently alters the DNA of the infected cell. Second, the proviral DNA contains several genetic elements which are able to activate nearby genes either by promoter insertion or by enhancement of expression via the LTR enhancer (9). This capability has given rise to the insertion-activation model for mammary tumorigenesis (10). Outlined briefly: if the provirus integrates close to an oncogene, it will "turn on" the oncogene, leading to neoplasia. Lastly, each newly integrated provirus creates novel restriction fragments by the introduction of its own DNA into the host genome (4).

If the proviruses truly integrate randomly, the detection of new host genome/virus genome junction restriction fragments would be impossible. In the polyclonal mouse lactating mammary gland novel junction fragments cannot be detected (8). On the other hand, if the progeny from a single cell expands to dominate the population, the novel junction fragments become detectable (8). These novel junction fragments become markers for following changes in cell subpopulations during the progression of neoplasia.

Figure 1

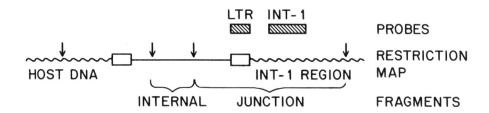

The Technology

Most of the evidence discussed here is based on restriction endonuclease mapping using the Southern blot technique and either viral specific or host specific probes which identify novel host genome/virus genome junction fragments (Fig. 1) (5).

A brief synopsis of this technology is supplied here for the uninitiated. High molecular weight DNA is extracted from various tissues. The DNA is digested with a restriction endonuclease which cleaves the DNA at the specific sites dictated by the nucleotide sequence recognized by the enzyme. The digestion cuts the DNA strands into a set of specific fragments referred to as restriction fragments.

The restriction fragments are separated according to their relative molecular weights by electrophoresis into an agarose gel. The fragments are denatured and then transferred by capillary action to nitrocellulose filters where they bind. Radioactive "probes" derived from cloned proviral DNA or host DNA are then applied to the filters. Those restriction fragments which contain homologous DNA will hybridize with the probe and after appropriate processing may be identified as distinctive bands upon autoradiography.

The System

The introduction of MuMTV into most inbred mice results in a productive infection and an increased tumor incidence (6). In addition, MuMTV infection results in an increased incidence of hyperplastic alveolar nodules (HANs), premalignant precursors from which tumors arise (5,6).

Normal mammary ducts can be transplanted into gland cleared mammary fat pads for a limited number of passages. These transplants rarely develop tumors. On the other hand, transplantation of HANs leads to the establishment of hyperplastic outgrowth lines which can be indefinitely passaged and very frequently develop tumors.

The HAN is, thus, considered an immortalized preneoplastic lesion, an intermediate between normal tissue and a malignant tumor (11,12). We have analyzed the progression of HANs to malignant tumors using the Southern blot technique (5,13).

The Rules

The rules are quite simple to follow, if the reader remembers that all mouse tumors have endogenous proviral DNA which can also be detected in uninfected tissues such as the liver or the spleen. These endogenous proviruses provide "germ line" restriction fragment patterns. Infection can be detected at the DNA level by the identification of novel restriction fragments which are not present in uninfected tissues (8).

If the tissue is infected but not clonal, the novel acquired host/virus junction fragments (Fig. 1) will not be detected. The tissue that is infected and has demonstrable acquired junction fragments is designated as <u>homogeneous</u> (14). By Southern blot analysis, when the intensity of the novel fragment bands approach half that of the endogenous germ line restriction fragment bands, the chances are high that the tissue originated from a single cell and is designated <u>clonal</u> (5). The limitations and nuances of this technique have been discussed elsewhere (5).

Using these techniques, this system and these rules can provide tumor cell genotypes and facilitate identification of their progenitors. The newly acquired MuMTV DNA is used as a novel and useful marker, much like sex-linked enzymatic polymorphisms or restriction fragment length polymorphisms (1). As will be discussed, understanding tumor progression can also assist in understanding the mechanisms of transformation.

<u>Are MuMTV Induced Tumors Clonal?</u>

A large number of Southern blot analyses have now been published which demonstrate that MuMTV-induced mouse mammary tumors are clonal (4,5). The occasional exceptions could be due to the utilization of restriction enzymes which do not clearly resolve the novel junction fragments from the background germ line restriction pattern, failure to take the stromal contribution to the total tumor cell population into account and, finally, inability to distinguish between newly integrated proviruses acquired at or prior to transformation and those acquired by subpopulations during tumor growth (5).

Again, with rare exceptions each spontaneous tumor has a unique MuMTV genotype with no fragments in common with other tumors. However, two host genes, int-1 and int-2, each of which is activated by provirus integration have been identified (15,16). Integrations in these regions are not site specific but rather, occur in clusters upstream and downstream from the coding sequences of the genes. When a provirus integrates into the int-1 or int-2 domain, it causes a rearrangement of the restriction pattern from that area of the genome. Probes developed from those specific areas of the mouse genome can be used to detect the rearranged DNA (15). This has provided further molecular evidence that many tumors are clonal. Since the provirus integrates into only one of the two homologous chromosomes, one chromosome maintains the germ line restriction site configuration (15). Many tumors have equimolar germ line and rearranged "int" domain fragments. This could occur only if most of the cells in the tumor are from the same origin, i.e., the tumor is a clonal proliferation.

Are HANs Clonal?

As can be imagined, the individual HANs are so small that it is difficult to extract sufficient DNA for restriction analysis.

However, DNAs from several HANs have been analyzed and contain novel host/virus junction fragments (13,17).

The most extensively studied hyperplastic tissues are the transplantable hyperplastic outgrowth (HPO) lines derived from HANs. By the rules given above, the HPOs are clonal (14). However, several reservations must be mentioned. MuMTV genotype analyses of HPO sublines derived from the same HAN or same HPO demonstrate genetically divergent populations (13,14). In some cases restriction analyses revealed that HPOs from the same HAN did not share a common genotype, although at least one common restriction fragment could always be identified (13). Therefore, the bulk of our data is consistent with a clonal origin but, considerable genetic polymorphism occurs in hyperplastic tissues. One interpretation would be that hyperplasias are composed of pluripotential populations of rapidly evolving cells. This interpretation is consistent with the biology of these tissues (5).

Are Tumors Subclones of Hyperplasias?

The transplantation experiments already tell us that tumors come from hyperplastic tissue (11). But, do these tumors emerge because of a pool of inapparent malignant cells spread throughout the hyperplastic population or by a series of subsequent transforming events?

All tumors studied retain the MuMTV genotype of the hyperplasia in which they arise (13). In most cases, the tumors have additional restriction fragments demonstrating that they come from a subset of the hyperplastic population. All tumors from the same HPO line have unique tumor specific restriction fragments (5,13). Therefore, it is likely that each tumor arises as an independent clone and does not represent a hidden pool of tumor cells spread throughout the population. This evidence suggests that tumors arise as the result of independent events subsequent to noduligenesis.

An additional type of genotypic relationship between hyperplasias and tumors merits special mention. A limited number of tumors have no significant MuMTV genoptypic differences from their hyperplasias (13). The virtual genotypic identity between tumor and hyperplasia has led us to postulate that the most important host/virus interactions occur early in neoplastic progression. With this in mind we have suggested that the virus is actually the mammary hyperplasia virus and not a mammary tumor virus (5). This is meant to imply that the molecular events leading to a malignant phenotype occur independently of the virus.

Does MuMTV Genotype Determine Phenotype?

Mammary tumors are known to be composed of heterogeneous, divergent populations (18). In some cases these divergent populations have different MuMTV genotypes. However, in at least one experiment, the divergent tumor populations had identical MuMTV genotypes (13). In this latter case, two tumors were serially transplanted, each divergent transplant was maintained as a separate transplant line. Five lines with unique patterns of growth, MuMTV expression and morphology were developed. All five lines had the same genotype. Thus, tumors may evolve independent of changes in the MuMTV genotype.

Markers versus Mechanism

One of the fundamental problems in tumor biology is the tremendous heterogeneity of the neoplastic population. The presence of clonal populations implies that the initiating event is a very rare event. Can the phenomena initiating the neoplasm be determined by examining the end stage? The tendency for tumors to diverge probably precludes our pinpointing the critical event by examination of only the end stage. The most profitable approach has come from seeking phenomena that are shared by all tumors in a given class. Even here, one may be determining only those characteristics of the terminal stage of a neoplasm.

Knowing the genetic evolution of a neoplasm can prevent over-interpretation of the phenomena observed at any given stage. For example, we detected a rearrangement of the int-1 locus in a BALB/cfC3H HPO (unpublished observation). As might be predicted, the tumors from that HPO had the same rearrangement. One might conclude that the integration of MuMTV into the int-1 site had caused the hyperplasia. This hypothesis was directly tested by examining three other sublines derived from the same HAN (Fig. 2). Since none of the other sublines contained rearranged int-1 DNA, the integration of provirus at the int-1 locus did not cause the hyperplasia. Rather the insertion of MuMTV occurred subsequent to noduligenesis and did not cause any observable changes in the growth properties or tumor potential of the subline.

Figure 2

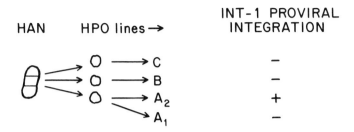

HAN   HPO lines →

INT-1 PROVIRAL
INTEGRATION

Conclusion

From the above data, mouse mammary hyperplasias are clearly genetically altered, immortalized populations. With the genotype data it is clear that the hyperplasias fit most reasonable definitions of neoplasias, albeit benign neoplasias. As a result we have proposed that the term protoneoplasia be applied to these forms of early neoplasia (5).

The mouse mammary tumor model is the first solid tumor in which marker systems for following the genetic evolution of neoplasia have been developed. However, we suggest that the model can be applied to all solid tumors. When the appropriate marker systems are developed we will be able to accurately characterize each step in neoplastic progression at the molecular level and to distinguish between physiological hyperplasias and true neoplasias. The concept of protoneoplasia promulgated here is important in that it defines the types of events that should be sought in other solid tumor systems and suggests strategies for detecting these events.

166

Acknowledgements: The work described from our laboratory was supported in part by grant CD-235 from the American Cancer Society and grant R01-CA-21454 from the National Cancer Institute. The authors gratefully acknowledge the contributions of Dr. L.J. Faulkin, Dr. R.L. Ashley, Dr. T.G. Fanning, V. Pathak, and D.W. Mitchell to this work.

References

1. Nowell, P.C. Science. 194:23-28, 1976.
2. Land, H., Parada, L.F., and Weinberg. Nature. 304:596-602, 1983.
3. Cooper, G.H. Science. 218:801-806, 1982.

4. Fanning, T.G., and Cardiff, R.D. Adv. in Viral Onco. 4: 71-94, 1984.
5. Cardiff, R.D. Adv. in Cancer Res. 42:167-190, 1984.
6. Nandi, S., and McGrath, C.M. Adv. Cancer Res. 17:353-414, 1973.
7. Varmus, H.E., and Swanstrom, R. In: RNA Tumor Viruses, edited by R. Weiss, N. Leich, H.E. Varmus, and J. Coffin. pp 369-512, Cold Spring Harbor Lab., N.Y.
8. Cohen, J.C., Shank, P.R., Morris, V.L., Cardiff, R.D., and Varmus, H.E. Cell. 16:333-345, 1979.
9. Varmus, H.E. Science. 216:812-820, 1982.
10. Varmus, H.E. Cancer Surveys. 1:309-319, 1982.
11. Cardiff, R.D., Wellings, S.R., and Faulkin, L.J. Cancer. 39:2734-2746, 1977.
12. Medina, D. Methods Cancer Res. 7:3-53, 1973.
13. Cardiff, R.D., Morris, D.W., and Young, L.J.T. J. Natl. Cancer Inst. 71:1011-1019, 1983.
14. Cardiff, R.D., Fanning, T.G., Morris, D.W., Ashley, R.L., and Faulkin, L.J. Cancer Res. 41:3024-3029, 1981.
15. Nusse, R., and Varmus, H.E. Cell. 31:99-109, 1982.
16. Peters, G., Brookes, S., Smith, R., and Dickson C. Cell. 33:369-377, 1983.
17. Fanning, T.G., Vassos, A., and Cardiff, R.D. J. Virol. 41:1007-1013, 1982.
18. Heppner, G.H., Shapiro, W.R., and Rankin, J.K. Pediatr. Oncol. 1:99-116, 1981

13

STRUCTURAL AND BIOLOGICAL PROPERTIES OF THE INT-1 MAMMARY ONCOGENE

R. NUSSE, A. VAN OOYEN, E. SCHUURING, M. VAN LOHUIZEN AND F. RIJSEWIJK

Departement of Molecular Biology, The Netherlands Cancer Institute (Antoni van Leeuwenhoekhuis), Plesmanlaan 121, 1066 CX Amsterdam, The Netherlands

INTRODUCTION

We are interested in defining genes implicated in the development of mammary tumors. In mice, mammary tumors can be induced by a variety of methods, including hormones, chemical carcinogens, gene transfer into germ line and a retrovirus (1.2).A direct view on specific genetic alterations in mammary tumorigenesis is nevertheless not always obtained. The identification of oncogenes specific for mammary tumors could eventually be helpful in, for example, examining what the mechanism of action of hormonal carcinogenesis is. The large majority of the cellular oncogenes has been discovered with the aid of retroviruses (3, 4); thus, the Mouse Mammary Tumor Virus (MMTV) could be the system of choice to define mammary oncogenes.

MMTV is a replicating retrovirus of the B type morphology. The virus is found in the milk of high mammary tumor incidence mouse strains (5). It is, as an endogenous provirus, present in the germ line of every inbred strain of mice, but most endogenous proviruses are expressed at a low level and are not thought to play a role in tumorigenesis. The GR strain forms an exception: an endogenous virus present on chromosome 18 is expressed at high levels and is the cause of the high tumor incidence (6).

The MMTV genome carries genes typical of every replicating retrovirus: gag for the viral core proteins, pol for the reverse transcriptase, and env for the viral glycoproteins on the envelope.In addition, the virus has a gene on the long terminal repeat (LTR) encoding a protein of 36,000 daltons (7, 8, 9, 10). This gene, orf, has no counterpart in the normal mouse DNA, making it unlikely that orf is derived from a cellular oncogene such as the viral oncogenes of acutely transforming retroviruses. A role for orf in oncogenesis is not excluded, however.

MMTV does not transform cells in culture, and it induces tumors only after a long period of latency, ranging from 4 to 12 months. The tumors

are clonal with respect to the integrated proviral copies, suggesting
that the tumors were outgrowths of cells with proviruses integrated at
sites that predispose to tumorigenesis (10). Experimental support for this
model came from the startling discovery that another slowly oncogenic retrovirus, Avian Leukosis Virus (ALV), integrates near the cellular myc
gene, and activates myc transcription (11). Transcriptional activation of
c-myc can occur either by promoter insertion or by stimulation of the myc
promoter by an enhancer on the ALV LTR (11-13).

The proposal that retroviruses lacking viral oncogenes induce tumors
by activating host cell oncogenes suggests a general strategy to uncover
novel oncogenes (4). Host cell DNA adjacent to an integrated provirus,
preferentially from a tumor with a single acquired provirus is cloned as
recombinant DNA in E.coli. The host genomic sequences are then examined
for more independent proviral integrations. This would indicate that cells
with a provirus in that particular domain have a selective growth advantage over cells with proviruses at other regions. The model also predicts
that a gene within the common integration domain is transcriptionally active as a consequence of proviral activation. Ultimately, a biological
assay in which the gene of interest is introduced into other cells may
tell whether a gene with oncogenic potential has been identified.

In this paper we shall review our efforts to isolate oncogenes activated by the MMTV provirus in murine mammary cancers. We show that a gene,
called int-1, has been found that conforms to many of the predictions listed above, and we report on the structure of the gene.

Finding a common integration site for MMTV proviruses in mammary tumors

Mammary tumors induced by MMTV contain variable numbers of integrated
proviruses, as revealed by digesting tumor DNA with EcoRI and hybridization with a probe specific for the right half of the provirus. EcoRI cuts
in the middle of the proviral element, so that every hybridizing fragment
corresponds to one provirus. A set of 26 tumors from the C3H strain was
screened for integrated proviruses; all of them contained 3 endogenous
proviral units and one of them contained a single acquired provirus. The
right half of this provirus was, with its adjacent cell DNA, cloned into
a bacteriophage vector. From the cellular sequences we selected a single
copy DNA fragment and used that as a probe to isolate a number of overlapping phage clones from a library of normal cell DNA. Thus we obtained

over 30 Kb of cloned DNA of the locus, which we called int-1 (14). It appeared that many tumors contained novel restriction fragments hybridizing to int-1 probes. The fragments also annealed to probes from the MMTV provirus, indicating that they arose due to proviral insertion.

In fig. 1 we present the int-1 restriction map, including the position and orientation of the integrated MMTV proviruses (16). The insertions are found over a distance of about 20 Kb, surrounding the portion of the locus that is transcribed into polyadenylated RNA in mammary tumors (see below). Proviruses integrated downstream from the transcriptional unit, which is from left to right on this map, are all in the same orientation as the int-1 gene; proviruses found upstream from the gene are in the opposite orientation (15). One exception has been found: tumor 102 contains an MMTV provirus upstream from int-1 in the same transcriptional orientation (Fig. 1). By means of somatic cell genetics, we have mapped int-1 on mouse chromosome 15 (ref. 15).

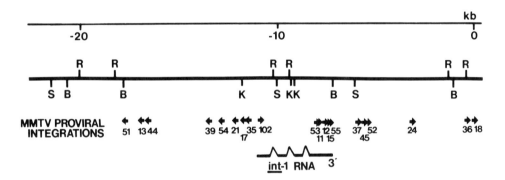

Fig. 1   Map of the int-1 region and integrated proviruses in different tumors. The restriction map is compiled from previous studies (14, 15) with minor modifications. Transcription is from left to right. Sites of proviral integrations and direction of transcription of the proviruses are indicated.
R: EcoRI; B: BglII; S: SacI; K: KpnI.

Transcription of int-1, and the mechanism of activation

Most tumors with proviral integrations surrounding the int-1 gene
contain a polyadenylated transcript of 2.6 Kb (Fig. 2). This RNA has thus
far not been found in normal tissues of the mouse, including normal mammary glands. In the tumors with insertions near the polyadenylation site,
int-1 RNA is appreciably longer (Fig. 2). We have used the "sandwich hybridization" method to show that these transcripts are longer because they
include sequences from the MMTV LTR (15). In these instances, transcription of int-1 appears to proceed into the U3 region of the 5' LTR of MMTV
proviruses so that polyadenylation occurs at the site provided by the LTR.
The tumors with the atypical int-1 transcript do not manifest the normal
transcript of 2.6 Kb. Apparently, only the mutated allele of int-1 is
transcribed, indicating that activation occurs in cis.

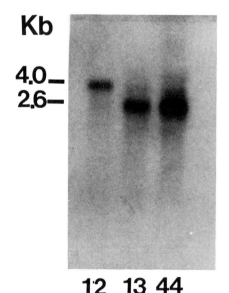

Fig. 2   Hybridization of
int-1 probe to RNA from
mammary tumors
3 µg poyladenylated RNA
was subjected to electro-
phoresis in 1% agarose gels
containing formaldehyde,
transferred to nitrocellulose paper and hybridized
to an int-1 probe. The
autoradiogram shows RNA from
mammary tumors 12, 13 and
44.

The mechanism of transcriptional activation of int-1 seems to be enhancement rather than promoter insertion. The latter mechanism is prevalent in myc activation by Avian Leukosis Virus in chicken bursal lymphomas: proviral insertion upstream from the gene and in the same transcriptional orientation (11, 12, 13). The MMTV insertions at int-1 are, in the large majority of tumors always pointing away from the gene. This configuration may also be relevant for the mechanisms of enhancement: if the enhancer is located in the U3 region of viral LTR, the orientation away from the int-1 gene would avoid the interposition of the MMTV promoter between the viral enhancer and the int-1 promoter. Since enhancers are thought to act only on a proximal promoter, a proviral insertion pointing towards int-1 cannot activate the gene. The insertion in tumor 102, as it replaces the int-1 promoter, is compatible with this notion.

The growing evidence that the MMTV enhancer overlaps the glucocorticoid receptor binding site on the viral LTR (17, 18, 19, 20) suggests the interesting possibility that int-1 transcription in mammary tumors is under the control of steroid hormones. Preliminary experiments with cell lines obtained from mammary tumors suggest that steroid hormones indeed stimulate int-1 transcription.

The structure of the gene

The transcriptionally active region is located in the middle of the proviral insertion clusters, giving an indication of the position of the gene. The exact structure of int-1 was determined by DNA sequencing and nuclease S1 mapping (16).

Fig. 3 summarizes the configuration of int-1 as it has emerged from our studies (16). The protein-encoding domain is contained within four exons which are bracketed by typical eukaryotic transcription regulating sequences. The last exon contains a polyadenylation signal and long trailer sequence with stop codons in all three reading frames.

The int-1 protein

In order to deduce the amino acid sequence of the protein encoded by int-1 we aligned the nucleotide sequence of the four exons, searched for translational start and stop signals and translated the nucleotide sequence in the three possible open reading frames. The second AUG, which conforms to the consensus sequence for eukaryotic initation sites (CC$_G^A$CCAUGG,

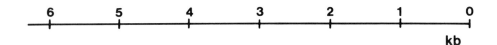

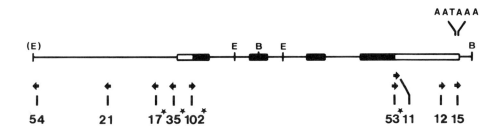

Fig. 3   Structure of the int-1 gene
The intron-exon structure as determined by nuclease S1 mapping and DNA
sequencing is shown (26). Exons are indicated by blocks; coding sequences
are black. Sites and orientations of proviral integrations in tumors having
an integration in the depicted area are represented by arrows (cf. Fig. 2).
Tumor numbers are below arrows. B: BamHI; R: EcoRI.

(21)) is followed by a large open reading frame traversing the four aligned exons. This frame encodes a protein of 370 amino acids, stops at a
UGA stop codon within the last exon and is followed by a relatively large
untranslated trailer sequence.

Comparison of the amino acid sequence of the deduced protein with
over 2000 sequences present in the database of the University of California at San Diego did not reveal any significant similarities (R.F. Doo-
little, personal communication), so that little can be predicted about the
function of the int-1 protein. Interesting, however, is the high content
of hydrophobic amino acids at the NH2 terminus suggesting an interaction
of the protein with cellular membranes during its translation or function.

Proviral integrations within the int-1 gene leave the protein encoding
domain intact
After having established that proviral insertions at the int-1 locus

sometimes occurred in the exons of the gene, we were intrigued to find out whether integrations sometimes disrupted the protein-encoding domain. Accordingly, we cloned some host-proviral DNA junction fragments from mammary tumors in which restriction mapping had indicated that insertion had occurred close to the gene.

Near the 5' end of the transcriptional unit proviruses are most proximal to the gene in tumors 17, 35, and 102. Restriction enzyme fragments containing part of the MMTV provirus and neighbouring int-1 gene sequences were cloned from these tumors and the precise insertion sites were determined. The integrated proviruses of tumors 17 and 35 were located in front of the first exon (Fig. 3). The proviral integration in tumor 102, which is in the same transcriptional orientation as the int-1 gene, was found within the first exon, but before the AUG start codon of the int-1 protein.

Many mammary tumors have a provirus integrated close to the 3' end of the int-1 transcripts, all in the same orientation as the gene. In addition to the tumors shown in Fig. 3, we have found five others with an insertion within the last exon. Restriction site mapping showed that of all these tumors no. 53 has it provirus closest to the central portion of the int-1 gene. DNA sequencing of the cloned host-proviral DNA junction showed that integration of MMTV in this tumor was only five nucleotides downstream from the TGA stop codon of the int-1 protein. We conclude from this preservation of the int-1 protein-encoding domain in mammary tumors that the proviral insertions at the locus are dominant mutations leading to growth advantage of the cells; if int-1 was merely a preferred insertion domain for MMTV proviruses we would not expect selection for an intact gene product.

Transfection and transformation studies with int-1 constructs

We have attempted to obtain direct evidence for the oncogenic nature for int-1 by gene transfer experiments. High expression of int-1 was accomplished by constructing a strong promoter in front of the gene. Two constructs were made, one with an LTR from Moloney Leukemia Virus, and another one having an MMTV promoter with an additional enhancer. Initial experiments showed that int-1 was not able to transform NIH/3T3 cells. We therefore turned to primary rat embryo cell assay developed by Land et al. (22) to detect the combined oncogenic action of two genes that are thought to contribute to separate steps on carcinogenesis. Primary rat embryo cells transfected with the pEJ Ha-ras gene alone do not become transformed; only if a "stage I" or immortalizing gene is cotransfected, the cells grow into tumorigenic cell lines. Both int-1 constructs that we made were active in this assay. Cotransfection with ras on the primary rat embryo cells gave rise to foci of transformed cells. These foci are tumorigenic in nude mice and contain large amounts of acquired int-1 gene copies and large amounts of int-1 RNA.

Thus, int-1 shares biological properties with myc and other nuclear oncogene products, but its structure does not point to a nuclear location. Its mode of activation, by insertion of a provirus,also points to a function early in oncogenesis, although it remains to be established whether int-1 activation is an immortalizing event.

Molecular cloning of human int-1

Probes from the transcriptional domain of int-1 detect, at reduced hybridization stringency, homologous sequences in various other organisms including man and Drosophila. We have employed this high degree of conservation to isolate a molecular clone of the human int-1 homologue (23) from a library of human placental DNA constructed in the bacteriophage vector Charon 4A.

The extent of homology between the mouse and human int-1 sequences was determined by examination of heteroduplex structures in the electron microscope. Examination of the molecules in the electron microscope revealed heteroduplex structures as shown in Fig. 4. A typical heteroduplex contained four regions of homology between the mouse and the human gene. The location and length of the double stranded regions corresponded to the exon sequences of the mouse gene. The human int-1 gene has been mapped on chromosome 12 (23).

Recently, we have established the nucleotide sequence of the human int-1 homologue. The conservation between mouse and man is, as expected, maximal in the protein encoding domain of the gene. Only four amino acid changes were found, all in the hydrophobic leader of the int-1 protein. None of these substitutions, however, influence the hydrophobic nature of the leader domain. The remainder of the protein is completely conserved.

Surprisingly, the conservation of int-1 is not limited to the coding domain. Parts of the introns are more than 75% conserved, and so is the region upstream from the gene. Evolutionary conservation of non-coding DNA may indicate some function in regulation. For int-1, this prediction cannot be tested unless the normal function of the gene in normal cells has been elucidated.

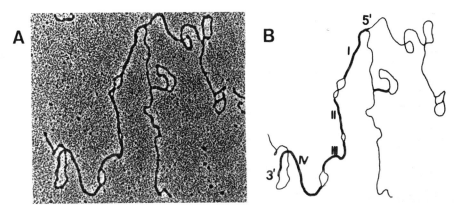

Fig. 4   Heteroduplex analysis of the mouse and the human int-1 DNA, with a tracing of the molecule (23).

Concluding remarks

We have presented a molecular and biological analysis of the int-1 oncogene. The gene has unique properties: its transcription has only been found in mammary tumors with MMTV proviruses inserted nearby the locus; it has no homology with other oncogenes; it is highly conserved between mouse and man. In gene transfer studies on early passage embryo cells, int-1 behaves as a stage I oncogene.

A gene termed int-2 has been isolated by Peters et al. (24, 25) from tumors in the BR6 strain. Int-1 and int-2 are apparently not related to each other (unpublished observations), are on different chromosomes (26), but do have quite similar properties. For example, the configuration of proviruses surrounding these loci is virtually identical -proviruses inserted at both sides and pointing away from the gene, and the tumors with int-1 or int-2 insertions are histologically similar. In collaboration with Drs. Peters and Dickson we have screened many virally induced mammary tumors for insertions at the two different loci and have found that they are, except for one case, mutually exclusive, that is tumors have either an int-1 or an int-2 insertion. Nonetheless, quite some tumors are negative for these loci, suggesting that more genes can be involved. The transgenic mice studies of Stewart et al. (2) show that myc activation gives similar mammary tumors. We have surveyed our int-1 and int-2 negative tumors for myc activation by insertion of MMTV but we have detected none. Thus, more than three loci are implicated in mammary tumorigenesis. Whether this spectrum of oncogenes correlates with yet unrecognized differences in tumor cell properties is worth investigating in view of the diversity in phenotypes of breast cancer cells.

Acknowledgements

We thank Marjon Paape and Vivian Kwee for technical analysis, and Jos Olijve for typing this manuscript. The work on int-1 was started in the lab of Harold Varmus, whom we thank for his continued interest and discussions.

References

1. Hilgers, J. and Bentvelzen, P. Adv. Cancer Res. 26: 143-195, 1979.
2. Stewart, T.A., Pattengale, P.K. and Leder, P. Cell 38: 627-637, 1984.
3. Bishop, J.M. Ann. Rev. Biochem. 52: 301-354, 1983.
4. Varmus, H.E. Ann. Rev. Genet. 18: 553-612, 1984.
5. Teich, N., Wyke, J., Mak, T., Bernstein, A. and Hardy, W. In: RNA Tumor Viruses (Eds. R. Weiss, N. Teich, H. Varmus, J. Coffin), Cold Spring Harbor Laboratory, 1982).
6. Michalides, R., Van Nie, R., Nusse, R., Hynes, N.E. and Groner, B. Cell 23: 165-173, 1981.
7. Donehower, L.A., Huang, A.L. and Hager, G.L. J. Virol. 37: 226-238, 1981.
8. Kennedy, N., Knedlitschek, G., Groner, B., Hynes, N.E., Herrlich, P., Michalides, R. and Van Ooyen, A.J.J. Nature 295: 622-624, 1982.
9. Dickson, C. and Peters, G. J. Virol. 37: 36-47, 1981.
10. Cohen, J.C., Shank, P.R., Morris, V.L., Cardiff, R. and Varmus, H.E. Cell 16: 333-345, 1979.
11. Hayward, W.G., Neel, B.E. and Astrin, S.M. Nature 290: 475-480, 1981.
12. Neel, H.G., Hayward, W.G., Robinson, H.L., Fang, J. and Astrin, S.M. Cell 23: 323-334, 1981.
13. Payne, G.S., Bishop, J.M. and Varmus, H.E. Nature 295: 209-213, 1982.
14. Nusse, R. and Varmus, H.E. Cell 31: 99-109, 1982.
15. Nusse, R., Van Ooyen, A., Cox, D., Fung, Y.K.T. and Varmus, H.E. Nature 307: 131-136, 1984.
16. Van Ooyen, A. and Nusse, R. Cell 39: 233-240, 1984.
17. Majors, J. and Varmus, H.E. Proc. Natl. Acad. Sci. USA 80: 5866-5870, 1983.
18. Chandler, V.L., Maler, B.A. and Yamamoto, K.R. Cell 33: 489-499, 1983.

19. Zaret, K.S., Yamamoto, K.R. Cell 38: 29-38, 1984.
20. Hynes, N., Van Ooyen, A., Kennedy, N., Herrlich, P., Ponta, H. and Groner, B. Proc. Natl. Acad. Sci. USA 80: 3637-3641, 1983.
21. Kozak, M. Nature 308: 241-246, 1984.
22. Land, H., Parada, L.F. and Weinberg, R.A. Nature 304: 596-602, 1983.
23. Van 't Veer, L., Geurts van Kessel, A., Van Heerikhuizen, H., Van Ooyen, A. and Nusse, R. Mol Cell Biol. 4: 2532-2534, 1984.
24. Peters, G., Brookes, S., Smith, R. and Dickson, C. Cell 33: 369-377, 1983.
25. Dickson, C., Smith, R., Brookes, S. and Peters, G. Cell 37: 529-536, 1984.
26. Peters, G., Kozak, C. and Dickson, C. Mol. Cell Biol. 4: 375-378, 1984.

14

THE ROLE OF SPECIFIC REGIONS FOR PROVIRAL INTEGRATION IN MOUSE MAMMARY TUMOR VIRUS (MMTV) INDUCED TUMORS

H. DIGGELMANN

Swiss Institute for Experimental Cancer Research - 1066 Epalinges (Switzerland)

In the workshop entitled "Viruses and Oncogenes" an effort was made to summarize the current knowledge on specific chromosomal regions involved in MMTV-induced mammary tumor formation. Two such regions, int-1 and int-2 have been isolated and characterized previously (1-4). A new region, int-41, has been identified and molecularly cloned from a Balb/c mammary tumor containing two exogenous proviruses (5). The three loci, located on three different chromosomes (3, 5, 6), have several features in common : they are transcriptionally inactive in normal mammary gland, in lactating mammary gland and in other normal mouse tissues so far examined. However they are expressed in those tumors in which the locus is rearranged by proviral integration. The pattern of proviral integration in int-1 and int-2 is very characteristic, with intact proviruses generally being integrated upstream or downstream, in the transcriptional orientation pointing away from the active int-gene. Integrations into the int-1 or int-2 transcription unit have occasionally been observed, but these do not interrupt the coding region of the gene. int-1 and int-2 genomic DNA's and cDNA's have been sequenced. Both mRNAs contain unusually long 5' and 3' untranslated regions and a long open reading frame. The sequences of the predicted proteins show no significant homology to known proteins, particularly to no known oncogene products (7, 8). So far the int-gene products have not been isolated and nothing is known about their function.

All three int-loci have been highly conserved during evolution and are present in human DNA as single copy genes. int-1 and int-2 human genes have been cloned (8, 9) and a high degree of conservation between the murine and human amino acid sequences has been demonstrated. In the case of int-1 the two proteins differ by only 4 amino acids (8). The int-41 locus (5) was reported to have unique properties : this chromosomal region seems to be involved in kidney adenocarcinomas caused by MMTV in the Balb/c/cf/Cd substrain of mice (10, 11, 12). Garcia et al. (5) examined a small number of primary tumors, serially transplanted tumors and a tissue culture cell line derived from one of them for rearrangements in int-1, int-2 and int-41 as well as for transcriptional activity of the three loci. Neither the int-1 nor the int-2 loci were rearranged nor transcriptionally active. However using the int-41 specific probe one of the primary kidney tumors showed a DNA rearrangement. Transcriptional activation of the int-41 domain was detected in this primary tumor as well as in the transplanted tumors. In the kidney tumor cell line a strong glucocorticoid stimulation of a 5.2 kb int-41 specific mRNA was observed and sandwich hybridization techniques defined this mRNA as a hybrid molecule composed of MMTV-LTR sequences covalently linked to host cell RNA. The int-41 chromosomal domain might therefore not only be implicated in mammary gland tumorigenesis, but generally involved in transformation of epithelial cells of different organs.

int-domains have frequently been considered to represent new cellular oncogenes. The direct proof that they are transforming genes was still missing. Attempts to transform NIH-3T3 cells with these loci have failed. Redmond (13) transformed normal mammary gland cells with tumor DNA containing an activated int-2 region but found that tumorigenicity was not accompanied by the transfer of the int-2 region. Nusse reported transformation of primary rat embryo fribroblasts with a MuLV-LTR-int-1 DNA construct in conjunction with an activated ras oncogene (8). In these transformants int-1 DNA was present and expressed, suggesting that the int-1 gene product can complement the ras-oncogene and that the combined action allows transformation of primary rat embryo fibroblasts. No such data is available on int-2 or int-41. Sonnenberg (14) presented interesting experiments which might shed some light on the int-2 function in mammary tumor cells. These authors studied the in vitro progression of mouse mammary adenocarcinomas to carcinosarcomas (in a tumor with a rearrangement in the int-2 chromosomal domain). They described a unidirectional pathway of progression from polygonal to cuboidal to elongated cells. In polygonal tumor cells expression of MMTV, int-2 and certain cytokeratin genes was observed. These cells give rise to adenocarcinomas in vivo. The cuboidal cells which are non tumorgenic do not express these three markers. The elongated cells cause carcinosarcomas when transferred into animals, but no MMTV or int-2 expression was detected. Expression of actin, vimentin and myc genes was identical in all three cell types. These data suggest that expression of int-2 is related to the adenocarcinoma phenotype and not involved in the progression to carcinosarcomas.

The data available today suggest that the int genes are involved in the formation of mammary and kidney adenocarcinomas in the mouse. The expression pattern, the high degree of conservation during evolution, and preliminary transformation data suggest that they are members of the cellular oncogene group. The apparent difficulty in demonstrating their oncogenic potential in tissue culture assays might reflect the limited types of target cells tested so far. It also suggests that the int-domains might cooperate with other cellular oncogenes in tumor forma-tion. In contrast to the situation in avian lymphomas, the MMTV pro-viruses generally found integrated in the vicinity of the int chromosom-al domains are intact. It is therefore possible that viral gene pro-ducts, eg. the orf protein coded for by the viral LTR, participate in some phases of the transformation process. It is also possible that transient activation of int genes plays a role in the pathway leading to epithelial cell transformation.

REFERENCES
1. Nusse, R. and Varmus, H.E. Cell 31:99-109, 1982.
2. Peters, G., Brookes, S., Smith, R. and Dickson, C. Cell 33:369-377, 1983.
3. Nusse, R., van Ooyen, A., Cox, D., Fung, Y.K.T., and Varmus, H.E. Nature 307:131-136, 1984.
4. Dickson, C., Smith, R., Brookes, S. and Peters, G. Cell 37:529-536, 1984.
5. Garcia, M., Vessaz, A., Wellinger, R., Marcoli, R. and Diggelmann, H. Data presented at this meeting.
6. Peters, G., Kozak, C. and Dickson, C. Mol. Cell. Biol. 4:375-378, 1984.
7. Moore, R., Dixon, M., Casey, G., Brookes, S., Peters, G. and Dickson, C. Data presented at this meeting.
8. Nusse, R., van Ooyen, A. and Rijsewijk, F. Data presented at this meeting.
9. Casey, G., Smith, R., Brookes, S., McGillivray, D., Dickson, C. and Peters, G. Data presented at this meeting.
10. Claude, A. J. Ultrastruct. Res. 6:1-18, 1962.
11. Felluga, B., Claude, A. and Mrena, E. J. Nat. Cancer Inst. 43:319-333, 1969.

12. Hilgers, J., Haverman, J., Nusse, R., van Blitersvijk, W.J., Cleton, F.J., Hageman, P.C., van Nie, R. and Calafat, J. J. Nat. Cancer Inst. 54:1323-1342, 1975.
13. Redmond, S., Hynes, N. and Groner, B. Data presented at this meeting.
14. Sonnenberg, A., Nusse, R. and Hilgers, J. Data presented at this meeting.

15

NOVEL ENDOGENOUS RETROVIRAL GENOMES IN HUMAN GENOMIC DNA

J.D. FETHERSTON, TOBY HORN, RENATO MARIANI-COSTANTINI, IQBAL ALI, JEFFREY
SCHLOM, and ROBERT CALLAHAN

Laboratory of Tumor Immunology and Biology, National Cancer Institute,
National Institutes of Health, Bethesda, Maryland, 20205, USA

INTRODUCTION

Human breast neoplasia remains the major cause of cancer related
deaths in women. Unfortunately little information is available
about the causes and nature of this disease. Several laboratories have
searched for a common element associated with human breast cancer (1).
Early studies suggested that a retrovirus resembling the mouse mammary
tumor virus (MMTV) might be expressed in human mammary tumors. However,
attempts to identify RNA related to MMTV in human breast tumor tissue
met with variable success (2,3) due to the poor quality of available DNA
probes and the insensitivity of the techniques used to quantitate or
detect DNA/RNA hybrids. In recent years using recombinant MMTV DNA
(4,5) and low stringency blot hybridization conditions (6,7), sequences
homologous to MMTV have been detected in human DNA (7,8). Here we describe
the isolation and characterization of a human recombinant clone (HLM-2)
which contains sequences related to the MMTV genome. Analysis of HLM-2
and other related clones has shown the following: (a) the human MMTV
related sequences are organized in a manner expected for a genetically
transmitted provirus; (b) the human proviral genome contains a mosaic
of sequences characteristic of different retroviral genera; (c) the
HLM-2 proviral genome is representative of a large family of endogenous
retroviral genomes; and (d) this class of endogenous retroviruses has been
intimately associated with primates throughout much of their evolution.

RESULTS

Preliminary attempts to detect MMTV related sequences in restriction
endonuclease digests of human genomic DNA using stringent hybridization
conditions were unsuccessful. However, under low stringency conditions
labeled (9) MMTV proviral DNA detected four major bands (3.6, 3.5, 2.9 and
1.9 kbp) as well as additional minor bands (2.1, 1.8, 1.6 and 1.4 kbp) in

EcoRI restricted DNA from human breast tumors and normal tissues.
Subgenomic fragments corresponding to the gag-pol and env region of MMTV
were used as probes to further evaluate EcoRI digests of human DNA. The
gag-pol probe reacted primarily with the 3.6 and 3.5 kbp bands and, to a
lesser extent, with the 2.9 and 1.9 kbp fragments while the env region
hybridized to the 2.1, 1.9, 1.8, 1.6 and 1.4 kbp bands. Similar observations
have been made by other laboratories (8 and Sweet et al., personnal
communication) using low stringency blot hybridization conditions.

To isolate human recombinant clones containing MMTV related sequences
a lambda Charon 4A (10) library of human fetal liver DNA (11) was screened,
under low stringency hybridization conditions, with cloned MMTV proviral DNA.
Fifty-five plaques (out of $5x10^5$ plaques screened) reacted specifically
with labeled MMTV DNA. One of these clones, designated HLM-2, was chosen
for further study. A partial restriction map of HLM-2 DNA is illustrated
in Fig. 1. EcoRI restriction fragments (8.2, 3.6, 1.8 and 1.4 kbp) of
HLM-2 DNA were hybridized to the gag, pol, env and long terminal repeat (LTR)
regions of the MMTV genome. Most striking was the intensity with which
the MMTV pol probe hybridized to the 3.6 kbp EcoRI fragment. Upon longer
exposure, sequence homology was detectable between the MMTV gag probe and
the 3.6 kbp EcoRI fragment as well as between labelled MMTV env DNA and
the 8.2 and 1.8 kbp EcoRI fragments. The MMTV LTR probe did not hybridize
with HLM-2 DNA.

The organization of the MMTV related sequences in HLM-2 has been
defined by additional restriction mapping using the MMTV gag, pol and env
probes. These data are summarized in Fig. 1. Two unexpected observations
emerged from this analysis. First, two regions at the opposite ends of
HLM-2 DNA contain MMTV env related sequences. Second, the MMTV pol and
env related sequences are interrupted by sequences unrelated to MMTV
(between map position 12 and 13) which are repeated between map position
4 and 5. Based on these and other results which are presented below, we
speculate that the MMTV gag and pol related sequences in HLM-2 are
organized in a manner expected for a genetically transmitted or endogenous
proviral genome. The repeated sequences which bound the gag-pol related
regions probably correspond to proviral LTRs.

184

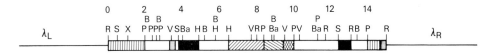

λ **HLM-2**

E, ECO RI; S, SST I; P, PST I; B, BGL II; Ba, BAM HI; H, HIND III; V, ECO RV; X, XBA I

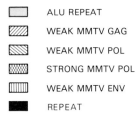

ALU REPEAT
WEAK MMTV GAG
WEAK MMTV POL
STRONG MMTV POL
WEAK MMTV ENV
REPEAT

Fig. 1. Partial restriction enzyme map of the human recombinant clone, HLM-2.
Restriction sites as well as regions of HLM-2 related to MMTV are indicated.
$_L$ and $_R$ designate the long and short arms of lambda Charon 4A, respectively.

Recently, using low stringency blot hybridization and nucleotide
sequence analysis, we have established the existence of two major pol
gene families in the evolution of retroviruses (12). One family consists
of mammalian type C viruses. Two laboratories have shown that a class
of human endogenous retroviral-like sequences is related to known mammalian
type C viruses (13, 14). The second family includes type A (M432), B (MMTV),
D (Squirrel Monkey Retrovirus, SMRV) and avian type C viruses (Rous
sarcoma virus, RSV, and avian myeloblastosis associated virus, MAV).
Based on blot hybridization analysis, the pol region of HLM-2 demonstrated
a high degree of sequence homology to the MMTV pol gene. Since the pol
region of MMTV is related to type A, D and avian type C retroviral pol genes,

we explored the possibility that other members of the Retroviridae might also share homology with HLM-2. The results of reciprocal low stringency blot hybridization experiments using recombinant proviral DNA corresponding to prototypes of the different retroviral genera are illustrated in Fig. 2.

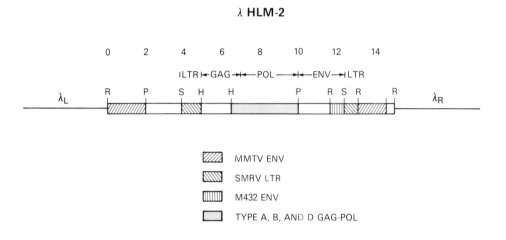

Fig. 2. Homologous regions between HLM-2 and different classes of the Retroviridae family. Regions of homology were determined by low stringency blot hybridization. Abbreviations for restriction enzymes are the same as in Fig.1.

A major region of homology exists between the type A, B, and D retroviral pol genes and the pol region of HLM-2 DNA. In the case of SMRV, a type D retrovirus, the homology includes the 3' half of the gag gene as well as the entire pol gene. The SMRV LTR also hybridizes weakly with the HLM-2 LTR-like elements. In addition to the pol region, the M432 viral genome hybridizes to an area of HLM-2 immediately adjacent to the 3' LTR. No homology was detected with a number of different mammalian type C proviral genomes. To more precisely identify the conserved regions of the HLM-2

pol gene, the nucleotide sequence of the 3.6 kbp EcoRI fragment was
determined. A comparison of a portion of this nucleotide sequence (9.5-
10.0 HLM-2 map units) with those of pol genes from other infectious
retroviruses revealed regions of significant homology between HLM-2 and
MMTV (51%), SMRV (50%), RSV (44%) and the human T-cell leukemia virus,
HTLV-I (37%). Similar results were obtained by comparing the translated
amino acid sequence of this region. No comparable homology could be
detected between this region of HLM-2 and the Moloney murine leukemia
virus pol gene. These findings show that the HLM-2 pol gene probably
arose from the same progenitor that gave rise to pol genes of the infectious
type A, B, D and avian type C retrovirus genera. Thus, the HLM-2 genome
appears to be a mosaic of sequences related to different classes of the
Retroviridae family.

Additional MMTV related human recombinant clones have been analyzed
by restriction enzyme mapping and heteroduplex formation. The
results show that the MMTV related sequences defined in HLM-2 are members
of a highly diverged family of retroviral-like sequences. This is
demonstrated by the large number of restriction site polymorphisms observed
between different clones. Heteroduplex analysis of several combinations
of recombinant clones showed no homology under stringent spreading conditions.
As the conditions were relaxed, long stretches of homology were observed.
In addition, each of the recombinant clones contained the LTR-like sequences
observed in HLM-2 which were always found flanking the MMTV gag-pol
related sequences.

We have begun to assess the organization of HLM-2 sequences in human
cellular DNA using the 3.6 kbp EcoRI fragment to probe restricted human
genomic DNA under stringent hybridization conditions. Consistent with
the restriction site polymorphisms noted in the analysis of the recombinant
clones, families of discrete restriction fragments containing sequences
related to the HLM-2 pol gene fragment were detected. Significantly, the
major EcoRI fragments observed (3.6, 3.5, 2.9 and 1.9 kbp) are similar to
those seen using the entire MMTV genome as a probe under low stringency
hybridization conditions. Restriction digests with other enzymes revealed
the present of cellular DNA fragments identical in size to those found
in the different human recombinant clones. The results suggest that our
collection of recombinant clones is representative of this human retroviral
related family.

The frequency of these clones in the human recombinant DNA library suggests that there are several copies of these sequences in human cellular DNA. Quantitative dot blot (15) analysis of human genomic DNA with HLM-2 probes is consistent with 50 copies of the pol and 1,000 copies of the LTR sequences. This result raised the possibility that a significant number of LTR-like elements are not associated with retroviral related structural genes. To test this, we have rescreened the human fetal liver DNA library using the HLM-2 LTR as a probe. Three clones were selected for further analysis. Partial restriction maps of two of the recombinant clones which hybridized to the LTR region but not to viral related structural gene sequences are illustrated in Fig. 3. Both clones (3B3 and 4-1)

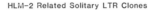

HLM-2 Related Solitary LTR Clones

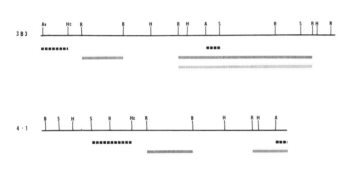

Fig. 3. Human recombinant clones containing HLM-2 related LTR sequences. The following restriction enzymes were used: EcoRI (R), SstI (S), HindIII (H), BamHI (B), ApaI (A), AvaI (Av), and HincII (Hc). Not all restriction enzyme sites are shown. Regions which hybridize to the HLM-2 LTR as well as members of the KpnI and Alu families of repetitive DNA are indicated.

contain two LTR-like elements separated by approximately 8 kbp of cellular DNA. The third clone (46-1.4) contains a single LTR. All of the LTR-like sequences are embedded in highly repetitive DNA.

The origin of these elements and the mechanism by which they have been amplified is unknown. One possibility is that during the evolution of the species, the LTRs became separated from the viral structural genes by cellular recombinational events and then subsequently amplified. Such a mechanism seems likely for the origin of solitary type C retroviral LTRs in murine DNA (16). Alternatively, viral RNA may have been inappropriately spliced such that the structural genes were lost but the signals for reverse transcription were preserved. This structure might then have reinserted into the germ line. A similar phenomenon may have occurred with the MMTV LTR in Balb/c mice (17, 18). In either case, these solitary LTRs may act as itinerant sequences or transposons.

The large sequence divergence of the different recombinant clones described earlier suggests that, in evolutionary terms, this family of retroviral genes was not recently introduced into the human cellular genome. To assess the conservation of these retroviral related sequences in other primate species, EcoRI restricted cellular DNAs from a variety of primates were analyzed by blot hybridization. Using the pol gene and LTR of HLM-2 DNA as probes, strong homology was readily evident between the DNAs of the two hominoid primates, Homo sapiens and Pan troglodytes. In contrast, under stringent hybridization conditions, only the pol region of HLM-2 reacted with all the monkey DNA samples tested. These included representatives of the two subfamilies of old world monkeys, Cercopithecinae (Erythrocebus patas and Macaca mulatta) and Colobinae (Presbytis and Colobus spp.) as well as subfamilies of the new world monkeys, Cebinae (Saimiri sciurea) and Aotinae (Aotes trivirgatus). The observed patterns of hybridization in old and new world monkey DNAs may reflect the presence of either an HLM-2-like endogenous retrovirus or an unrelated retroviral genome which shares homology to the HLM-2 pol gene. The striking similarity in the hybridization of human and chimpanzee (Pan troglodytes) DNAs to all the HLM-2 probes tested, is consistent with the long common evolutionary history of these two species (19-22). These results suggest that HLM-2 retroviral genes were introduced in the human lineage at a time preceding the divergence between Homo and Pan (21) but probably postdating the split between Cercopithecoidea (old world monkeys) and Hominoidea (21,22).

In summary, we have identified MMTV related sequences in human cellular DNA which are members of a large family of endogenous retroviral genomes. Based on our current information, we conclude that these sequences are not the human analogue of MMTV but instead represent a novel class of primate endogenous retroviruses.

REFERENCES

1. Sarkar, N. (1980) in The Role of Viruses in Human Cancer, Giraldo, G. and Beth, E. (eds.) pp. 207-235, Elsevier/North Holland, New York.
2. Axel, R., Schlom, J., and Spiegelman, S. (1972) Nature 235, 32.
3. Vaidya, A.B., Black, M.M., Dion, A.S., and Moore, D. (1974) Nature 249, 565.
4. Buetti, E. and Diggelman, H. (1981) Cell 23, 335.
5. Majors, J.E. and Varmus, H.E. (1981) Nature 289, 253.
6. Southern, E. (1975) J. Mol. Biol. 98, 503.
7. Callahan, R., Drohan, W., Tronick, S., and Schlom, J. (1982) Proc. Natl. Acad. Sci. (USA) 79, 5503.
8. May, F.E.B., Westley, B.R., Rochefort, H., Buetti, E., and Diggelman, H. (1983) Nuc. Acids Res. 11, 4127.
9. Rigby, P.W., Dieckmann, M., Rhodes, C., and Berg, P. (1977) J. Mol. Biol. 113, 237.
10. Blattner, F.R., Williams, B.G., Blechl, A.E., Denniston-Thompson, K., Faber, H.E., Furlong, L-A, Grunwald, D.J., Kiefer, D.O., Moore, D.D., Schumm, J.W., Sheldon, E.L., and Smithies, O. (1977) Science 196, 161.
11. Lawn. R.M., Fritsch, E.F., Parker, R.C., Blake, G., and Maniatis, T. (1978) Cell 15, 1157.
12. Chiu, I.M., Callahan, R., Tronick, S.R., Schlom, J., and Aaronson, S.A. (1984) Science 223, 364.
13. Martin, M.A., Bryan, T., Rasheed, S., and Khan, A.S. (1981) Proc. Natl. Acad. Sci. (USA) 78, 4892.
14. Bonner, T.I., O'Connell, C., and Cohen, M. (1982) Proc. Natl. Acad. Sci. (USA) 79, 4709.
15. Thomas, P.S. (1980) Proc. Natl. Acad. Sci. (USA) 77, 5201.
16. Wirth, T., Gloggler, K., Baumruker, T., Schmidt, M., and Horak, I. (1983) Proc. Natl. Acad. Sci. (USA) 80, 3327.
17. Wheeler, D.A., Butel, J.S., Medina, D., Cardiff, R.D., and Hager, G.L. (1983) J. Virol. 46, 42.
18. Van Ooyern, A.J.J., Michalides, R.J.A.M., and Nusse, R. (1983) J. Virol. 46, 362.
19. Simons, E.L. (1976) in Molecular Anthropology, Goodman, M. and Tashian, R.E. (eds.) pp. 35-62, Plenum Press, New York.
20. Walker, A. (1976) in Molecular Anthropology, Goodman, M. and Tashian, R.E. (eds.) pp. 63-77, Plenum Press, New York.
21. Sibley, C.G. and Ahlquist, J.E. (1984) J. Mol. Evol. 20, 2.
22. Gingerick, P.D. (1984) Yearbook of Physical Anthropology 27, 57.

16

EXPRESSION OF THE HUMAN HARVEY RAS ONCOGENE IN BREAST CANCER

Niki J. Agnantis[1] and Demetrios A. Spandidos[2,3]

[1] Hellenic Anticancer Institute, 171 Alexandras Ave., Athens, Greece

[2] Beatson Institute for Cancer Research, Garscube Estate, Bearsden, Glasgow G61 1BD

[3] Hellenic Institute Pasteur, 127 Vass. Sofias Ave., Athens, Greece

INTRODUCTION

The mechanism of cancer in humans remains elusive despite intensive research over the last few decades. Although few scientists doubt the role of environmental factors such as carcinogens and tumor promoters in influencing the incidence of different cancers, the identity and mode of action of these factors are still not known. In the past few years a different approach (gene transfer) has been ued to search for transforming genes present in tumor cells (1-3). These studies have resulted in the isolation and characterization of a number of transforming genes, named oncogenes, and have permitted an examination of their biological properties (for a review see ref. 4).

Transcriptional analysis of human oncogenes in a variety of tissues has revealed regulated expression of these genes (5-7). These results may help us to understand the deregulation of cell growth and differentiation.

In the present study we review our recent results on the relationship of Harvey-**ras** oncogene expression in malignant and normal breast tissue to the various clinicopathological properties of these tumors.

PATIENTS AND METHODS

Tissues were isolated from 24 female breast cancer patients who were operated on at the Breast Clinic of the Hellenic Anticancer Institute in Athens, Greece. During the preparation of frozen sections for the histopathological examination, tissue specimens for the RNA analysis were selected from tumors bigger than 1 cm in diameter and from normal breast tissue, located at a distance of approximately 2 cm from the tumor mass. All the material was stored at -70°C until RNA was isolated as previously described (5).

RESULTS

All histologically confirmed breast cancer tumours showed a significant elevation (2.5-15X) of Ha-**ras** transcripts when compared with the normal mammary tissue (7).

The following clinicopatholigical parameters were compared with the level of expression of the Ha-**ras** oncogene: p.T.N.M. stage of the disease, patient age, tumor topography, margin, tumor size, histological type of cancer, tumor grade, lymphocytic infiltration of the tumor mass, blood vessel invasion (in and out of the tumor mass), skin invasion of the breast, multicentricity of cancer (microscopic foci), associated cystic disease and axillary lymph node metastases (Agnantis, N.J., Parissi, P., Anagnostatis, D. and Spandidos, D.A. submitted).

The evaluation of the above parameters was made as follows:

1. According to the p.T.N.M. classification the stages of the disease, represented in the survey were T1, T2, T3 and T4 with various subdivisions.

2. Patient age was divided in three groups i.e. 23-50, 51-60 and 61-79 years old.

3. Most of the tumor mass were located in the four quadrants of the breast

but there were also some tumors located in the center of the mammary gland or in the centre of one of the four halves.

4. Tumor margin was divided in three groups, i.e. circumscribed, ill-defined and stellate.

5. Tumor size was divided into two groups, i.e. >2.5 cm and <2.5 cm.

6. The type of cancer was divided in five major histological categories viz. infiltrating duct, intraductal and infiltrating duct, infiltrating lobular, **in situ** and infiltrating lobular and mixed type (duct and lobular).

7. Only grades II and III were represented in the study since no grade I cases were available.

8. The lymphocytic infiltration of the tumor mass, skin and blood vessel invasion and multicentricity were assessed with a "yes" or a "no".

9. Associated cystic disease was divided into two groups, i.e. simple and complex. All negative cases were designated "no".

10. Each level was scanned for the axillary lymph node metastases, the evaluation was designated "yes" or "no".

Finally, for each parameter examined, the evaluation was compared with the mean value for the expression of the Ha-**ras** oncogene in that tumor.

The most significant results are summarised below:

1. Tumors for patients in the range between 50-60 years of age had the highest mean value of Ha-**ras** oncogene expression.

2. The stellate tumor margin and the larger tumor size had the lowest mean value.

3. The infiltrating duct histological type of tumor had the highest mean value.

4. Tumor Grade III had a lower mean value than Grade II.

5. The mean value was lower whenever lymphocytic infiltration was present

in the tumor.

6. Cases with lymph node metastases had a higher mean value.

DISCUSSION

In an attempt to explain our results on the elevated expression of the Ha-**ras** oncogene in malignant as compared to normal breast tissue we have considered the following:

The tumor samples were unselected and therefore we had a different number of patients in every stage of the disease (as defined by the pTNM system). This is probably why there was no correlation of Ha-**ras** expression with the stage of the disease. It has been suggested that tumor heterogeneity exists (for a review see ref. 8) and it is tempting to speculate that there may be different expression of the Ha-**ras** oncogene in different areas of the same tumor. Only 6 out of 24 cases had a pure histological type. All the others belonged to various subdivisions of the infiltrating duct type or were mixed types (duct and lobular). Thus it is possible that a degree of heterogeneity exists even in one tumor section.

The highest incidence of breast cancer was in the range of 51-60 years of age and this is probably why we found the highest level of Ha-**ras** expression here.

It is also possible that a cancer with large size stellate margins has more connective tissue stroma, more areas of necrosis or hemorrhage and fewer cancer cells than tumors with non stellate margins. This could explain the low expression of the Ha-**ras** oncogene in these cases.

Infiltrating duct breast cancer is the most common type (about 80%) and this could easily explain why this type of cancer had the highest mean value.

It is possible that cancers with a low differentiation, i.e. Grade III, have lower levels of expression of the Ha-**ras** oncogene. We have found similar results in a comparative study of hormone (estrogen and progesterone) receptor values with the histologic Grade of breast cancer (C. Petrakis, J. Yiotis and N.J. Agnantis, in preparation).

It is well known that lymphocytic infiltration of a tumour shows that an immune host reaction has taken place and this may lead to a decrease in oncogene expression. Whenever a lymph node metastasis is present, the disease is advanced and so the expression of an oncogene might be higher.

Finally, similar studies of oncogene expression in other breast conditions such as cystic disease (simple and complex), **in situ** cancers and fibroadenomas could be valuable in understanding oncogene activation in human tumors. Therefore we are currently studying quantitative and qualitative aspects of human Ha-**ras** oncogene expression in mammalian cells (9).

ACKNOWLEDGEMENTS:

We thank Dr. Peggy Anderson for critical appraisal of the manuscript.

REFERENCES

1. Spandidos, D.A. Anticancer Res. **3**, 121-125 (1983).

2. Cooper, G.M. Science **217**, 801-806 (1982).

3. Weinberg, R.A. Adv. Cancer Res. **36**, 149-156 (1982).

4. Vande Woude, G.F., Levine, A.J., Topp, W.C. and Watson, J.D. Cancer Cells, Vol. 2, Cold Spring Harbor Laboratory, New York (1984).

5. Spandidos, D.A. and Kerr, I.B. Br. J. Cancer **49**, 681-688 (1984).

6. Slamon, D.J., Dekernion, J.B., Verma, I.M. and Cline, M.J. Science 224, 269-272 (1984).

7. Spandidos, D.A. and Agnantis, N.J. Anticancer Res. **4**, 269-272 (1984).

8. Hart, I.R. and Fidler, I.J. Biochem. Biophys. Acta **651**, 37-50 (1981).

9. Spandidos, D.A. and Wilkie, N.M. Nature 310, 469-475 (1984).

17

THE SEARCH FOR ONCOGENES IN BREAST CANCER

B. GRONER, S. KOZMA, N.E. HYNES, S. REDMOND, R. JAGGI, W. GUNZBURG,
B. SALMONS, R. BALL, K. BUSER, E. REICHMANN AND A.C. ANDRES

Ludwig Institute for Cancer Research, Bern Branch, Inselspital
3010 Bern, Switzerland

INTRODUCTION

The concept of oncogenes has evolved impressively with the demonstration of the conferral onto cultured cells of a dominant transformed phenotype by tumor cell DNA mediated gene transfer (1-3). Genomic DNA transfection and the stable acquisition of transfected DNA by acceptor cells allows the distribution of tumor cell DNA into phenotypically normal cells. The rare transformation of a normal cell by the transfected DNA, i.e., at best 1 in 10^3 acceptor cells is able to stably acquire DNA and 1 in 10^3 stably transfected cells acquires a single specific gene, is accomplished by the uptake of oncogenes (4). This experimental protocol has led to the identification, molecular cloning and characterization of several cellular oncogenes and to the description of their mode of activation (5). The detection of oncogenes in primary tumor tissue, however, has not generally been successful (6). NIH/3T3 cells were originally chosen as acceptor cells because they can be efficiently transfected and it is possible to morphologically distinguish transformed from non-transformed cells. But there are certain limitations to the oncogene detection assay based on tumor DNA transfer into NIH/3T3 cells and focus formation of dense cells on the background of unaffected cells. a) Differentiation specific genes have been found to be restricted in their control of expression. Only specialized cell types are able to express certain genes upon gene transfer (7). The interaction of enhancer DNA sequences with cell type specific enhancer interacting proteins has been postulated to explain these transcriptional control mechanisms. Little is known about the tissue specific regulation of oncogene promoters. b) Oncogene products are thought to mediate their function through the interaction with cellular proteins. The cellular targets could be cell type or differentiation specific. The action of an oncogene could be post-transcription- and translationally-obscured by the absence of appropriate target molecules (8). c) It is possible that certain oncogenes will not confer an easily detectable morphological change on NIH/3T3 cells. These considerations suggest that other cell types in addition to NIH/3T3 should be used for the detection of cellular oncogenes and/or the evaluation of their biological potentials.

The multistep character of malignant transformation suggests that several independent genetic alterations are responsible for the final phenotype. An extended definition of oncogenes might comprise all genes which contribute to tumorigenesis. Subtle phenotypic changes of normal cells could be used to define and characterize "intermediate" oncogenes (conferring, e.g., anchorage independent growth and reduced growth factor requirements) as opposed to "ultimate" oncogenes (conferring tumorigenicity). These considerations led us to introduce human breast tumor DNA into NIH/3T3 and NMuMG cells (9) (established normal mouse mammary gland epithelial cells) and test the transfectants for tumorigenicity, soft agar growth and reduced growth factor requirements. This experimental scheme is outlined in Figure 1.

Figure 1   Detection of "Ultimate" and "Intermediate" Oncogenes by
           DNA-mediated Gene Transfer

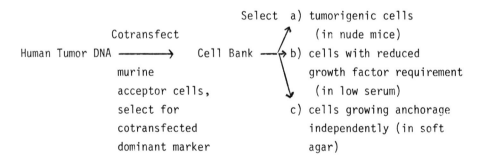

The introduction of oncogenes contained in retroviruses often results in the change of the growth properties and the differentiated functions of the infected cells (10). Little is known about the effects of oncogenes on mammary epithelial cells. To investigate the influence of oncogene expression on mammary epithelial cells two approaches were

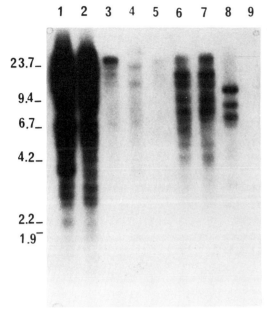

Figure 2: Southern blot analysis of DNA from tumors induced in nude mice by injection of NIH cells transfected with MDA-MB231 DNA. Primary tumor DNA: lanes 1 and 2. Secondary tumor DNA: lanes 3 to 5. NIH cells transfected with HM347 DNA. Primary tumor DNA: lanes 6 and 7. NIH cells transfected with human colon carcinoma DNA (lane 8) and control NIH DNA (lane 9). The DNA was digested with EcoRI and nick translated total human DNA was used as a hybridization probe.

taken: a) Mammary epithelial cells were cultured in vitro and the fgr oncogene (11) was introduced by microinjection. b) The EJ oncogene (5) was introduced into the germ line of mice under the control of the whey acidic protein gene promoter (12).

RESULTS AND DISCUSSION
Detection of "ultimate" and "intermediate" oncogenes in the DNA of human mammary tumor cells
Conferral of tumorigenicity

NIH/3T3 cells were transfected with DNA from an established human breast carcinoma line (MDA-MB 231) and DNA from primary cells of a human breast tumor metastasis (HM 347). Cell banks were established by cotransfection with pSV2neo and selection of transfected cells in G418. Several thousand individually transfected cells assure the representative transfer of each tumor DNA gene into the acceptor cells. The population of transfected acceptor cells is called a "cell bank" (4). The cell banks were grown to 10^6 cells and injected into nude mice. Two independent tumors developed in mice injected with NIH cells

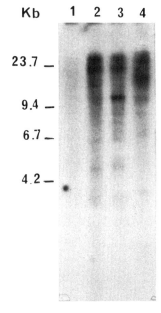

Kb 1 2 3 4

23.7 —

9.4 —

6.7 —

4.2 —

Figure 3: Southern blot analysis of NMuMG cell DNA of clones transfected with human breast tumor metastasis DNA and able to grow in soft agar. Lane 1: NMuMG DNA. Lanes 2 and 3: Soft agar clone DNA of NMuMG-HM347. Lane 4: Soft agar clone DNA of NMuMG-HM1596. The DNAs were digested with EcoRI and hybridized to a nick translated probe of total human DNA.

transfected with MDA-MB231 DNA (NIH-MB231). The acquisition of repetitive human DNA by the tumor cells is shown in Figure 2 by hybridization with a human DNA probe (lanes 1 and 2). DNA from tumor No. 2 was used for a secondary transfection of NIH/3T3 cells and this cell bank (2° NIH/MB231) also gave rise to tumors after injection into nude mice. The repetitive human DNA pattern (Fig. 2, lanes 3 to 5) is reduced in its complexity in comparison to the tumor DNA of primary transfectants (lanes 1 and 2). Subsequent analysis of the tumor DNA with cloned human ras probes (not shown) indicates that tumor No. 1 from NIH/MB231 contains several copies of the human Ki-ras gene. This amplification cannot be seen in the donor MDA-MB231 DNA. Tumor No. 2 of NIH/MB231 and the secondary tumors do not appear to contain a member of the human ras family.

A cell bank arising from the transfection of the human breast tumor metastasis HM347 into NIH/3T3 cells (NIH-HM347) is also tumorigenic. The tumorigenicity is most likely due to the acquisition of human tumor DNA which can be shown by the presence of human repetitive sequences (Fig. 2, lanes 6 and 7). Analysis of the NIH/HM347 tumor DNA with a human N-ras probe (not shown) revealed the presence of a single human N-ras gene copy in the nude mouse tumor DNA.

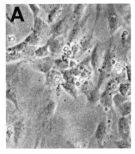 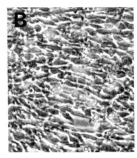

Figure 4: Photomicrograph of NIH cells grown in medium containing 1% fetal calf serum. A) Control NIH/3T3 cells. B) NIH/3T3 cells transfected with HM347 DNA. A clonal growth can be seen.

These results show that at least three different "ultimate oncogenes" contained in human breast tumor DNA can be transferred to NIH/3T3 cells and cause their tumorigenicity (Ki-ras, N-ras and an unknown gene). It is obviously of great interest to determine the mode of activation of the ras genes, their involvement in the transformation of the original tumor cells and the identity of the human gene transferred to NIH-MB231 tumor No. 2. The N-ras gene and two additional genes (mcf 2 and mcf 3) have been detected by Fasano et al. (13) in a similar assay in which DNA from the MCF-7 cell line was introduced into NIH/3T3 cells. An activated H-ras oncogene was found by Kraus et al. (14) in the mammary carcinosarcoma line HS578 T.

Conferral of anchorage independent growth

Normal murine mammary epithelial cells (NMuMG) were used to establish a cell bank by transfection with primary human breast tumor metastasis DNA (NMuMG-HM347). Introduction of this cell bank into mude mice did not result in tumor growth. We have shown previously that the activated human Ha-ras gene confers tumorigenicity to these cells (4), i.e., that a single "ultimate" oncogene is sufficient for this process. NMuMG cells do not form soft agar colonies when cultivated in 0.4% soft agar containing DMEM and 10% fetal calf serum. When the NMuMG-HM347 cell bank was plated in soft agar medium colonies grew with a frequency of about 5×10^{-4}. This is consistent with the interpretation that the transfer of a single human gene is responsible for this growth phenotype. The hybridization of the DNA of these anchorage independently growing NMuMG cells with a human repetitive DNA probe is shown (Fig. 3, lanes 2 and 3). Soft agar growth was also observed in a second cell bank of NMuMG cells transfected with the human metastasis HM1596 (Fig. 3, lane 4). Investigation into the identity of the transfected human gene indicated that it is not a member of the ras family (not shown). The DNA of HM347 was thus shown to contain two different genes possibly related to the transformed phenotype. The N-ras gene confers tumorigenicity to NIH/3T3 cells and a gene of unknown identity confers anchorage independent growth to NMuMG cells.

Conferral of low growth factor requirements

The genetic relationship between certain oncogenes and genes coding for growth factors or growth factor receptors has provided a direct mechanistic link for the observations which show that oncogenes can confer growth factor autonomy to cells (15). Oncogenes, however, don't have to be growth factors or receptors but can act through amplification of the mitotic signals generated by a growth factor at its receptor. Reduction of the growth requirements may be one of the intermediate steps distinguishing normal from transformed cells. The cell bank NIH-HM 347 was screened for cells with reduced serum requirements for growth. Normal NIH/3T3 still divide in medium supplemented with 5% serum but are not able to divide in only 1% serum. The cell bank was plated in 10% serum at an intermediate density and after one round of replication the serum was reduced to 1%. A small number of colonies developed in transfected NIH cells but not in untransfected controls (Fig. 4). Since this selection procedure is based on a different principle than that of the two described above (tumorigenicity and anchorage independent growth) it is possible that a different human gene is responsible. The nature of the gene conferring the low growth factor requirement to NIH/3T3 cells is under investigation.

Introduction of oncogenes into the mouse germ line and cultured mammary epithelial cells.

Transgenic WAP-ras mice

A definitive test for the role of oncogenes in the transformation of specific cell types in vivo can be approached by the introduction of activated oncogenes into the fertilized eggs of mice (16). A small percentage of eggs stably acquire the injected DNA. Mice which result carry the injected DNA in all somatic cells. Recent progress in the introduction and analysis of genes which are expressed in a tissue specific manner has shown that a short DNA sequence is sufficient to direct the organ and cell type specific expression in transgenic mice

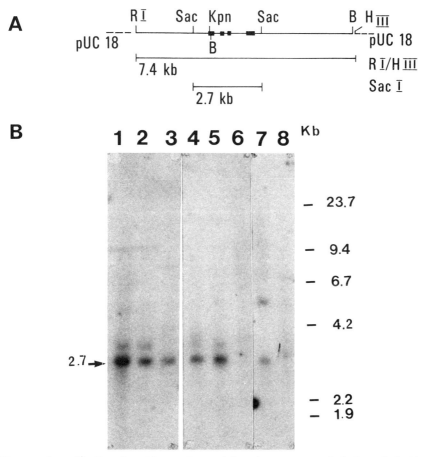

Figure 5: A) Construction of a chimeric gene containing 2.5 kb 5'
sequence (RI to Kpn I) contributed by the whey acidic protein and 4.9 kb
(Kpn I to Bam H1) contributed by the structural region of the activated
c-Ha ras oncogene. B) Southern blot analysis of DNA derived from the
tails of transgenic mice. Lanes 1 to 5 show the DNA of 5 positive mice.
Lane 6 is from an injected, but negative, mouse. Lane 7 is human DNA
and lane 8 wild type mouse DNA. The DNA was digested with Sac I and
hybridized to a nick translated human Ha-ras probe.

(17). Based on these observations we have constructed a chimeric
oncogene which is potentially able to be expressed in mammary epithelial
cells and subjected to the signals governing lactation. The whey acidic
protein (WAP) is the major whey protein in the milk of rodents (12). It
is synthesized under the influence of lactogenic hormones in
differentiated breast epithelial cells. A molecular clone of the WAP
gene was obtained and the WAP promoter region (RI-KpnI, about 2.5 kb,

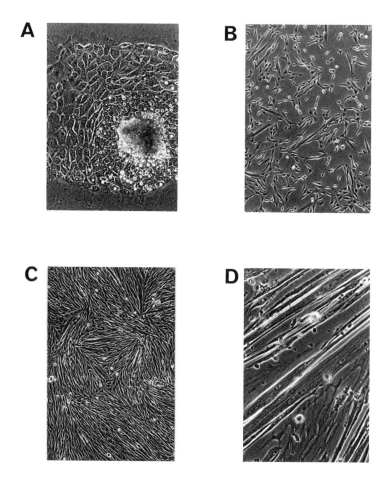

Figure 6: Photomicrographs of primary mouse mammary gland epithelial cells microinjected with the fgr oncogene: A) Organoids attached to plastic surface after two days of culture. B) Proliferating cells after microinjection with the fgr oncogene. C) Dense elongated cells. D) Fused, multinucleated, striated cells which show frequent spontaneous contractions.

Fig. 5) was linked to the structural part of the EJ oncogene (B-B, about 4 kb, Fig. 5). This construct might provide the putative transcriptional regulation sequences in the DNA located 5' of the WAP gene RNA initiation site to the EJ oncogene. 560 fertilized eggs were injected, 71 mice were born and 5 were found to have acquired the

WAP-ras oncogene in their somatic cells. The transgene is characterized by a 2.7 kb Sac I restriction fragment which is visualized in the tail DNA of the positive mice in Figure 6. The tissue specific expression of the WAP-ras oncogene and the mammary tumor incidence of the transgenic mice will be of great interest.

Oncogene introduction into primary mammary epithelial cells

The effect of oncogenes on defined differentiated cells can also be studied in vitro (18). The introduction of cloned oncogenes into primary cultures of mammary epithelial cells was used to investigate their susceptibility to transformation and measure the influence of oncogenes on cell proliferation and differentiation functions. Such experiments have been described by Butel et al. (19) utilizing the SV 40 genome. Organoids were prepared (19) from mid-pregnant Balb/c mice by mechanical and enzymatic dissection of mammary gland tissue and were then separated by sieving out aggregates between 53 and 840 um in diameter. After two days in culture the peripherally attached cells (Fig. 6, A) were injected with a molecular clone of the FeSV genome (11) containing the fgr oncogene. Focal outgrowth of injected cells was observed and the rapidly proliferating cells could be transferred several times (Fig. 6, B). When the cells were allowed to grow to high density (Fig. 6, C) fusion of cells was observed. Elongated, multinucleated cells underwent irregular spontaneous contractions (Fig. 6, D). These cells have the appearance of myotubes. Our experiments suggest that a progran resembling skeletal muscle differentiation is turned on in the injected epithelial cells. This observation is reminiscent of skeletal muscle elements produced by cell lines derived from neoplastic rat mammary epithelial stem cells (20). The initial response to the oncogene is proliferation and if cells are kept below a certain density they keep proliferating and seem to be immortalized. Upon fusion into myotube-like structures, however, they stop dividing.

The experiments described here are based on two principles: a) Introduction of genomic DNA from mammary tumors into NIH and NMuMG cells which allows the selection of transformation related phenotypes in the acceptor cells and the molecular characterization of the responsible genes. The cloned genes can then be tested for their involvement in the etiology of breast cancer. To date, members of the ras family of oncogenes as well as other, as yet unidentified, genes have been detected. b) The effect of oncogenes on mammary epithelial cells is being studied by the introduction of defined oncogenes into these cells in vivo and in vitro. Transgenic mice allow an in vivo analysis of the expression of oncogenes targeted by provision with a tissue specific promoter (WAP-ras).

REFERENCES
1. Krontiris, T.G. and Cooper, G.M. Proc. Natl. Acad. Sci. USA 78:1181-1184, 1981.
2. Shih, C., Padby, L.C., Murray, M. and Weinberg, R.A. Nature 290:261-264, 1981.
3. Perucho, M., Goldfarb, M., Shimizu, K., Lama, C., Fogh, J. and Wigler, M. Cell 27:467-476, 1981.
4. Hynes, N.E., Jaggi, R., Kozma, S.C., Ball, R., Müllener, D., Wetherall, N.T., Davis, B.W. and Groner, B. Mol. Cell. Biol. 5:268-272, 1985.
5. Tabin, C.J., Bradley, S.M., Bargmann, C.I., Weinberg, R.A., Papageorge, A.G., Scolnick, E.M., Dhar, R., Lowy, D.R. and Chang, E.H., 1982.
6. Pulciani, S., Santos, E., Lauver, A.V., Long, L.K., Aaronson, S.A. and Barbacid, M. Nature 300:539-542, 1982.
7. Walker, M.D., Edlund, T., Boulet, E.R. and Rutter, W.J. Nature 306:557-561, 1983.
8. Lipsich, L., Brugge, J.S. and Boettiger, D. Mol. Cell. Biol. 4:1420-1424, 1984.
9. Owens, R.B., Smith, H.S. and Hackett, A.J. J. Natl, Cancer Inst. 53:261-266, 1974.
10. Weiss, R.A., Teich, N., Varmus, H.E. and Coffin, J.M. (eds) Molecular Biology of Tumor Viruses. RNA Tumor Viruses. Cold Spring Harbor Laboratory, New York, 1982.
11. Naharro, G., Robbins, K.C. and Reddy, E.P. Science 223:63-66, 1984.
12. Campbell, S.M., Rosen, J.M., Henninghausen, L.G., Strech-Jurk, U. and Sippel, A.E. Nuc. Acids Res. 12:8685-8697, 1984.
13. Fasano, O., Birnbaum, D., Edlund, L. Fogh, J. and Wigler, M. Mol. Cell. Biol. 4:1695-1705, 1984.
14. Kraus, M.H., Yuasa, Y. and Aaronson, S.A. Proc. Natl. Acad. Sci. USA 81:5384-5388, 1984.
15. Sporn, M.B. and Roberts, A.B. Nature 313:745-747, 1985.
16. Stewart, T.A., Pattengale, P.K. and Leder, P. Cell 38:627-637, 1984.
17. Ornitz, D.M., Palmiter, R.D., Hammer, R.E., Brinster, R.L., Swift, G.H. and MacDonald, R.J. Nature 313:600-602, 1985.
18. Falcone, G., Tato, F and Alema, S. Proc. Natl. Acad. Sci. USA 82:426-430, 1985.
19. Butel, J.S., Wong, C. and Medina, D. Experim. Mol. Path. 40:79-108, 1984.
20. Rudland, P.S., Dunnington, D.J., Gusterson, B., Monaghan, P. and Hughes, C.M. Cancer Res. 44:2089-2102, 1984.

18

IN VITRO TRANSFORMATION OF HUMAN BREAST EPITHELIAL CELLS

SIDNEY E. CHANG

Marie Curie Memorial Foundation, Research Institute, The Chart, Oxted, Surrey, UK

INTRODUCTION

One approach to investigating the relationship between cell lineage, differentiation and cancer of the human breast is to study breast epithelial cells in culture, and to use immunological markers and molecular biology techniques to classify these cells and to follow the biological changes that accompany their interconversion or differentiation and their transformation in vitro.

In the last few years a range of polyclonal and monoclonal antibodies have been developed to membrane and cytoskeletal antigens of epithelial cells and to the extracellular matrix components which these cells produce. These markers are invaluable in distinguishing between epithelial cells at different stages of differentiation in the breast and are indispensable in experiments which try to relate cell types in vitro with specific mammary cells in vivo (1,2).

The above advances in immunology have been matched by equally sophisticated developments in molecular biology and virology and one consequence of this has been a growing pool of evidence to show that most cancers involve multiple steps and that oncogenes may be responsible for each step (reviewed in 3,4). The availability of cloned oncogenes and methods to introduce these genes into cells opens up a whole new field of study viz. the genesis of cancer in epithelial cells and how this is related to differentiation.

BREAST EPITHELIAL CULTURES

The two major sources of normal human breast tissue are organoids from reduction mammoplasty tissue (5,6) and milk. The studies described in this review have utilized the latter source. When milk is expressed from the breast, clumps of secretory lumenal epithelia are shed into the

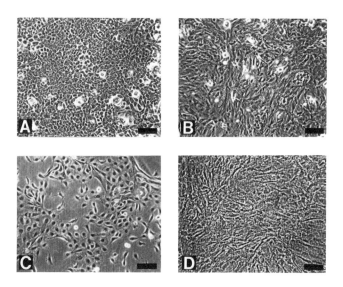

Fig. 1. Milk epithelial cell types. (A.B) Closed colony phenotypes
containing (A) cuboidal or (B) elongate cells. (C) Open colony type.
(D) Late milks. Bars represent 100 μm.

secretions (7) and it is these clumps that can be recovered and cultured
in vitro (8-10).   Primary milk cultures differ from cultures derived
from mammary organoids in several respects. First they are not contam-
inated with fibroblasts as mammary organoid cultures often are. Second,
they appear to have few basal (myoepithelial) cells, an advantage since
there has been no reliable positive marker for this cell type in vitro.
Finally, since milk is obtained from a fully functioning mammary gland
it could be argued that cultures derived from it should display a wider
range of differentiated epithelial phenotypes than do organoid cultures.
      Characteristically, primary milk cultures are dominated by closed
colony phenotypes containing either cuboidal or elongate cells (Fig. 1
A and B) or mixtures of them both (9). A minor but nevertheless distinctive colony type is the open colony type containing polygonal cells separated from each other (Fig. 1C). In low serum concentrations this colony
type proliferates more rapidly than the closed colony phenotypes (9) and

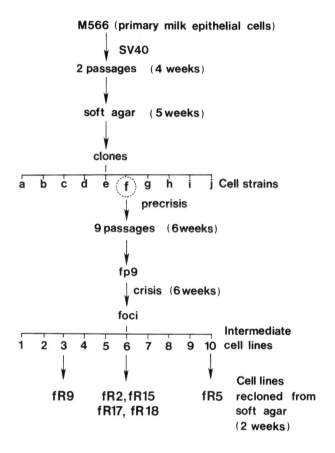

Fig. 2.   Isolation of the fR series of SV40 transformed breast epithelial
cell lines.   Epithelial cells cultured from milk pool M566 and infected
with SV40 were plated in soft agar after 2 passages.   Ten cell strains
(a to j) were established from soft-agar clones, and of these, a, c, e,
f, h, and i were the most viable.   Strain f went into crisis at passage
9 (fp9: the passage number is prefixed by p).   After 6 weeks, foci
appeared in the fp9 cultures, and 10 of these were picked.   These foci
formed the intermediate cell lines (f1 to f10).   When these cell lines
were recloned in soft agar, many clones were obtained.   Several of these
clones were chosen, and these gave rise to the fR cell lines.
(Reprinted with permission from ref. 14).

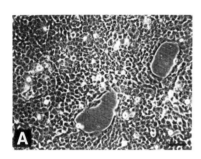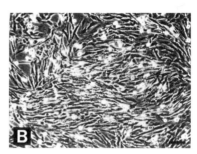

Fig. 3.   SV40 transformed milk epithelial cells.   (A) fR2 (cuboidal)
and (B) fR5 (elongate).   Bars represent 100 μm.   (Reprinted with permission from ref. 14).

when they touch and become close packed, they often resemble the closed
colony phenotype containing cuboidal cells (9-12).

    Experiments that try to relate the different colony types in milk
cultures with specific cell types in the mammary gland (10) have been
limited to primary cultures since with passage the original morphological
types disappear and a new cell type emerges which by morphological and
other criteria is different not only from the epithelial types found in
primary milk cultures but also from mammary fibroblasts (1,12,13).   The
origin of these "late milk" (LM) cells (Fig. 1D) is unclear but it is
conceivable that they may be an _in vitro_ counterpart to the rare basal
stellate cells which are found as a discontinuous layer in the terminal
ductal lobular units (TDLUs) of lactating human breast (1,2).

ESTABLISHMENT OF SV40 TRANSFORMED BREAST EPITHELIAL CELL LINES
    To obtain permanent cell lines of mammary epithelial origin which
express some properties characteristic of the original cell types, cells
from primary milk cultures were transformed with SV40 by Chang et al (14).
SV40 was chosen as the tool to "establish" the milk cells as there had
been reports that showed that this DNA virus was capable of extending the
lifespan of some human epithelial cells _in vitro_ (15,16,17), and in the
case of human epidermal keratinocytes, SV40 transformed cell lines with
apparently unlimited lifespan had been isolated (18,19).

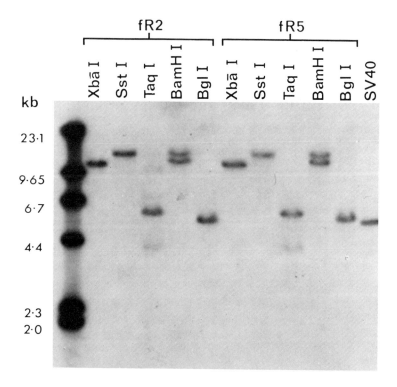

Fig. 4.   Detection, by autoradiography, of the SV40-containing sequences
in DNA isolated from fR2 and fR5 cells. DNA from the two lines were
digested with restriction enzymes which cut SV40 once (TaqI, BamHI and
BglI) or not at all (XbaI and SstI), then electrophoresed on a 0.8% (w/v)
agarose gel and then finally blotted onto nitrocellulose filter (68).
The filter was probed with nick-translated ^{32}P-labelled SV40 DNA.

   Although it was relatively easy to obtain SV40-transformed milk epithelial cell strains with an extended lifespan in vitro (Fig. 2), these
strains eventually entered crisis (20) and died. One strain (M566f),
however, after entering a quiescent state for about 6 weeks, spontaneously
gave rise to viable foci. These post-crisis foci were cultivated and
after being cloned in soft agar gave rise to the fR series of SV40 transformed breast epithelial cell lines with apparently unlimited lifespan
(14). Whereas morphologically the M566f cell strain was unlike the dom-

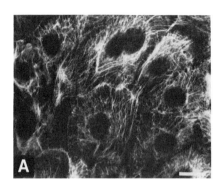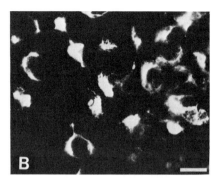

Fig. 5.   Immunofluorescence staining for the cytokeratin antigen recognized by LE61 (36).   (A) Milk epithelial cells.   (B)   SV40 transformed
milk epithelial cell line fR2. Bars represent 20 μm. (Reprinted with
permission from ref. 14).

inant cell types seen in primary milk cultures the cloned fR lines had
either a cuboidal (majority) or elongate morphology. The two lines that
have been studied in depth are fR2 (cuboidal) and fR5 (elongate) (Fig. 3)
which closely resemble the cuboidal and elongate colony phenotypes seen
in milk cultures   (Fig. 1 A and B).   These morphologically different
lines must have shared a common precursor cell since their karyotypes
are similar and besides being hypotetraploid, include several rearrangements involving chromosomes 1 and 11 (21). Rearrangements in these two
chromosomes, particularly with chromosome 1, are often found in breast
carcinomas and lines derived from metastatic pleural effusions (22-32).

     Southern blots of fR2 and fR5 DNA probed with radiolabelled SV40 show
that the viral genome is integrated in a simple and similar fashion in
both cell lines (Fig. 4; S. Chang and K. Dixon). Only one SV40-containing
band is obtained with the restriction enzymes XbāI and SstI which do not
cut SV40 and two bands are obtained with BamHI and BglI which normally cut
SV40 once. The appearance of multi-bands with TaqI (a one cutter) and
other data (not shown) suggests that there may be some duplication of
parts of the SV40 genome in the fR cells.

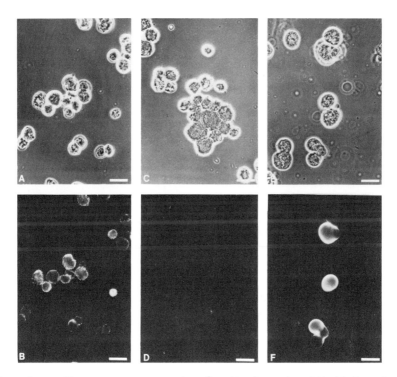

Fig. 6. Immunofluorescence screening for the breast epithelial membrane differentiation antigen HMFG-1 (38,39) on live cells. (A,B) fR2. (C,D) fR5. (E,F) Milk epithelial cells. Bars represent 20 μm. (Reprinted with permission from ref. 14).

CHARACTERIZATION OF THE fR LINES

Once the fR lines were established it was important to show that they were SV40 transformed and were of breast epithelial origin. Using an indirect immunofluorescence test and monoclonal antibody (mAb) PAb 205 (33), SV40 large T-antigen was detected in the nuclei of the fR cells (14). The T-antigen in fR cells is probably similar to authentic T-antigen since it co-electrophoreses with the latter on SDS-polyacrylamide gels (S. Chang).

Cytokeratins are the intermediate filaments of epithelial cells and are not found in other cell types (34,35). The presence, therefore, of

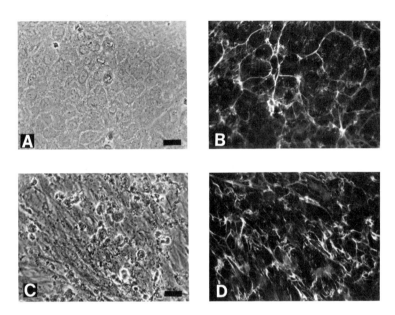

Fig. 7. Immunofluorescence staining for the fibronectin antigen FN4 on fR2 cells (A,B) and FN3 on fR5 cells (C,D). Bars represent 30 μm.

cytokeratin antigens can be used as a diagnostic test for epithelial cells. By indirect immunofluorescence and using the mAb LE61 (36), which recognizes a keratin 18 antigen (B. Lane, personal communication), the epithelial nature of the fR cells was confirmed. In primary cultures of milk cells this cytokeratin antigen is seen to be distributed as a delicate basketwork throughout the cytoplasm,with filaments anchored in desmosomes at the cell periphery (Fig. 5A). This cytokeratin distribution is typical of a wide variety of cultured epithelial cells. In contrast the LE61 antigen in fR cells is seen as a distorted, collapsed and irregular filament system, often present only as a perinuclear ring or "cap" (Fig. 5B). The fR5 line with fusiform morphology was almost completely negative with LE61, as also were 3 fusiform cell lines (S1.3, S1.10 and S2.9) which were isolated as cloned variants from the LE61 positive cuboidal fR9 cell line. It is possible that the lack of expression of the LE61 antigen and fusiform morphology of fR cells may be causally related. In this context it is of interest that after 70 passages (at least 210 doublings), rare colonies of cuboidal cells were found in cultures of fR5 cells. These colonies were LE61 positive (S. Chang).

During lactation fat is released from the secretory lumenal cells of the breast as droplets surrounded by a piece of the apical plasma membrane. These milk fat globule (MFG) membranes which come from fully differentiated normal mammary epithelia have been used extensively for the production of polyclonal and monoclonal antibodies (see 1 for some references). The most immunogenic components of human MFG are glycoproteins especially those associated with a large mucin-like product (>400K) consisting of at least 50% carbohydrate (37). Among the mAbs developed to this component and directed to oligosaccharide determinants are HMFG-1 and HMFG-2 (1.10.F3 and 14.A3 respectively), isolated and characterized by Taylor-Papadimitriou and colleagues (1,2,38-41). The determinant recognized by HMFG-1 is found in larger numbers than the HMFG-2 site in the lactating breast whilst the reverse is commonly the case on breast cancer cells (1,40). Both HMFG-1 and 2 determinants are only weakly expressed in the non-lactating breast (38).

Using the HMFG-1 mAb it was evident that the fR cells do express antigens normally associated with the fully differentiated breast (14). In both a radiolabelled binding assay and by indirect immunofluorescence, live fR cells were found to express, to different degrees, the HMFG-1 determinant. The highest level was expressed by fR2 cells (Fig. 6A,B) and the lowest by the fusiform fR5 line (Fig. 6C,D). The lack of HMFG-1 expression on fR5 cells is not related to its fusiform shape since the fusiform cells (S1.3, S1.10, and S2.9) mentioned above do express this antigen. The range of HMFG-1 expression on the fR lines is perhaps not surprising since milk cultures themselves express this antigen in a heterogenous manner (Fig. 6E,F; 14).

Fibronectins are high molecular glycoproteins which are found in plasma, in cell and basement membranes and in stromal matrices (42). Two forms of fibronectin have been identified: plasma (43) and cellular (44). Using the fR5 line as immunogen, two monoclonal antibodies, FN3 and FN4 (also known as 5G6) have been isolated and characterized (45). FN3 recognizes a determinant on human cellular but not plasma fibronectin whereas FN4 recognizes a determinant on both. The FN3 and FN4 antigens are expressed in an extracellular matrix in fR cells (Fig. 7; 45), in contrast

to a punctate pattern in primary milk cultures (45), a distribution also
observed with polyclonal antisera to purified human plasma fibronectin
(46). The extracellular fibronectin matrix on the fR cells is similar
to, though less extensive, than that seen with the same reagents (45) on
breast fibroblasts, the late milk cells (12) and the unique carcinosarcoma derived breast cancer cell line Hs578T (47). The FN3 and FN4
reagents do not stain breast carcinoma cell lines like T47D, in agree-
ment with other experiments utilizing conventional polyclonal antisera
(45,48).

MODULATION OF THE HMFG-1 ANTIGEN IN MILK CULTURES AND RELATIONSHIP OF
ITS EXPRESSION TO GROWTH AND SV40 TRANSFORMATION

The observation that the HMFG-1 antigen is only expressed by 55-60%
of cells in primary milk cultures and that there is no simple correlation
between cell morphology and expression of this antigen (14) prompted a
series of experiments by Chang and Taylor-Papadimitriou (12) to see if
the HMFG-1 antigen is modulated in vitro.

Using a fluorescence-activated cell sorter (FACS) milk cells were
separated into HMFG-1 plus (+) and minus (-) fractions and their behaviour in vitro observed. Over a two week period the HMFG-1 (-) cells
showed more growth than the (+) cells and when stained for HMFG-1 the
two types of cultures were shown to contain some cells that expressed
this antigen, confirming that modulation of the antigen did occur in
vitro. A further cell sort of the original minus and plus populations
into HMFG-1 (+) and (-) cells followed by another round of growth experiments showed that in terms of HMFG-1 expression and growth
(-/-) >> (+/-) > (-/+) > (+/+). In other words not only was the HMFG-1
antigen modulated in vitro but also its expression was coupled with loss
in growth potential (12). This observation that expression of the
HMFG-1 antigen on normal breast cells is associated with decreased growth
rate is interesting for if this were also true for tumour cells it could
explain why those patients with infiltrating breast carcinomas secreting
a matrix component with many HMFG-1 sites have a good prognosis (49).

Both HMFG-1 (+) and (-) cultures contained closed colonies of epithelial cells. In addition the HMFG-1 (-) cultures contained colonies of
the open type (Fig. 1C), the colony type which is known to proliferate
fastest in low serum concentrations (9). It is likely that it was these

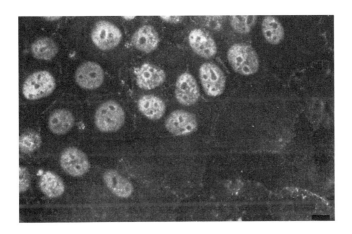

Fig. 8.   Immunofluorescence staining for SV40 large T-antigen with
monoclonal antibody PAb205 (33) on FACS separated HMFG-1 negative milk
cells two weeks after infection with SV40 virus. Bar represents 20 μm.

open colonies that gave the HMFG-1 (-) cultures their growth advantage
over the (+) cultures. Besides containing the ubiquitous closed colonies,
the HMFG-1 (+) cultures were unique in that they only contained colonies
of the late milk cells (Fig. 1D).

When FACS sorted HMFG-1 (+) and (-) cells were infected with SV40
and then stained for SV40 large T-antigen two weeks later it was observed
that only the (-) cultures contained colonies of T-antigen positive cells
(Fig. 8; S. Chang). In view of the observations that open cells, whilst
rapidly dividing, express little of the HMFG-1 antigen (12), and that
SV40 transformed milk epithelial cell strains including M566f, the precursor to the fR lines, express only low levels of this antigen (14), it
is possible that the cells that were transformed by SV40 were of the open
colony type. If this were the case then it could explain why so few
SV40 transformed milk epithelial cell strains were isolated (14), the
reason being that the number of cells in open colonies in milk cultures
is usually very small.

It is also possible that the HMFG-1 (+) milk cells are equally susceptible to transformation by SV40 but are not because they possess a
physical barrier through which the SV40 virus cannot penetrate. Surface
mucins are known to protect epithelial cells in vivo and it is possible
that the mucin-like extracellular matrix in which most of the HMFG-1 antigen is localized on milk cells (40) could help protect the HMFG-1 (+)
cells from SV40 infection.

WHAT ARE THE fR CELLS?

Our current hypothesis is that fR cells are derived from a LE61 (+)
cell in the secretory lineage (1,2) which, in culture, may have been an
open colony type expressing low levels of the HMFG-1 antigen. Recently
it has been found that the fR cells do not react with BA16 (50), a mAb
which recognizes the 40 Kd human keratin (51) classified as keratin 19
(52).   This observation is potentially important since in vivo it is
found that BA16 (-) cells form a minor proportion of the epithelial cells
in the breast and have a distribution which would be expected of a cell
with the proliferative potential to give rise to new TDLUs or branching
within TDLUs at pregnancy (50). In addition, BA16 (-) cells also constitute a minor population (10-20% of colonies) in milk cultures and
here they are usually found as large colonies of cuboidal cells, the
colony phenotype which often derive from the open colony type (9,12).
Together these observations suggest that the fR lines are related to a
minor epithelial cell type (with a proliferative potential) that is found
in the breast and in milk cultures.

The fR cells are unique in that they are one of the few examples of
SV40 transformed human epithelial cells that show an apparently unlimited
lifespan in vitro.   The fR2 and fR5 cells have been passaged over 80
times (at least 240 doublings), and are anchorage independent (i.e. they
grow in soft agar) but are non-tumorigenic in nude mice. Because of the
long time span (6 months) involved in the evolution of the fR cells and
the apparent multistep sequence involved in their selection it is possible
that cellular oncogenes may have been activated in these cells. Experiments are in progress to see if this is the case. If there are any cellular oncogenes activated in the fR cells it will be interesting to see if
they are related to those identified in MCF-7 cells (N-Ras, mcf2 and mcf3;
53) or the carcinosarcoma Hs578T line (H-Ras; 54).

DNA TRANSFECTION OF MILK EPITHELIAL CELLS

One possible reason why milk cells are transformed by SV40 virus at a very low frequency is that most of the cells may be protected from viral infection by a mucin-like matrix over their cell membranes (see above). In view of this, alternative ways of transforming milk cells in vitro have been explored and in particular the calcium-phosphate mediated DNA transfection technique (55) has been tried since this method has proven to be efficient for introducing cloned oncogenes into rodent fibroblast cells (e.g. 56,57).

Among the few reports describing successful attempts to introduce DNA by transfection into epithelial cells (58) is that by Griffin and Karran (59) which showed that certain cloned fragments of EBV (p13/p33 and p31) can immortalize African Green Monkey Kidney (AGMK) epithelial cells. Since EBV is unique among the DNA tumour viruses by virtue of its association with two human malignancies, Burkitt's lymphoma and naso-pharyngeal carcinoma, it is important to see whether the fragments of EBV DNA which can immortalize AGMK and Marmoset (Callithrix jacchus) kidney epithelial cells (60; D. King, L. Karran and B. Griffin) can do likewise in human epithelia. Experiments in progress (60; S. Chang and B. Griffin) suggest that the lifespan of milk epithelial cells in culture can be extended by at least one of the EBV cloned DNA fragments (p31) but whether immortality can indeed be induced in these cells is still not clear.

Milk cells have also been transfected with SV40 DNA and about 4 weeks post-transfection foci of viable cells were observed emerging from and in between quiescent colonies of milk epithelial cells (S. Chang). At 6 weeks these foci were big enough to be removed and were cultured independently. Most of the foci selected gave rise to cells that eventually reach a crisis stage from which, to date, none have survived. However, one focus termed "B" has been cultured for over 3 months (8 passages) without it passing through any obvious crisis stage. It is still too early to say whether these cells, like the fR lines, can be cultured indefinitely.

The uncloned B cells are morphologically heterogenous (Fig. 9) and do not resemble any of the fR lines or the pre-crisis SV40 transformed milk cell strains previously isolated (14). By indirect immunofluorescence SV40 large T-antigen is seen to be expressed in the nuclei of B cells

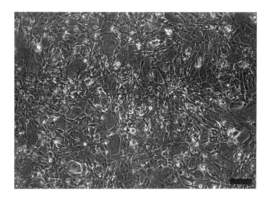

Fig. 9.   SV40 transfected milk epithelial cells B at passage 5.
Bar represents 50 μm.

showing that they are SV40 transformed.   The epithelial nature of the
cells is demonstrated by the presence of the LE61 keratin 18 antigen in
their cytoplasm (Fig. 10A).   In addition these cells express the keratin
19 antigen detected by BA16 (Fig. 10B).   As in many of the fR lines, the
keratin antigens in the B cells are condensed and often appear as a
perinuclear ring in contrast to the filamentous network seen in primary
milk cultures (Fig. 4A;   14) and breast cancer lines (1).   There is only
a limited expression of the fibronectin antigens recognized by FN3 or
FN4 and in early passages this is seen primarily as a punctate pattern
(data not shown) similar to that observed on primary milk cultures (45).
Finally, the B cells do express the breast differentiation HMFG-1 antigen
(Fig. 11) and at levels apparently greater than that on any of the fR
lines (data not shown).

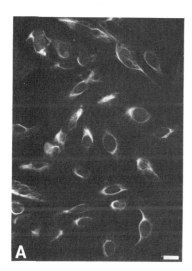 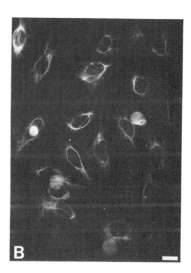

Fig. 10.   Immunofluorescence staining of B cells for the cytokeratin
antigen recognized by (A) LE61 (36) and (B) BA16 (50).   Bars
represent 20 μm.

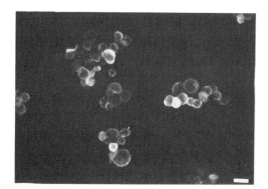

Fig. 11.   Immunofluorescence screening for the breast epithelial
membrane differentiation antigen HMFG-1 (38,39) on live B cells.
Bar represents 20 μm.

CONCLUSIONS

It is evident from the above summary that the recently isolated B cells (although not yet fully characterized nor cloned) represent an SV40 transformed milk epithelial cell phenotype that is quite different from the fR lines (14).   These differences are summarized in Table 1. In expressing the BA16 keratin 19 antigen it is likely that the B cells are related not only to the major proportion (80-90%) of colonies in primary milk cultures which are known to express this antigen (50) but also to malignant breast carcinomas which show a homogenously positive reaction with the BA16 reagent (61).   The fR cells, in contrast, seem to be related to a minor colony population (10-20%) in milk cultures and to isolated and small groups of lumenal epithelial cells in the breast which do not express the BA16 antigen.   In addition it is also possible that the fR cells may be related to some of the cells found in fibroadenomas since a large percentage (5-50%) of cells in these benign tumours are usually BA16 negative (61).

In considering possible models for the relationship between BA16 negative (-) and positive (+) cells in the secretory lineage, Bartek et al (61) have postulated that the 19(-) cell is a precursor to the 19(+) cell which is at a later stage of differentiation and has less growth potential than the 19(-) cell.   If this were the case then it would be expected that the presence of 19(-) cells would be correlated with good growth potential, explaining why it is much easier to culture epithelial cells from normal breast and benign lesions (fibroadenomas) than it is to culture cells from primary breast tumours (62,63).   In this context it may be relevant that the fR cells (19-) have a shorter doubling time than the B cells (19+).

The data presented in this paper demonstrates how invaluable immuno-logical markers are for establishing the relationship between different breast epithelial cells _in vivo_ and _in vitro_.   With the markers currently available it could be argued that the fR and B cells are related to cells in milk cultures and in normal and malignant breast tissue as is shown in Fig. 12.

The _in vitro_ transformation studies described in this paper raise an important point, namely that the target cell for transformation _in vivo_ may be determined by circumstance and the type of transforming agent or

Table 1.	Monoclonal Antibodies			
	Human milk fat globule	Cytokeratins		Fibronectins
Cells	HMFG-1	18 (LE61)	19 (BA16)	FN3 and FN4
Primary Milks (heterogenous)	+++ (55-60%)	+++	+++ (85% of colonies)	(+) (punctate)
SV40 Transformed Milk Cells				
⌐fR2 (cuboidal)	+++	++	-	++ (ECM)
└fR5 (elongate)	-	- odd +	-	++ (ECM)
B (passage 5) (heterogenous)	+++	+++	++	(+) (punctate) (some ECM)
Normal Breast	-	+++	+++ odd - (singly & in groups)	ND
Fibroadenomas (benign tumour)	- ➔ +	+++	- (5-50%)	ND
Malignant Breast Tumours	+ ➔ +++	+++	+++ (>95%)	ND
Breast Cancer Cell Lines	++ ➔ +++	+++	+++	+ (punctate)

Reaction of monoclonal antibodies with breast cells in vitro and in vivo. Monoclonal antibodies: HMFG-1 (38,39); LE61 (36); BA16 (50); FN3 and FN4 (45). Data compiled from following publications: 1,2,12,14,38, 39,40,45,50 and 61. ECM: extracellular matrix.

222

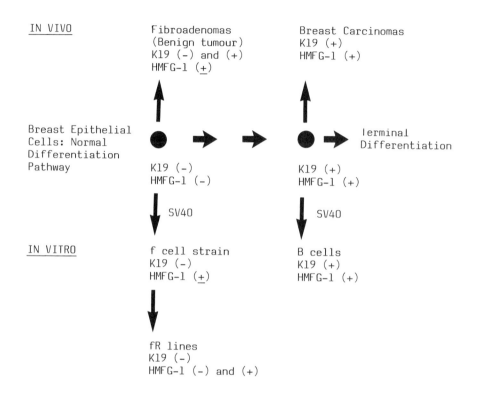

IN VIVO   Fibroadenomas   Breast Carcinomas
                 (Benign tumour)   K19 (+)
                 K19 (−) and (+)   HMFG-1 (+)
                 HMFG-1 (+)

Breast Epithelial   Terminal
Cells: Normal   Differentiation
Differentiation
Pathway   K19 (−)   K19 (+)
                 HMFG-1 (−)   HMFG-1 (+)

                    SV40   SV40

IN VITRO   f cell strain   B cells
                 K19 (−)   K19 (+)
                 HMFG-1 (+)   HMFG-1 (+)

                 fR lines
                 K19 (−)
                 HMFG-1 (−) and (+)

Fig. 12.   A model of the possible relationship between the SV40
transformed milk epithelial fR lines and B cells and epithelial cells
in the secretory lineage of the breast.

event. By using the same transforming agent (SV40) and two different approaches (viral infection and DNA transfection) two different types, 19(-) and 19(+), of SV40 transformed breast epithelial cells have been isolated. In making this point, however, it should be noted that when the fR lines were being isolated putative SV40 transformed BA16 keratin 19(+) cells may have been lost during the first soft agar selection step (Fig. 2). This is an important consideration since the B cells, to date, do not grow in soft agar (i.e. they are not anchorage independent) in contrast to the fR lines which grow efficiently in agar. It is quite possible, therefore, that the B cells, although expressing SV40 large T-antigen as detected by indirect immunofluorescence, may only be partially transformed i.e. immortalized. If this is the case it would be interesting to compare their behaviour with that of the two lines isolated from reduction mammoplasty organoids following benzo(a)pyrene treatment (64). These two lines show an apparently unlimited growth potential in vitro and do not exhibit any "transformed" characteristics.

The B cells, if immortal, could prove to be a suitable recipient human epithelial cell type into which one might introduce cloned onco-genes e.g. Harvey ras, adenovirus E1B, etc., which have been classified as "transforming" by experiments using immortal rodent fibroblast cells (e.g. 3,56,57,65). Assuming that fully transformed B cells would be anchorage independent we could use growth in soft agar as a selective procedure for isolating these cells. In addition it would be interesting to see what effects oncogenes have on differentiation and growth properties of the B cells, particularly in collagen matrixes where full expression of differentiated functions by human mammary epithelial cells is more likely to be obtained than on plastic (2,66,67).

When this project was conceived the aim of it was to establish in vitro cell lines which clearly expressed characteristics typical of the different cell types found in milk cultures. This paper summarizes our work and shows that it has been possible to achieve our objectives and in the process we may have developed an approach which could help us tackle the difficult problem of how epithelial differentiation and can-cer are related in the human breast.

ACKNOWLEDGEMENTS

I thank Jacqueline Keen (ICRF) and Kathy Dixon (MCMF) for their technical assistance, Patricia Purkis and Angela Lewin for milk samples and Jean Marr for typing this manuscript. I also thank Birgitte Lane, Jiri Bartek, Joy Burchell and Margaret Knowles for their helpful discussions and gifts of monoclonal antibodies, and Joyce Taylor-Papadimitriou for her support and encouragement.

REFERENCES

1. Taylor-Papadimitriou, J., Lane, E.B. and Chang, S.E. In: Understanding Breast Cancer (Eds. M.A. Rich, J.C. Hager and P. Furmanski), Marcel Dekker, Inc., 1983, pp. 215-246.
2. Taylor-Papadimitriou, J., Bartek, J., Durban, E., Burchell, J., Hallowes, R.C., Lane, E.B. and Millis, R. Martinus Nijhoff, in press, 1985.
3. Land, H., Parada, L.F. and Weinberg, R.A. Science 222: 771-778, 1983.
4. Bishop, J.M. Ann. Rev. Biochem. 52: 301-354, 1983.
5. Stampfer, M., Hallowes, R.C. and Hackett, A.J. In Vitro 16: 415-425, 1980.
6. Hallowes, R.C., Bone, E.J. and Jones, W. In: Tissue Culture in Medical Research II (Eds. R.J. Richards and K.T. Kajan) 1980, pp. 213-220.
7. Holquist, D.G. and Papanicolou, G.N. Ann. N. Y. Acad. Sci. 63: 1422-1435, 1956.
8. Buehring, G.C. J. Natl. Cancer Inst. 49: 1433-1434, 1972.
9. Taylor-Papadimitriou, J., Shearer, M. and Tilley, R. J. Natl. Cancer Inst. 58: 1563-1571, 1977.
10. Taylor-Papadimitriou, J., Fentiman, I.S. and Burchell, J. In: Cell Biology of Breast Cancer (Eds. C.M. McGrath, M.J. Brennan and M.A. Rich) Academic Press, 1980, pp. 347-362.
11. Stoker, M., Perryman, M. and Eeles, R. Proc. Soc. London. Ser. B 215: 231-240, 1982.
12. Chang, S.E. and Taylor-Papadimitriou, J., Cell Diff. 12: 143-154, 1983.
13. McKay, I. and Taylor-Papadimitriou, J. Exp. Cell Res. 134: 465-470, 1981.
14. Chang, S.E., Keen, J., Lane, E.B. and Taylor-Papadimitriou, J. Cancer Res. 42: 2040-2053, 1982.
15. Rafferty, K.A., Ruben, R.L. and Young, S.K. In Vitro. 14: 227-235, 1978.
16. Ruben, R.L. and Rafferty, K.A. Growth. 42: 357-368, 1978.
17. Kaighn, M.E., Narayan, K.S., Ohnuki, Y., Jones, L.W. and Lechner, J.F. Carcinogenesis. 1: 635-645, 1980.
18. Steinberg, M.L. and Defendi, V. Proc. Natl. Acad. Sci. USA. 76: 801-805, 1979.
19. Taylor-Papadimitriou, J., Purkis, P., Lane, E.B., McKay, I. and Chang, S. Cell Differentiation. 11: 169-180, 1982.
20. Giradi, A.J., Jensen, F.C. and Koprowski, H. J. Cell. Comp. Physiol. 65: 69-84, 1965.

21. Rodgers, C.S., Hill, S.M., Hulten, M.A., Chang, S.E., Keen, J. and Taylor-Papadimitriou, J. Cancer Genetics and Cytogenetics. **8**: 213-221, 1983.
22. Nelson-Rees, W.A., Flandermeyer, R.R., Hawthorne, P.K. Int. J. Cancer. **16:** 74-82, 1975.
23. Cruciger, Q.V.J., Pathak, S., Cailleau, R. Cytogenet. Cell Genet. **17**, 231-25, 1976.
24. Kakati, S., Hayata, I., Sandberg, A.A. Cancer. **37**: 776-782, 1976.
25. Seman, G., Hunter, S.J., Miller, R.C., Dmochowski, L. Cancer **37**: 1814-1824, 1976.
26. Kovacs, G. Int. J. Cancer **21**: 688-694, 1978.
27. Kovacs, G. Cancer Genet. Cytogenet. **3**: 125-129, 1981.
28. Rowley, J.D. Virchows Arch. (Cell Pathol.) **29**: 139-144, 1978.
29. Pathak, S. Cancer Genet. Cytogenet. **1**: 281-289, 1980.
30. Satya-Prakash, K.L., Pathak, S., Hsu, T.C., Olive, M., Cailleau, R. Cancer Genet. Cytogenet. **3**, 61-73, 1981.
31. Rodgers, C.S., Hill, S.M. and Hulten, M.A. Cancer Genetics and Cytogenetics **13**: 95-119, 1984.
32. Rodgers, C.S., Hill, S.M. and Hulten, M.A. Cancer Genetics and Cytogenetics **15**: 113-117, 1985.
33. Clark, R., Lane, D.P. and Tjian, R. J. Biol. Chem. **256**: 11854-11858, 1981.
34. Franke, W. W., Appelhans, B., Schmid, E., Freudenstein, C., Osborn, M. and Weber, K. Differentiation **15**: 7-25, 1979.
35. Sun, T.-T., Shih, C. and Green, H. Proc. Natl. Acad. Sci. USA. **76**: 2813-2817, 1979.
36. Lane, E.B. J. Cell Biol. **92**: 665-673, 1982.
37. Shimizu, M. and Yamauchi, K. J. Biochem. **91**: 515-524, 1982.
38. Arklie, J., Taylor-Papadimitriou, J., Bodmer, W., Egan, M. and Millis, R. Int. J. Cancer **28**: 23-29, 1981.
39. Taylor-Papadimitriou, J., Peterson, J.A., Arklie, J., Burchell, J., Ceriani, R.L. and Bodmer, W.F. Int. J. Cancer **28**: 17-21, 1981.
40. Taylor-Papadimitriou, J., Burchell, J. and Chang, S. In: Monoclonal Antibodies and Cancer (Eds. Boss, B.D., Langman, R., Trowbridge, I. and Dulbecco, R.) Academic Press, 1983, pp 227-238.
41. Burchell, J., Durbin, H. and Taylor-Papadimitriou, J. J. Immunol. **131**: 508-513, 1983.
42. Yamada, K.M. and Olden, K. Nature **275**: 179-184, 1978.
43. Tamkun, J.W. and Hynes, R. O. J. Biol. Chem. **258**: 4641-4647, 1983.
44. Hynes, R. O. and Destree, A.T. Proc. Nat. Acad. Sci. USA. **74**: 2855-2859, 1977.
45. Keen, J., Chang, S.E. and Taylor-Papadimitriou, J. Mol. Biol. Med. **2**: 15-27, 1984.
46. Taylor-Papadimitriou, J., Burchell, J. and Hurst, J. Cancer Res. **41**: 2491-2500, 1981.
47. Hackett, A.J., Smith, H.S., Springer, E. L., Owens, R. B., Nelson-Rees, W. A., Riggs, J. L. and Gardner, M. B. J. Natl. Cancer Inst. **58**: 1795-1806, 1977.
48. Shibata, H. and Taylor-Papadimitriou, J. Int. J. Cancer **28**: 447-453, 1981.
49. Wilkinson, M. J. S., Howell, A., Harris, M., Taylor-Papadimitriou, J., Swindell, R. and Sellwood, R.A. Int. J. Cancer **33**: 299-304, 1984.
50. Bartek, J., Durban, E.M., Hallowes, R.C. and Taylor-Papadimitriou, J. J. Cell Sci., in press, 1984.

51. Wu, U.-J. and Rheinwald, J.G. Cell 25: 627-635, 1981.
52. Moll, R., Franke, W. W., Schiller, D.L., Geiger, B. and Krepler, R. Cell 31: 11-24, 1982.
53. Fasano, O., Birnbaum, D., Edlund, L., Fogh, J. and Wigler, M. Mol. and Cell Biol. 4: 1695-1705, 1984.
54. Kraus, M.H., Yuasa, Y. and Aaronson, S.A. Proc. Natl. Acad. Sci. USA. 81: 5384-5388, 1984.
55. Graham, F.L. and Van der Eb, A.J. Virology 52: 456-467, 1973.
56. Land, H., Parada, L.F. and Weinberg, R.A. Nature 304: 596-602, 1983.
57. Ruley, H.E. Nature 304: 602-606, 1983.
58. Hynes, N.E., Jaggi, R., Kozma, S.C., Ball, R., Muellener, D., Wetherall, N.T., Davis, B.W. and Groner, B. Mol. and Cell. Biol. 5: 268-272, 1985.
59. Griffin, B.E. and Karran, L. Nature 309: 78-82, 1984.
60. Griffin, B.E., Karran, L., King, D. and Chang, S.E. In: Viruses and Cancer (Eds. P.W.J. Rigby and N.M. Wilkie). Soc. for General Micro-biology, Sym. 37. Cambridge Univ. Press, 1985, pp93-110.
61. Bartek, J., Taylor-Papadimitriou, J., Miller, N. and Millis, R. Submitted for publication, 1985.
62. Hallowes, R.C., Millis, R., Pigott, D., Shearer, M., Stoker, M.G.P. and Taylor-Papadimitriou, J. Clin. Oncol. 3: 81-90, 1977.
63. Taylor-Papadimitriou, J. and Fentiman, I.S. In: Commentaries on Research in Breast Disease 2. (Eds. Bulbrook, R.D. and Taylor, D.J.) Alan R. Liss, N.Y., 1981, pp87-107.
64. Stampfer, M.R. and Bartley, J.C. Proc. Nat. Acad. Sci. USA. In press, 1985.
65. Newbold, R.F. and Overell, R.W. Nature 304: 648-651, 1983.
66. Foster, C.S., Smith, C.A., Dinsdale, E.A., Monaghan, P. and Neville, A.M. Developmental Biol. 96: 197-216, 1983.
67. Durban, E., Butel, J.S., Bartek, J. and Taylor-Papadimitriou, J. Elsewhere in this volume.
68. Southern, E.M., J. Molec. Biol. 98: 503-517, 1975.

19

OF MICE AND WOMEN: GENETIC ANALYSIS OF BREAST CANCER IN FAMILIES

MARY-CLAIRE KING

School of Public Health, University of California, Berkeley, California, 94720, U.S.A.

Breast cancer is genetic, in the sense that breast tumor development is initiated by alterations--mutations, somatic recombinations, duplications, and so on--of DNA sequences in breast epithelial cells. These alterations may be inherited in the germ line, or may be due to somatic events induced by environmental mutagens. If an alteration is inherited in the germ line in a family, then an unusually large number of breast cancer cases are likely to appear in that family. If inherited alterations are common, then breast cancer will tend to cluster in families.

Familial clustering of breast cancer has been confirmed for a wide variety of populations at low and high risk (1, 2). Familial clustering probably reflects the presence of several different forms of inherited susceptibility to breast cancer in a population, as well as familial clusters of cases caused by common environmental exposures or shared ways of life increasing breast cancer risk. If different susceptibility genes or combinations of genes occur in different families, this genetic heterogeneity may appear at the epidemiological level as clustering of breast cancer with specific other cancers in the same family, as increased risk associated with particular ages, by the presence of male breast cancer, by frequent bilateral tumors, by particular histologic type, by anomalous hormonal profiles, or by other risk factors specific to a subset of susceptible families (3).

DNA Sequences in Breast Carcinogenesis

The DNA sequences involved in the expression of breast cancer at the cellular level may be the same whether the sequence is inherited in altered form or is altered in somatic cells by environmental carcinogens. Thus, families in which inherited genetic alterations increase susceptibility to breast cancer may serve as "human models" for identifying genes involved in the development of either familial or non-familial breast cancer. That is, families with inherited breast cancer susceptibility provide the chance to test the role in human tumorigenesis of inherited alterations in sequences potentially related to breast cancer development (4). Oncogenes and human sequences related to mouse mammary tumor virus (MMTV) are two classes of candidates for such inherited alterations.

In the past few years, more than 20 oncogenes have been isolated from human tumor cell lines (5). The normal human genome contains DNA sequences homologous to these oncogenes. For several oncogenes, the difference between DNA from normal individuals vs tumor appears to be one nucleotide substitution in an oncogene sequence. For example, for a patient with lung carcinoma associated with cigarette smoking (and not inherited susceptibility), a single mutation in $\underline{ras}^K$ appears in tumor tissue but not normal tissue of the same patient (6). Similarly, ovarian carcinoma tissue contains an activated $\underline{ras}^K$ gene, whereas normal cells from the same patient lack transforming activity (7). Mammary tumors in rats induced by nitrosomethylurea yield DNA which transforms 3T3 cells. The oncogenes from these mammary tumors appear to be members of the $\underline{ras}$ family (8). However, a DNA transforming sequence has not been isolated from human breast adenocarcinoma. The key to the role of oncogenes in human breast cancer may be the amount of normal $\underline{ras}$ protein in tumor tissue. Elevated levels of the p21 $\underline{ras}$ protein have been detected in 11 of 15 human breast intraductal carcinomas (Schlom, pers comm.). Elevation of normal p21 levels specifically in breast tumors could reflect alterations in integration sites or flanking sequences of oncogenes, which unlike transforming sequences could be inherited without immediate consequences for the carrier. The $\underline{c-myc}$ oncogene sequence itself appears to be amplified in one of five human breast cancer cell lines (9), supporting both the possible role of $\underline{myc}$ in some breast cancer development and the genetic heterogeneity of breast cancer. Thus, alterations in sequences regulating oncogene amplification or expression are candidates for inherited sequences increasing susceptibility to breast cancer.

The mouse mammary tumor virus is, of course, implicated in mammary carcinogenesis in mice. Though viral particles do not appear to be associated with human breast carcinogenesis, sequences homologous to regions of MMTV, integrated into the human genome, may play a role. The gp 52 protein of MMTV appears to be a receptor for progesterone and dexamethasone in mice (10). Antibodies reactive with MMTV have been found in sera of human breast cancer patients more frequently than in controls, and in sera of healthy members of families with high incidence of breast cancer (11). It is therefore reasonable to ask whether mutations altering the regulation of human sequences homologous to MMTV may be associated with inherited susceptibility to human breast cancer. A human sequence homologous to the MMTV int-1 sequence whose integration is associated with C3H mouse mammary carcinogenesis has been identified and mapped to human chromosome 12 (12). In BR6 mice, newly integrated proviruses induced by MMTV consistently appear adjacent to a different sequence, int-2 (13). Int-2 is not homologous to either MMTV or int-1. The human sequence homologous to int-2 maps to chromosome 11q13 (14). Int-2 expression appears in vitro to be associated with differentiation of mouse mammary tumor cells (15). Finally, the human sequence homologous to the gp 52 region of MMTV has been isolated and cloned (16). The circumstances under which this hlm sequence is expressed in humans are not yet understood, but multiple copies appear in the human genome, none adjacent to an int sequence (17).

Genetics of Breast Cancer in Families

What is the relevance of these sequences, all expressed either in tumor tissue or tumor cell lines, to breast cancer in human families? In large families with many cases of breast cancer, it is possible to test statistically whether the pattern of cancer occurrence is consistent with genetic inheritance of susceptibility (18). If inherited susceptibility to breast cancer exists in the family, it is possible--at least in principle--to locate the sequence responsible through genetic linkage analysis (1,19).

The hypothetical family in the figure illustrates linkage analysis. Suppose the observed pattern of breast cancer occurrence in this family is consistent with autosomal dominant inheritance of breast cancer susceptibility, although the sequence conferring susceptibility maybe unknown. In order to try to identify the susceptibility sequence in this family, we first obtain, for every person in the pedigree, the current age or age at death, whether the individual had cancer, and if so, at what site. We also obtain blood samples for genetic marker analysis from each living member of the family. Red cells and plasma are used to type protein markers; lymphocytes are immortalized and DNA extracted from each subject's cell line for analysis of DNA polymorphisms. Possible results for a marker with three common alleles A, B, and C might be as illustrated in the figure. The marker could be detected at either the DNA or protein level; the principle of linkage is the same.

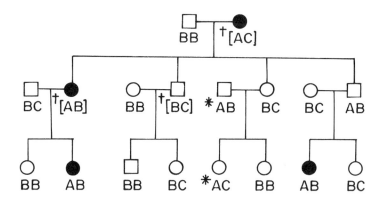

Hypothetical family with breast cancer, analyzed at a
marker locus with three alleles. Dark circles represent women
with breast cancer, whose disease susceptibility is consistent
with autosomal dominant inheritance, and crosses indicate
deceased individuals, whose genotypes at marker loci can be
assigned probabilistically, based on the marker genotypes of
their relatives. Such "reconstructed" genotypes are in
brackets.

The putative autosomal dominant allele increasing susceptibility to breast cancer among women in the family shown in the figure above may be linked to allele A on one of the grandmother's chromosomes. A larger family than this one (or several families with the same pattern) would be required to confirm the linkage. Other families in which linkage of breast cancer susceptibility to this marker appears likely would not necessarily show linkage to allele A. Furthermore, allele A does not in itself indicate breast cancer susceptibility in this family: only if allele A represents the grandmother's chromosome and recombination between the susceptibility allele and the marker locus has not occurred. In other words, linkage between a susceptibility allele and a marker locus does not imply that any particular genotype at the marker locus will be associated with disease susceptibility in the general population or even among a group of high-risk families.

Oncogenes and MMTV-related sequences are good candidates for genetic markers for linkage analysis of breast cancer in families. Suppose breast tumor development involves alterations at two genetic loci. In highly susceptible families, one of these alterations could be inherited, with the alteration at the other locus a somatic event. By itself the inherited alteration is innocuous. However, an environmentally induced or spontaneous mutation, translocation, or transposition might occur in breast epithelial cells in some women in this family in a different critical sequence. In this speculation, at least two mutations, in different genes, are required for cancer development (20). Inheritance of susceptibility in this case would be linked to a polymorphism near the sequence with the inherited alteration. In order to detect linkage, it would not be necessary to know the exact inherited alteration, or even to identify the sequences involved in the subsequent somatic events. Thus, linkage provides an approach for detecting the involvement of more than one locus in carcinogenesis, when one alteration is inherited and other changes result from somatic mutation.

In screening ocogene sequences for linkage to breast cancer susceptibility, we would not expect to detect inherited alterations crucial to tumor development in ras sequences themselves, because such ras alterations are probably lethal. However, altered integration of normal ras sequences that lead to elevated expression could be heritable in normal cells. Altered integration could be detected by linkage analysis, either as a change in a flanking sequence or associated with an innocuous polymorphism in a ras sequence in that family.

As the hypothetical family in the figure indicates, a marker will only be useful for genetic analysis if several alleles can be distinguished. Thus, sequences of importance to mammary carcinogenesis can be used as markers only if they are polymorphic. The polymorphisms need not occur at sites involved in the sequence's function. It is only necessary to be able to test for coinheritance of any one form of the sequence with breast cancer in the family. If one allelic form of the sequence is consistently inherited with breast cancer susceptibility, then that sequence can be isolated and the specific alterations responsible for susceptibility can be identified.

Detecting polymorphism in a known sequence, for the purpose of using the sequence in linkage analysis, is straightforward. DNA from five to ten unrelated individuals is extracted from white cells. Each sample is digested with several restriction enzymes. For each enzyme, banding patterns of all samples probed with the sequence are compared. If more than one pattern appears among the few individuals for a particular enzyme-probe combination, a polymorphism is possible. To confirm that the variation is genetic, it is most efficient to test the inheritance of the patterns in healthy families with several children. The informative families will be those in which the parents differ in restriction pattern. By comparing parents and children, the genetics of the polymorphism can be determined (21).

Suppose that none of the oncogenes or MMTV-like sequences are linked to breast cancer in a family with many cases of the disease. Genetic linkage analysis in such families can nevertheless be used to identify sequences responsible for inherited susceptibility, even if the function of the sequence is completely unknown. The genetic analysis of retenoblastoma in families is an example of this approach. (22, 23). Inherited susceptibility to retinoblastoma occurs in some families as a result of two alterations at the same locus, one inherited and one somatic. That is, susceptibility is inherited as a dominant trait, but the alleles responsible for malignant transformation are recessive at the cellular level. The function of the sequence is unknown. Transformation assays would not detect susceptibility genes of this sort. However, such a sequence would lie somewhere in the human genome and must therefore be linked to a genetic marker. Thus, linkage analysis can detect the sequence. The analogous pattern for breast cancer could occur in a family in which susceptibility is consistent with segregation of a dominant susceptibility gene. This susceptibility might not necessarily be linked to any oncogene or other known sequence potentially involved in breast cancer development, but could be located by screening probes throughout the genome.

Success in locating a susceptibility gene of completely unknown function is "simply" a matter of testing enough highly polymorphic markers in extremely informative families. Even if a breast cancer susceptibility allele is segregating in a family, it is only possible to demonstrate linkage to a marker locus if such a polymorphic marker locus happens to be on the same chromosome as the susceptibility gene, and to be reasonably close to it. Since not all genetic markers are segregating in informative patterns in all families, a great many markers are requred to "cover" the 23 chromosomes. While the human genome is by no means completely "covered" by markers at present, extraordinary progress has been made in the last two years so that many markers are now available at the DNA level (24).

The historical limitation of linkage analysis was the difficulty of developing adequate numbers of polymorphic genetic markers based on assays of protein products of marker genes. At least 150 markers are required to obtain a marker in reasonably close linkage with a gene of unknown location (say, 10% recombination); only about 30 protein markers are available today. The estimate of 150 is based on the knowledge that the human chromosome map is 3000 percentage units of recombination long, and that for a marker to be within 10% recombination of an unknown gene, the ideal set of 150 markers would be equally spaced at 20% recombination distance. If markers are less evenly spaced, many more are required to cover the genome (25).

As they become available, DNA probes obtained as random chromosome fragments that detect the presence of individual differences will supply enough genetic markers. There is a least one difference between two individuals (i.e. a polymorphism, hence potentially a marker) at a nucleotide site every 1000 nucleotides (26). Of the total 3 billion nucleotides in human haploid DNA there are therefore potentially 3 million polymorphisms, of which a substantial fraction can be detected using all known enzymes; about 10% are detectable using restriction enzymes easily and cheaply available. This yields roughly 300,000 potential markers in the human genome.

Today there are about 200 DNA probes known and potentially useful for testing for polymorphisms. However, these 200 probes are not equally spaced on the chromosomes but are more randomly scattered. When more knowledge is available about chromosomal locations of probes, markers too close together can be avoided. Additional mapping information will also permit us to fill long gaps in the human map from the markers available. Today, the collection of fully desirable markers is still incomplete but will improve rapidly, since a large number of laboratories around the world are working at this task (24).

Recent applications of recombinant DNA techniques to human genetics have already revolutionized linkage analysis of genetic disease. It is now possible, in priniciple, to obtain genetic markers arbitrarily close to a gene of known sequence. This procedure was first applied to the diagnosis of sickle cell anemia in utero (27, 28). The application of linkage analysis to breast cancer is far more difficult because genes responsible for inherited susceptibility to the disease have not been identified, because different genes are likely to be involved in different families, and because disease onset is fairly late in life. However, the approach of linkage analysis can now be extended to any disease for which individual genes influence susceptibility, by using random DNA segments (19). This approach has already been successfully applied for the case of Huntington's chorea (29), which like breast cancer is a late-onset disease of unknown etiology, for which very large families provided the critical information. The degree of probable etiologic heterogeneity of breast cancer makes the analysis of individual large families even more crucial.

By identifying genes responsible for breast cancer susceptibility in high-risk families, it becomes possible to determine the mode of expression of the susceptibility genes. Mechanisms of carcinogenesis for inherited breast cancer susceptibility are likely to explain breast cancer in the population as a whole. By investigating the expression of susceptibility genes in families, it may also be possible to identify particular ways of life, such as diet, childbearing practices, or hormone use, that decrease or exacerbate inherited risk.

Supported in part by N.I.H. grant CA27632.

REFERENCES

1. King MC, Lee GT, Spinner NR, Thomson G, Wrensch MR. 1984. Ann Rev Pub Hlth 5:1-52.

2. Schwartz AG, King MC, Belle SH, Satariano WA, Swanson GM. 1985. J Nat Cancer Inst (in press).

3. King MC, Elston RC. 1985. Genet Epid 2 (In press).

4. Weinberg RA. 1983. Scientific American 247:126-142.

5. Cooper GM. 1982. Science 217:801-806.

6. Santos E. Martin-Zanca D, Reddy EP, Pierotti MA, Della Porta G, Barbacid M. 1984. Science 223:661-664.

7. Feig LA, Bast RC, Knapp RC, Cooper GM. 1984. Science 223:698-701.

8. Sukumar S, Notario V, Martin-Zanca D, Barbacid M. 1983. Nature 306:658-661.

9. Kozbar D, Croce CM. 1984. Cancer Res 44:438-441.

10. Harris LF, Bates HA, Miller LL, Crutchfield CE, Henderson BA, Hickok DF. 1985. Int Assoc Breast Cancer Res Proceedings, p.74

11. Day NK, Witkin SS, Sarkar NH, Kinne D, Jussawalla DJ, Levin A, Hsia CC,ler N, Good RA. 1981. Proc Natl Acad Sci USA 78:2483-2487.

12. Nusse R, Varmus HE. 1982. Cell 31:99-109.

13. Peters G, Brookes S, Smith R, Dickson C. 1983. Cell 33:369-377.

14. Casey G, Smith R, Brookes S, McGillivray D, Dickson C, Peters G. 1985. Int Assoc Breast Cancer Res Proceedings, p. 173.

15. Sonnenberg A, Nuse R, Hilgers J. 1985. Int Assoc Breast Cancer Res Proceedings, p. 114.

16. Callahan R, Drohan W, Tronick S, Schlom J. 1982. Proc Natl Acad Sci USA 79:5503-5507.

17. Callahan R, Ali I, Bassin R, Horn T, Mariani-Costantini R, Robbins J, Schlom J. 1985. Int Assoc Breast Cancer Res Proceedings, p. 36.

18. Go RCP, King MC, Bailey-Wilson J, Elston RC, Lynch HT. 1983. J Nat Cancer Inst 71:455-461.

19. White R, Leppart M, Bishop DT, Barker D, Berkowitz J, Brown C, Callahan P, Holm T, Jerominski L. 1985. Nature 313:101:101-105.

20. Land MA, Parada LF, Weinberg RA. 1983. Science 222:771-778.

21. Feder J, Yen L, Wijsman E, Wang L, Wilkins L, Schroder J, Spurr N, Cann H, Blumenberg M, Cavalli-Sforza L. 1985 Amer J Hum Genet. In press.

22. Cavanee WK, Dryja TP, Phillips RA, Benedict WF, Godbout R, Gallie B1, Murphree AL, Strong LC, White R1. 1983. Nature 305:779-784.

23. Cavanee WK, Hansen MF, Nordenskjold M, Kock E, Maumenee I, Squire JA, Phillips RA, Gallie BL. 1985. Science 228:501-503.

24. Human Gene Mapping 7. 1984. Cytogenet Cell Genet 37:Nos. 1-4.

25. Lange K, Boehnke M. 1982. Amer J Hum Genet 34:842-845.

26. Ewens WJ, Spielman RS, Harris H, 1981. Genetics 78:3748-3750.

27. Kan YW, Dozy AM. 1978. Lancet 2 (8096):910-912.

28. Chang JC, Kan YW. 1981. Lancet 2:1127-129.

29. Gusella JF, Wexler NS, Conneally PM , et al. 1983. Nature 306:234-238.

20

DIETARY FAT AND MAMMARY CARCINOGENESIS

CLEMENT IP

Department of Breast Surgery, Roswell Park Memorial Institute,
Buffalo, New York 14263, USA

INTRODUCTION

Nutritional modification of mammary carcinogenesis has been
a growing area of research in the past decade because of the
increasing awareness that dietary deficiencies, excesses, and
imbalances can play an important role in the pathogenesis of
cancer. This chapter will attempt to summarize the effects of
dietary fat on the development of mammary tumors in laboratory
animals. Because of limited space, a comprehensive treatment of
the subject has to be sacrificed; hopefully, it will not be at
the expense of succinctness and relevance. My approach is to
focus on certain significant observations in this area of
research, and where appropriate, to weave in some pertinent data
from our laboratory.

Evidence that a high fat diet increased the incidence of
spontaneous mammary tumors in mice was first reported by
Tannenbaum in 1942 (1). For the next 25 years, there were only a
few publications in the literature showing that chemically-
induced mammary carcinogenesis was also increased in rats with a
high fat intake. Starting in 1967, Carroll and co-workers
published a series of papers examining the influence of dietary
fat on DMBA-induced mammary tumorigenesis in female Sprague-
Dawley rats (2-6). These studies ignited a revival of interest
which has remained unabated as evidenced by the proliferation of
publications in recent years.

It should be noted that a diet rich in fat is also high in
calories, but pair-feeding experiments have indicated that
dietary fat has an effect that is independent of caloric
intake (7). Enhanced mammary tumorigenesis, as a result of
increasing dietary fat, has now been demonstrated in an

impressive array of spontaneous, carcinogen-induced, X-
irradiation-induced, transplantable, benign, and malignant
experimental mammary tumor models in both rats and mice. For a
comprehensive survey of these studies, the reader should refer to
a recent review by Welsch and Aylsworth (8). In general, when
animals are fed a high fat diet, total mammary tumor yield is
increased. This parameter, which is perhaps the most sensitive
indicator, is very often accompanied by an increased tumor
incidence and a reduced latency period of tumor appearance. An
accelerated growth rate is frequently observed in the
transplantable tumor model. Although the susceptibility of the
mammary gland to chemically-induced neoplasia is decreased in
older rats, Chan and Dao (9) as well as our own laboratory (10)
have demonstrated that a high fat diet enhances mammary
tumorigenesis in old as well as young rats.

Levels and Types of Fat

A high fat diet can be formulated in one of three ways. The
simpliest way is to add fat directly to a basal regimen. It is a
crude method which has the effect of diluting native nutrients in
the basal mix. The dilution method is unacceptable to
nutritionists and should not be practised in any animal
experiments. In the substitution protocol, fat is substituted
for an equal weight of carbohydrate while protein, minerals,
vitamins, and fiber are maintained at a constant percentage by
weight. Adding fat to an animal diet increases the caloric
density of the diet. Rodents generally adjust their food
consumption so that similar energy intake is maintained even with
diets containing substantially different energy density.
Accordingly, with the substitution method, in addition to the
changes in fat and carbohydrate intake, the intake of protein,
minerals, vitamins, and fiber will all be lower in those animals
fed the high fat diet. This results in the comparison of the
effects of two different diets rather than the effect of dietary
fat. The correct way is the isocaloric method in which fat is
substituted for an equal weight of carbohydrate, while the

proportions of protein, minerals, vitamins, and fiber are
adjusted to maintain constant nutrient to calorie ratios. The
use of isocaloric diets has been discussed in detail by Visek and
Clinton (11), and should be adopted in all animal experimentation.

Investigators have examined different levels of fat in the
diet, ranging from a fat-free diet to one containing over 30% of
fat by weight. Comparisons of data among laboratories may become
difficult, since we are dealing here with two issues: that of
essential fatty acid (EFA) deficiency and excess fat intake. In
order to facilitate interpretation of results, I propose the use
of the AIN-76 semi-synthetic diet containing 5% corn oil as the
control. Studies involving a high fat diet can then be compared
against this standard formulation. When examining the effect of
a low fat diet, care should be exercised to insure that the diet
contains adequate EFA for growth of the animals.

In addition to quantity of fat, the type of fat also appears
to be important. Carroll and Khor (6) assessed the effect of ten
different fats present at the 20% level in the diet on the
occurrence of DMBA-induced mammary tumors in rats. They found
that in general, polyunsaturated fat diets gave a higher tumor
yield than did saturated fat diets. Similar observations have
been reported by other laboratories (12-17), including our
own (18). In further studies, Carroll and Hopkins (19)
demonstrated that diets containing 3% sunflower seed oil
(polyunsaturated fat) and 17% beef tallow or coconut oil
(saturated fats) enhanced tumorigenesis as much as did a diet
containing 20% sunflower seed oil. Rats on these diets developed
twice as many tumors as those fed diets containing 20% of the
saturated fats alone. These findings suggest that there may be a
requirement for polyunsaturated fat in mammary tumorigenesis,
which is not satisfied by fats such as coconut oil or beef
tallow. It is thought that linoleate may be the essential fatty
acid primarily responsible for the tumor promoting effect of
unsaturated fat (20). We were able to confirm the conclusion of
Carroll and Hopkins; however, the value we obtained for linoleate
requirement was around 4 to 5% based on regression analysis (21).

Human breast cancer mortality shows a strong positive correlation with total fat intake and little or no correlation with vegetable fat intake (22). In countries where fat intake is low, it is most likely that edible fats consist of predominantly polyunsaturates from plant sources. However, in countries where fat intake is high, a greater proportion tends to be saturated fat from animal sources. Unfortunately, epidemiological data cannot produce information on the EFA requirement for human breast cancer. Assuming such a requirement exists and is relatively low, most human diets are likely to supply enough EFA to permit an optimal tumor response. If this is the case, the conclusion of the above studies implies that once the EFA requirement for optimal tumor expression is met, further enhancement of development would depend on the amount and not on the type of dietary fat.

It is estimated that in the U.S., about 40% of dietary vegetable fats are partially hydrogenated during industrial processing in order to increase stability and to achieve the desired physical properties (23). Commercial hydrogenation of vegetable oils results in the introduction of trans fatty acids. We have investigated the effect of feeding a fat which contained approximately 38% trans isomers (designated trans fat) on the induction of mammary tumors by DMBA in rats (24). The corresponding control fat (designated as cis fat), which had a similar fatty acid composition, consisted of only cis isomers. Since both the trans and cis fats were rather saturated, a comparison was also made between these two types of fat and corn oil, which contains about 60% linoleic acid. Each fat was present in the diet at 2 levels, 5% and 20% by weight. It was found that diets containing either trans fat or cis fat were much less effective than were the corn oil diets in promoting the development of mammary neoplasia at either the 5 or 20% level. Our results thus suggest that trans fat behaves very much like a saturated fat in the modification of mammary tumorigenesis.

Most intriguing is the effect of fish oil. There are two recent reports, one dealing with the transplantable R3230AC mammary adenocarcinoma (25) and the other with the MNU-induced mammary tumor model (26), which show that a high intake of fish oil actually retarded tumor development. Fish oils are generally high in eicosapentaenoic acid and docosahexaenoic acid. These are long chain omega-3 polyunsaturated fatty acids with 5 and 6 double bonds, respectively. When the omega-3 fatty acids are ingested, they tend to replace omega-6 fatty acids in tissue lipids. The omega-3 fatty acids may exert their effects by competing with arachidonic acid for the cyclooxygenase enzyme, thereby lowering the formation of the 2-series prostaglandins. The significance of prostaglandins in carcinogenesis will be discussed in a little more detail in a later section.

Influence of dietary fat in the initiation versus promotion stage of mammary carcinogenesis

Carroll and Khor (5) have examined the effect of feeding a high corn oil diet before and after DMBA administration to rats at 50 days of age. They reported that fat intake prior to and at the time of carcinogenic injury had negligible effect, and it was the level of dietary fat given during the proliferative phase of tumorigenesis that determined the final tumor incidence. Borrowing from the two-stage carcinogenesis concept, it was suggested that dietary fat acts preferentially on the promotion phase. Using rats that were treated with DMBA at 150 days of age (these adult rats are more resistant to carcinogenesis) and the same protocol of fat feeding, we arrived at essentially the same conclusion (10). Furthermore, we found that an enhancement of mammary tumorigenesis could still be observed when the high corn oil diet was given as late as 20 weeks following carcinogen treatment. The hypothesis that fat has little influence on the initiation phase is supported by the finding of Gammal et al. (3) that the uptake and clearance of DMBA by the mammary gland was similar in rats fed either a high fat or a low fat diet.

However, the question remains as to the role of fat in the metabolism of DMBA, since fat intake is known to alter the hepatic microsomal mixed function oxygenase activity (27,28), an

enzyme system responsible for the activation and/or
detoxification of polycyclic hydrocarbons. In view of the
lipophilic nature of DMBA, any change in the body lipid
composition of the animal may also affect the distribution of the
carcinogen.

In order to obviate these variables that may influence the
initiation process, we performed an experiment in which mammary
gland explants from rats fed either a low fat or a high fat diet
were exposed to DMBA in organ culture before grafting to
recipients maintained on either one of two regimens. Results
indicated that tumor incidence was much lower in recipient rats
that were given a low fat diet, regardless of whether the transplant tissue came from donors that were fed either a low fat or a
high fat diet (29). Our experiment suggests that the action of
fat is primarily exerted at the promotion stage of carcinogenesis, and it is the fat intake of the host that governs the
subsequent neoplastic growth of transformed cells.

Rogers and co-workers (30) have examined the DNA labeling
index of terminal end buds, terminal ducts, alveolar buds and
lobules in the mammary glands of virgin rats fed either a 5% or a
20% corn oil diet. These parameters were measured at different
times ranging from weaning to about 150 days of age. No
significant differences were found between the two groups at any
time period examined. Whole mounts from the same rats actually
showed a slight but consistent increase in glandular
differentiation in rats fed the 5% fat diet. It appears from
these studies that a 20% corn oil diet retards differentiation
slightly but does not cause significant alteration in DNA
synthesis in the mammary gland in the time period during which
initiation and early growth of tumors occur.

All the studies described above have used corn oil as the
lipid source. We have also compared the effects of animal and
vegetable fats fed before and during DMBA administration on
mammary tumorigenesis. Weanling rats were divided into different
dietary treatment groups: 5% corn oil (reference control), 20%
corn oil, 20% palm oil, 20% beef tallow, or 20% lard. One week

following DMBA administration, all rats were switched to the 5%
corn oil control diet and were maintained on this diet until the
end of the experiment. Rats fed the 20% lard or beef tallow diet
during the treatment period showed a significant enhancement in
mammary tumor incidence and yield when compared with all other
dietary treatment groups (unpublished results). Mammary tumor
development in rats fed the 20% corn oil or palm oil diets did
not differ from the 5% corn oil control. It remains to be
determined whether animal fats contain certain carcinogenic or
co-carcinogenic agents that may potentiate the action of DMBA.

Is the effect of dietary fat mediated by a hormonal mechanism?

Several hormones have been implicated in the maintenance and
growth of mammary tumors in experimental animals, including
prolactin, estrogen, progesterone, glucocorticoids, growth
hormone, insulin and thyroxin. Of these hormones, prolactin and
estrogen have received the most attention. Mammary tumors do not
develop in animals that are either hypophysectomized or ovariectomized early in life. Similarly, injection of antagonists that
either inhibit the release of the hormone or interfere with the
intracellular action of the hormone very often leads to regression of existing tumors (31).

Reports from the laboratories of Chan (32) and Ip (33) have
shown that a high dietary fat intake increases serum prolactin
levels during proestrus-estrus. In contrast, results from the
laboratories of Cave (34), Carroll (35), Meites (36) and
Rogers (37) have failed to confirm these earlier findings. It is
interesting to point out that in those studies demonstrating an
increased circulating level of prolactin by dietary fat, comparisons were made between rats fed either a 0.5% or a 20% fat diet.
Blood was collected from anesthetized animals in both cases.
Those laboratories reporting no effect used rats that were feed
either a normal fat diet (3-5% fat) or a 20% fat diet. Diets
containing only 0.5% fat may be marginally deficient in essential
fatty acids, hence the differences in prolactin levels observed

by Chan and Ip may be due to depressed secretion in a nutritional deficient state. In the studies from the laboratories of Meites (36) and Rogers (37), the animals were fitted with atrial cannulas that allowed frequent blood sampling throughout the estrus cycle with minimal stress to the animals.

Chan et al. (38) have reported a slight but significant increase in total serum estrogens during metestrus-diestrus in rats fed a 20% lard diet, compared to those on a 5% lard diet. We have measured circulating estradiol levels during proestrus in rats fed 0.5%, 5% or 20% corn oil diets and found that the steroid was reduced only in rats fed the 0.5% fat diet (39). Hopkins et al. (35) and Wetsel et al. (37) have subsequently reported that high dietary fat does not influence serum estradiol or progesterone levels in the rat. Overall, there is little evidence to support the conclusion that high dietary fat intake increases prolactin and ovarian hormone secretion.

In an attempt to determine if the hormonal responsiveness of a target tissue can be modified by dietary fat through changes in receptor content, we have also examined estrogen and progesterone receptor levels in DMBA-induced mammary carcinomas (39). Estrogen receptor levels in the tumor were the same in the groups given 5% and 20% corn oil, but were slightly lower in the group given 0.5% corn oil. No differences was detected in the progesterone receptor concentration. In a subsequent study, we also found that the induction of progesterone receptor by estrogen in the uterus and in the MT-W9B transplantable mammary tumor was not altered by dietary fat intake (40). These data suggest that dietary fat does not influence the sensitivity of normal or neoplastic tissue to estrogen action.

Cave and Erickson-Lucas (41) observed that the concentration of prolactin receptors was increased in mammary tumors of rats fed a 20% corn oil diet when compared to those on a 0.5% corn oil diet. Using animals that were fed either a 5% or a 20% corn oil diet, Wetsel and Rogers (42) failed to detect any difference in hepatic prolactin binding. In a more recent study, Cave and Jurkowski (43) showed that there was no change in prolactin binding capacity in both mammary tumor and liver if the control diet contained at least 3% corn oil. As in the estrogen receptor data, it appears that animals fed a very low level of dietary fat have reduced prolactin receptors. But when normal fat intake is compared with high fat consumption, the difference is not readily apparent.

The evidence that the enhancing effect of a high fat diet is independent of altered secretion of estrogen and prolactin is clearly demonstrated in a recent article by Aylsworth et al. (44). In their study, sham-operated rats and ovariectomized rats were injected daily with haloperidol to increase prolactin secretion, bromocryptine to decrease prolactin secretion, and/or estradiol benzoate. They showed that a high fat diet was still capable of stimulating DMBA-induced mammary tumorigenesis even under conditions when the circulating levels of estradiol and prolactin were strictly controlled. The conclusion of this experiment is consistent with our earlier observation that the differential effect between a high and a low fat diet in promoting mammary tumorigenesis was still apparent in rats which were lesioned in the median eminence of the hypothalamus to increase the prolactin output in these animals (33).

We have also carried out a vehicle-controlled experiment to determine whether high dietary fat intake could affect the development of hormone-independent mammary tumors in rats that were made deficient in estrogen and prolactin by tamoxifen and bromocryptine injection during the first week after DMBA administration. At the end of the treatment period, rats were placed on either a 5% or a 20% corn oil diet for the duration of the experiment. Vehicle-treated rats were ovariectomized 27 weeks and drug-treated rats 47 weeks after DMBA to determine hormone dependency. Approximately 80% of tumors in the first group and 25% in the second group were hormone dependent, regardless of the fat intake of the host; however, a high fat diet stimulated tumorigenesis in both groups of animals (45). These results demonstrate that high dietary fat promotes the development of both hormone-dependent and hormone-independent tumors, and does not influence the hormonal responsiveness of these tumors.

Direct effect of fatty acids on mammary epithelial cells
in vitro

Kidwell and co-workers (46,47) have provided the most
convincing evidence that the growth of both normal and neoplastic
rat mammary epithelial cells was stimulated by the addition of
unsaturated fatty acids to a hormone enriched medium, but was
inhibited by the addition of saturated fatty acids. Linoleic
acid was found to reduce doubling time and to stimulate thymidine
incorporation, whereas stearic acid had the reverse effect. If
substitution of unsaturated fatty acids in the membrane phospholipids is a response to mitogenic stimulation of the mammary
cells, then analysis of the membranes from proliferating versus
nonproliferating epithelium should reveal these changes.
Injection of perphenazine, which caused a rapid proliferation of
the mammary epithelium, was associated with a decrease in total
amount of mammary fat and an increase in the relative abundance
of unsaturated fatty acids. The phospholipids of epithelial cell
membranes from the glands of perphenazine treated animals contained twice as much linoleic acid as those from the untreated
controls (47).

Administration of perphenazine is known to elevate serum
prolactin levels. When mammary explants were incubated with
prolactin, there was a release of free fatty acids into the
medium (47). The question is how does prolactin affect the
release of free fatty acids and what is the source? The evidence
points to the adipocytes that are adjacent to the epithelium.
First, the magnitude of the change in total fatty acid composition of the gland is so large that it must involve the mammary
adipocytes which contain over 90% of the total mammary lipids as
triglycerides. Secondly, prolactin addition to isolated mammary
epithelial cells actually enhanced the selective uptake of
unsaturated fatty acids into these cells rather than their
release, so that the total fatty acids concentration of the
growth medium was lowered.

Based on these experimental data, Kidwell and Shaffer (48)
advanced the following hypothesis to integrate the relationship
between mammary epithelium and mammary fat cells, mediated by a

third cell type, the mast cells. According to these authors, when the glandular epithelium is stimulated to proliferate by a hormone such as prolactin, the epithelium transmits a signal of undefined nature to the mast cells in the near vicinity. The mast cells then release histamine which in turn causes hydrolysis of triglycerides from the adipocytes. The saturated fatty acids are removed from the gland by the venous effluent. On the other hand, the unsaturated fatty acids are either reassimilated into triglycerides in fat cells or are taken up by the epithelial cells, supplanting the saturated fatty acids in membrane phospholipids.

Other mechanisms of action

The role of polyunsaturated fatty acids in regulating tumor development has not yet been elucidated. However, it is known that linoleate, via the intermediate arachidonic acid, can serve as the precursor of the prostaglandins and related compounds of both the cyclooxygenase and lipoxygenase pathways. Abraham and co-workers have published a series of papers on the inhibitory effect of prostaglandin synthesis antagonists on the growth of several transplantable mammary tumors in rats with a high fat intake (20,49,50). A similar observation has also been reported by Carter et al. in the DMBA-induced mammary tumor system (51). Prostaglandins have been known to play a role in the regulation of both humoral and cell-mediated immunity (52). It is beyond the scope of this chapter to review the involvement of prostaglandins in carcinogenesis. The underlying interaction between dietary fat, prostaglandins and the host defense mechanism in controlling neoplastic growth is not clear at the present time.

Since the growth promoting effect of fat on mammary tumorigenesis is more closely associated with polyunsaturated fats than with saturated fats, it is conceivable that certain unsaturated fatty acid metabolites, such as epoxides or peroxides, may be important in neoplastic cell proliferation. Slaga et al. (53) have recently reported that benzoyl peroxide is a promoter in the DMBA-induced skin tumor model. Shamberger (54) has also shown that the skin of mice treated with DMBA and croton oil exhibited greater peroxidation and produced more tumors than the skin treated with DMBA and croton resin. Extensive peroxidation is known to lead to structural and functional alterations in cellular components, and has been postulated to play a role in carcinogenesis (55). Malondialdehyde, a product of lipid peroxidation, has been shown to react with proteins and nucleic acids (56,57). Lipid peroxidation, although a normal occurrence in animal tissues, can lead to a host of deleterious effects in cells if it remains unchecked.

It has been proposed that intercellular communication may play a key role in tumor promotion. Aylsworth et al. (58) have recently shown that palmitoleic, linoleic, and arachidonic acids inhibited metabolic cooperation of Chinese hamster V79 cells, whereas stearic and palmitic acids were without effect. Thus, unsaturated but not saturated fatty acids appear to inhibit cell-to-cell communication in vitro. They suggest the possibility that incorporation of unsaturated fatty acids may alter the structural and biophysical properties of the membrane to cause a destabilization of gap junctions and resulting in the blockade of passage of materials (signals) between cells, i.e. inhibition of metabolic cooperation.

It is more than likely that the effect of dietary fat is mediated by several mechanisms, some of which may yet await discovery. Metabolic adaptation as a result of changes in nutrient intake is a well documented phenomenon. The consumption of a high fat diet no doubt culminates in the integration of a host of factors in the endogenous milieu that are favorable to the growth of neoplastic tissue. In view of the overwhelming epidemiological and experimental evidence linking dietary fat and breast cancer, further research focused on defining the conditions under which fat is most effective in stimulating mammary neoplasia should be an area of high priority towards realizing our goal of reducing breast cancer morbidity.

REFERENCES

1. Tannenbaum, A. Cancer Res. 2:468-475, 1942.
2. gammal, E.B., Carroll, K.K. and Plunkett, E.R. Cancer Res. 27:1737-1742, 1967.
3. Gammal, E.B., Carroll, K.K. and Plunkett, E.R. Cancer Res. 28:384-385, 1968.
4. Carroll, K.K., Gammal, E.B. and Plunkett, E.R. Can Med. Assoc. J. 98:590-594, 1968.
5. Carroll, K.K. and Khor, H.T. Cancer Res. 30:2260-2264, 1970.
6. Carroll, K.K. and Khor, H.T. Lipids 6:415-420, 1971.
7. Tannenbaum, A. Cancer Res. 5:616-625, 1945.
8. Welsch, C.W. and Aylsworth, C.F. J. Natl. Cancer Inst. 70:215-221, 1983.
9. Chan, P.C. and Dao, T.L. Cancer Letter 18:245-249, 1983.
10. Ip, C. Cancer Res. 40:2785-2789, 1980.
11. Visek, W.J. and Clinton, S.K. In: Dietary Fats and Health (Eds. E.G. Perkins and W.J. Visek), AOCS Monograph 10, Champaign, IL., 1983, chapter 46.
12. Rao, G.A. and Abraham, S. J. Natl. Cancer Inst. 56:431-432, 1976.
13. Hopkins, G.J. and West, C.E. J. Natl. Cancer Inst. 58:753-756, 1977.
14. King, M.M., Bailey, D.M., Gibson, D.D., Pitha, J.V. and McCay, P.B. J. Natl. Cancer Inst. 63:657-663, 1979.
15. Tinsley, I.J., Schmitz, J.A. and Pierce, D.A. Cancer Res. 41:1460-1465, 1981.
16. Lee, S.Y. and Rogers, A.E. Nutr. Res. 3:361-371, 1983.
17. Chan, P.C., Ferguson, K.A. and Dao, T.L. Cancer Res. 43:1079-1083, 1983.
18. Ip, C. and Sinha, D. Cancer Res. 41:31-34, 1981.
19. Carroll, K.K. and Hopkins, G.J. Lipids 14:155-158, 1979.
20. Hillyard, L.A. and Abraham, S. Cancer Res. 39:4430-4437, 1979.
21. Ip, C., Carter, C. and Ip, M.M. Cancer Res. in press, 1985.
22. Carroll, K.K. Cancer Res. 35:3374-3383, 1975.
23. Emken, E.A. In: World Soybean Research Conference II Proceedings (Ed. F.T. Corbin), Westview Press, 1980, pp. 667-679.
24. Selenkas, S.L., Ip, M.M. and Ip, C. Cancer Res. 44:1321-1326, 1984.
25. Karmali, R., Marsh, J. and Fuchs, C. J. Natl. Cancer Inst. 73:457-461, 1984.
26. Jurkowski, J.J. and Cave, W.T. J. Natl. Cancer Inst., in press, 1985.
27. Campbell, T.C. and Hayes, J. Pharmacol. Reviews 26:171-197, 1974.
28. Cheng, K.C., Ragland, W.L. and Wade, A.E. J. Environ. Pathol. Toxicol. 4:219-235, 1980.
29. Ip, C. and Sinha, D. Cancer Letters 11:277-283, 1981.
30. Rogers, A.E., Fernstrom, J.D., Ge, K., McConnell, R.G., Leavitt, W.W., Wetsel, W.C., Yang, S.O. and Camelio, E.A.

In: Molecular Interactions of Nutrition and Cancer (Eds. M.S. Arnott, J. Van Eys and Y.M. Wang), Raven Press, New York, 1982, pp. 381-399.

31. Leung, B.S. Progress in Cancer Research and Therapy 10: 219-261, 1978.
32. Chan, P.C., Didato, F. and Cohen, L.A. Proc. Soc. Exp. Biol. Med. 149:133-135, 1975.
33. Ip, C., Yip, P. and Bernardis, L.L. Cancer Res. 40:374-378, 1980.
34. Cave, W.T., Dunn, J.T. and MacLeod, R.M. Cancer Res. 39: 729-733, 1979.
35. Hopkins, G.J., Kennedy, T.G. and Carroll, K.K. J. Natl. Cancer Inst. 66:517-522, 1981.
36. Aylsworth, C.F., Van Vugt, D.A., Sylvester, P. and Meites, J. Proc. Soc. Exp. Biol. Med. 175:25-29, 1984.
37. Wetsel, W.C., Rogers, A.E., Rutledge, A. and Leavitt, W.W. Cancer Res. 44:1420-1425, 1984.
38. Chan, P.C., Head, J.F., Cohen, L.A. and Wynder, E.L. J. Natl. Cancer Inst. 59:1279-1283, 1977.
39. Ip, C. and Ip, M.M. J. Natl. Cancer Inst. 66:291-295, 1981.
40. Ip, M. and Ip, C. Nutrition and Cancer 3:27-34, 1981.
41. Cave, W.T. and Erickson-Lucas, M.J. J. Natl. Cancer Inst. 68:319-324, 1982.
42. Wetsel, W.C. and Rogers, A.E. J. Natl. Cancer Inst. 73:531-536, 1984.
43. Cave, W.T. and Jurkowski, J.J. J. Natl. Cancer Inst. 73:185-191, 1984.
44. Aylsworth, C.F., Van Vugt, D.A., Sylvester, P.W. and Meites, J. Cancer Res. 44:2835-2840, 1984.
45. Sylvester, P.W., Ip, C. and Ip, M.M. Proc. Am. Assoc. Cancer Res. 25:131, 1984.
46. Wicha, M.S., Liotta, L.A. and Kidwell, W.R. Cancer Res. 39:426-435, 1979.
47. Kidwell, W.R., Knazek, R.A., Vonderharr, B.K. and Losonczy, I. In: Molecular Interactions of Nutrition and Cancer (Eds. M.S. Arnott, J. Van Eys and Y.M. Wang), Raven Press, New York, 1982, pp. 219-236.
48. Kidwell, W.R. and Shaffer, J. J. Am. Oil Chemists' Soc. 61:1900-1904, 1984.
49. Rao, G.A. and Abraham, S. J. Natl. Cancer Inst. 58:445-447, 1977.
50. Abraham, S. and Hillyard, L.A. J. Natl. Cancer Inst. 71: 601-605, 1983.
51. Carter, C.A., Milholland, R.J., Shea, W. and Ip, M.M. Cancer Res. 43:3559-3562, 1983.
52. Goodwin, J.S. and Webb, D.R. Clin. Immunol. Immuno-pathology 15:106-122, 1980.
53. Slaga, T.J., Klein-Szanto, A.J., Triplett, L.L., Yotti, L.P. and Trosko, J.E. Science 213:1023-1025, 1981.
54. Shamberger, R.J. J. Natl. Cancer Inst. 48:1491-1497, 1972.
55. Demopoulos, H.B., Pietronigro, D.D., Flamm, E.S. and Seligman, M.L. J. Environ. Pathol. Toxicol. 3:273-303, 1980.

56. Klamerth, O.L. and Levinsky, H. FEBS Letter 3:205-207, 1969.
57. Roubal, W.T. and Tappel, A.L. Arch. Biochem. Biophys. 113:150-155, 1966.
58. Aylsworth, C.F., Jone, C., Trosko, J.E., Meites, J. and Welsch, C.W. J. Natl. Cancer Inst. 72:637-645, 1984.

21

EXPERIMENTAL MODELS FOR MAMMARY CARCINOGENESIS AND FOR BREAST CANCER
THERAPY
A. HACKETT/G. HEPPNER
Peralta Cancer Research Institute, 3023 Summit, Oakland, CA 94609,
Michigan Cancer Foundation, 110 E. Warren, Detroit, MI 48201

The focus of this workshop was on the design of in vitro and animal
models to answer questions of relevance to the development and therapy
of human breast cancer. Throughout this lively session, several
members of the audience suggested that at a certain level no models
were adequate for the "real thing" and challenged the speakers to show
how their work could impact on understanding human breast cancer. Dr.
Joyce Taylor-Papadimitriou called attention to the quite different
relationships of epithelial and fat cells in human and rodent breast
tissue and also mentioned that, for practical and ethical reasons,
investigators studying human mammary glands often worked with adult
tissue whereas much work in rodents occurred with comparably younger
glands. She urged that such differences be better appreciated in
experimental design. Other investigators, such as Dr. Martha Stampfer,
stressed the differences in basic knowledge in rodent versus human
breast cancer development and pointed out that, as of yet, the human in
vitro systems were not up to a full integration with studies in rodent
carcinogenesis.

The workshop began with a discussion on in vitro systems to study
human mammary gland carcinogenesis. Dr. Stampfer described her work on
the development of an autogenic series of breast cell lines that
represent different "stages" in the neoplastic process. Rapidly
growing primary cultures of normal human mammary epithelial cells were
exposed to 1 μg/ml of benzo(a)pyrene (BaP) for 2 or 3, 24 hr periods.
The BaP treated populations displayed a longer period of active growth
in culture compared to the untreated control cells. Two continuous
epithelial cell lines have thus far emerged. The lines display several
properties which distinguish them from their normal progenitors,
including altered morphology and nutritional requirements, aberrations
in expression of certain differentiated properties and antigens, and

changes in X-ray sensitivity. One line is near diploid, with an aneuploid subline. The second line is quite heterogeneous in ploidy, suggesting that it may be useful in studying the onset of "genetic instability." Neither line forms tumors in nude mice, but transfection with the ras gene will induce tumorigenicity in one line and ras plus the T gene will induce tumorigenicity in the second line. However, Dr. Stampfer emphasized that we know very little about whether similar stages of malignant progression actually occur in human carcinogenesis.

A second in vitro system was described by Dr. Paul Janiaud. This consists of exposure of normal human mammary cultures to hormones (i.e., DES) and then carcinogens (i.e., DMBA) in the presence of rat liver cells. Metabolism of carcinogen to active species occurs in this system and is enhanced by physiological concentrations of hormone. A large number of morphologically transformed cell colonies are apparent about 1 month following carcinogen exposure. These colonies have a human karyotype and produce a low level of tumors in nude mice.

Discussion next shifted to work with animal model systems. Dr. Clement Ip presented data on establishing the fatty acid requirements for mammary carcinogenesis in rats. Mammary tumors were induced by 5 mg of DMBA given i.g. at 50-55 days of age. Semi-synthetic diets were fed to the animals starting 3 days after DMBA treatment and continuing until sacrifice. When rats were fed diets containing levels of linoleate ranging from 0.5% to 11.5% (each diet contained 20% fat by weight), tumor development increased proportionately in the range of 0.5% to 4.4%. Above this level, however, tumorigenesis appeared to plateau. When rats were fed diets containing 8% to 20% of fat (a constant of 8% of corn oil (4.8% linoleate) with additional fat coming from coconut oil), there was a linear enhancement in both tumor incidence and yield with increased levels of dietary fat. The incidence in rats fed the 8% fat diet was 40%. Linear regression analysis indicated that an increment of 2.6% in incidence was expected per 1% increase in the level of fat in the diet beyond the 8% level. Dr. Ip stressed that above a certain amount further enhancement of tumorigenesis depends upon the level not the type of fat. He also suggested that this model, if applicable to human cancer, could be used to calculate optimal dietary fat content.

Dr. Dan Medina then reviewed the current thinking on selenium in prevention of breast cancer. Dietary selenium has similar effects on development of mammary tumors in rats and mice of both viral and chemical etiology. Inhibition of tumor development depends upon the continuous presence of selenium in the diet and post-initiation events are inhibited independently of initiation itself. The major inhibitory effect is during the normal to preneoplastic stage of mammary tumor development. Selenium has very little effect on established tumors. Effects on metastasis have not yet been studied. The essential mechanism of selenium action is also not known, although there is some in vitro evidence for a direct effect on growth of mammary epithelial cells.

Dr. Robert Nicolson discussed the paradoxical actions of the anti-estrogen, tamoxifen, on the development of DMBA-induced carcinomas in rats. Accelerated growth of the mammary gland in Sprague-Dawley rats begins with the onset of ovarian activity at about 30 days of age. During the next 20 days there is rapid growth of the gland into the fat-pad by ductal extension and branching. The fine peripheral ductules end in bulbous terminal buds (TB). Oral administration of DMBA (20 mg) on day 50 causes proliferative cribiform lesions in TB within 4-6 weeks and palpable mammary adenocarcinomas in approximately 74% of animals by week 20. Ovariectomy on day 28 blocks mammary gland development, decreases the numbers of TB, and reduces the susceptibility of the gland to DMBA. Treatment of intact or ovariectomised animals with tamoxifen (300 µg/day) for 20 days beginning on day 30 is associated with normal ductal extension and TB activity. The mammary glands of intact tamoxifen-treated animals are, however, refractory to DMBA (0 tumors in 22 animals by week 20). Concurrent administration of α-ergobromocryptine (250 µg/day) and tamoxifen to ovariectomised animals, while abolishing the antiestrogen-induced stimulation of circulating prolactin levels, fails to prevent its induction of ductal extension and TB activity. These data indicate that although tamoxifen shows substantial estrogen activity on the developing mammary gland, it nevertheless inhibits mammary tumor development.

Discussion next moved to models for therapy of breast cancer. Dr. Ricardo Mesa-Tejada told of his work on treating the T47D breast cancer cell line with daunorubicin-conjugated monoclonal antibodies in treatment. He stressed an often over-looked aspect of this approach, namely the propensity of many tumor cells to nonspecifically adsorb and internalize immunoglobulins. Consequently, imaging of radiolabeled antibodies within tumors growing in vivo is not a good test for antibody specificity. Different monoclonal antibodies differ in their nonspecific affinity for tumor cells. Dr. Mesa-Tejada's results indicate the need for caution in planning experiments on uptake of monoclonal antibody by cancer cells.

Dr. Francis Balkwill used human breast cancer xenografts in nude mice as a model system to study the antitumor activity of interferons (IFN), both alone and in combination with cyclophosphamide (CY). Daily therapy with several types and subtypes of human IFN-α was both cytostatic and cytotoxic but IFN-β and γ had little activity. The effects of IFNs were on the xenograft cells and not the host immune system. Combinations of IFN-α or γ and CY were strongly synergistic and caused an increase in the number of tumor cells in S phase of the cell cycle. For maximal synergy daily IFN therapy and once weekly CY was necessary. As IFNs have been shown to increase the expression of some surface and tumor associated antigens, IFN plus monoclonal antibody therapy is also being investigated by Dr. Balkwill.

A rat model system for the evaluation of chemo-hormonal treatment was described by Dr. J.H. van Dierendonck. Mammary carcinomas arising after irradiation and/or prolonged treatment with estrogen in Wag/Rij rats were studied with respect to transplantability, growth rate, sensitivity to endocrine manipulation, ability to grow in tissue culture, DNA ploidy and hormone receptor content. Transplants from estrogen induced tumors did not grow without hormonal stimulation, in contrast to those induced by radiation. A well-differentiated, diploid, radiation-induced adenocarcinoma was selected for further study. It has a doubling time of 22.5 days in second passage and shows regression after ovariectomy and treatment with tamoxifen. Three lines are available from this tumor. The lines are somewhat heterogeneous in estrogen receptor (ER) levels and have higher progesterone receptor than ER levels. Preliminary results indicate that this tumor system might be a promising model for in vivo as well as in vitro studies.

Dr. Bonnie Miller discussed an in vitro assay to study the drug
sensitivity of heterogeneous tumors. Tumor cell subpopulations of
individual cancers may interact with each other so that the growth and
drug sensitivity of one subpopulation is changed by the presence of
another. These interactions are being modeled in assays designed to
study drug sensitivity of breast cancers. A bolus of tumor cells from
culture, or a small fragment of tumor, is embedded in collagen, and the
outgrowth is measured by planimetry. Cells growing in these cultures
have many characteristics in common with cells from in vivo tumors,
including increased percentage of cells in G_0G_1, areas of necrosis,
and decreased drug sensitivity in comparison with monolayer cultures.
In order to test the ability of cell subpopulations of different drug
sensitivities to interact with each other in collagen cultures,
contact-mediated communication between subpopulations of a single mouse
mammary tumor was measured in "metabolic cooperation" assays. The
results indicate that tumor subpopulations show differential and
specific abilities to influence each other's drug sensitivity and
suggest that the collagen assay may be useful to assess tumor drug
sensitivity in vitro.

The last presentation of the workshop was by Dr. F. Prop on the use
of feline mammary cancers as a therapeutic model for human breast
cancer. Feline mammary tumors share histopathological features with
human mammary carcinomas and have a comparable postoperative course and
prognosis. They are being used by Dr. Prop to carry out an in vivo -
in vitro correlation study on the sensitivity of feline cancer to
adjuvant therapy with Adriamycin (20 mg/M2 every second week). The in
vitro assay was developed for human cancers but its validity is being
tested in the cat for practical and ethical reasons. Collagenase is
used to obtain a suspension of tumor cell clumps that are seeded into
plastic culture flasks. Each clump settles to grow into a cell
island. Such islands often represent single subpopulations as shown in
nuclear DNA frequency distribution histograms. After treatment for 24
hrs with Adriamycin (conc. range from 0.25 to 2.0 µg/ml) the cells get
4 days recovery time in normal medium. The course of events is
recorded by periodical photographs of selected areas. After that
period the cultures are fixed and Feulgen-stained for DNA
cytophotometry. The culture system appears to be as efficient for

feline as for human breast cancers. Long term follow-up of the treated cats is now in progress in order to test the ability of the assay to predict response to drug.

It was clear from all the presentations that investigators are making a concerted effort to develop model systems that address problems in development and therapy of human breast cancer. Clearly, no one model is adequate by itself. The identification of which models are best suited for which specific facets of human disease remains a priority for future research.

22

TUMOUR AND PATIENT VARIABLES AS INDICATORS OF PROGNOSIS. THE SILENT PERIOD

R.D. BULBROOK, J.W. MOORE, B.S. THOMAS, D.Y. WANG, H.G. KWA[++], D.S. ALLEN & J.L. HAYWARD[+]

Clinical Endocrinology Laboratory, Imperial Cancer Research Fund, London, WC2A 3PX; Breast Unit, Guy's Hospital, London [+]; Antoni van Leeuwenhoekhuis, The Netherlands[++]

The word 'cure' was used in the title of Halstead's paper in 1894 in which he described his technique of radical mastectomy (1) and this had so powerful an effect that the treatment remained standard for the next 50 years. There appeared to be little practical point in investigating factors which might be related to prognosis since patients received identical treatment whether their outlook was good or bad. Clinical or pathological staging was used mainly to compare results between centres but was not used to determine treatment. Histological grading was used as an academic excercise.

Research was concentrated on patients with metastatic disease where the introduction of additive endocrine therapy followed by adrenalectomy or hypophysectomy meant that there appeared to be an element of choice for the clinician and the advantages of being able to predict responsiveness were obvious.

The greatest catalyst for change was the publication of two randomised trials of the use of adjuvant chemotherapy (2,3). Within the space of a few years a very large number of treatment options became available and since most of them were associated with side-effects, the problem of selecting patients who were likely to benefit became acute. In response to this need the literature became saturated with reports that a wide variety of host and tumour factors might be useful in predicting the outcome of treatment. With the possible exception of receptor-site assays, the thymidine-labelling index and, of course, stage and grade, none of these predictors has proved to be so reliable that their measurement influenced clinical decision-making. Rather than reviewing again a field in which progress is static (4) it might be more profitable to discuss a neglected topic, namely, the possibility of finding useful prognostic factors in the period before diagnosis (the silent period). It may very well be that the clinical course of the disease, in terms of disease-free interval, response to treatment, and survival, may have already been determined. The ideal method for such a study would be a prospective investigation of a normal population but the logistic difficulties are such that there has been a reluctance to commit resources to a field where the chance of failure is likely to be high. There are however, some preliminary data from two prospective studies (5,6) and more can be expected from a third experiment in progress (7).

The use of tumour markers for very early diagnosis need not be considered further. Present evidence indicates that the expression of measurable amounts of markers is a late event in the natural history of the disease and detection depends on a considerable tumour burden. As far as breast cancer is concerned, it appears that no marker of sufficient specificity or sensitivity has been discovered that a study of its distribution in an apparently normal population would be justifiable at present.

As for classic anamnestic variables, it has been reported that a late age at menarche or first birth and decreased parity are associated with a late age at diagnosis (8,9) but our own results cast some doubt on these findings because the changing pattern of reproductive history has not been taken into account (10). The role of height and weight in influencing age at diagnosis and clinical course is still controversial (11). As far as risk is concerned, the most powerful variables,in our experience, are nulliparity and a late age at first baby either of which increases risk two-fold but, in common with others, we have not found classical variables alone or in combination, to be of practical use in identifying a substantial high-risk group.

Intuitively, it might be expected that endocrine function would be of primary importance in the silent period (ie. between transformation and diagnosis). The number of breast cells at risk of the first and second "hits" (12) would be determined by hormonal stimuli early in life. The time taken for a transformed cell population to grow to a size where physical diagnosis was possible ($> 10^7$ cells) would again be most likely to be controlled by the endocrine environment and the biological diversity of a tumour at diagnosis might be similarly influenced.

Prospective and clinical studies of oestrogen status

Blood specimens have been collected from 5,000 normal women in Guernsey. Thirty-one of the volunteers have subsequently developed breast cancer. The proportions of their total serum oestradiol in the non-protein bound, the albumin-bound and the sex hormone-binding globulin (SHBG) fractions have been measured in the "pre-cancer cases" and in age-matched controls.

The pre-cancer cases had significantly more of their blood oestradiol in the free (non-protein bound) and albumin-bound fractions (the biologically available fractions) than did the controls. The abnormality was so pronounced that it might be a useful predictor of risk of breast cancer (13). The reasons for the high percentage of available oestradiol are, first, a decrease in the amount of SHBG in the blood of the pre-cancer cases, and second, an abnormality in binding in that there is more free oestradiol than would be expected from the SHBG concentration.

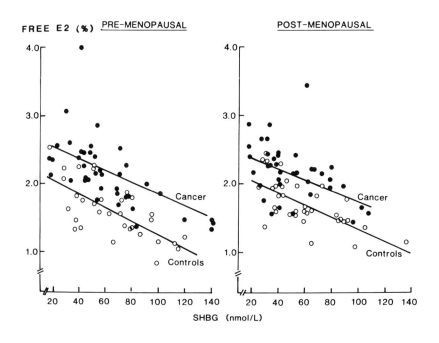

Fig. 1. Relation between free oestradiol and SHBG in women with operable breast cancer and controls
(● denotes patients with breast cancer; o, normal controls)

Abnormalities identical to those found in the pre-cancer cases can be demonstrated at diagnosis (Fig. 1). Women with operable breast cancer have a significantly raised fraction of their blood oestradiol in the non-protein-bound (free) compartment.

The question now is whether the enhanced oestrogenic stimulus found before and at diagnosis is associated with the subsequent clinical course of the disease.

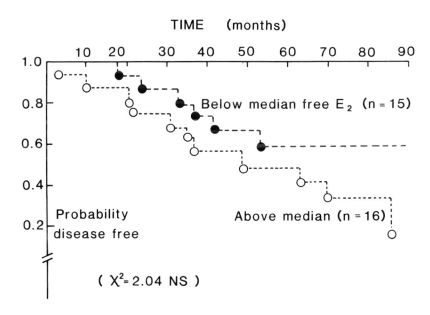

Fig. 2. Recurrence after mastectomy and free oestradiol levels in post-menopausal patients

The number of patients available for this phase of the study is small but in pre-menopausal patients there appears to be no difference in recurrence rates in women with high or low proportions of available oestradiol. In post-menopausal women (Fig. 2) there is a weak (and non-significant) trend for women with an increased proportion of free oestradiol to recur at a faster rate than those with a smaller proportion of available hormone. More data would be desirable.

Prospective and clinical studies of prolactin status

The linear regression of prolactin on age for the pre-menopausal women in our prospective study who subsequently developed breast cancer showed an abnormal relationship between these variables. Blood prolactin levels rose sharply between age 30 and the menopause (Fig. 3).

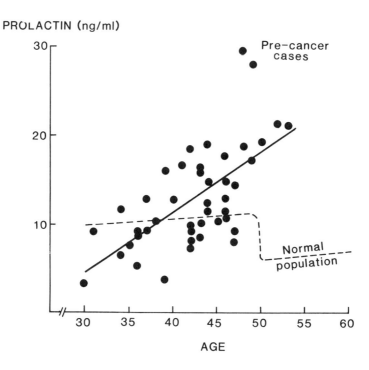

Fig. 3. Abnormal age relationship of prolactin in pre-menopausal pre-cancer cases. The curve for the normal population is taken from results for 4,866 women, described in (14).

One could speculate that the enhanced risk associated with a late menopause is related to the increased levels of prolactin in the 45-52 age group. There is a gradient of risk in this sub-group : the higher the prolactin level, the greater is the risk of breast cancer (see Fig. 4).

In post-menopausal women, the relation between risk and prolactin levels appears to be weak or non-existent.

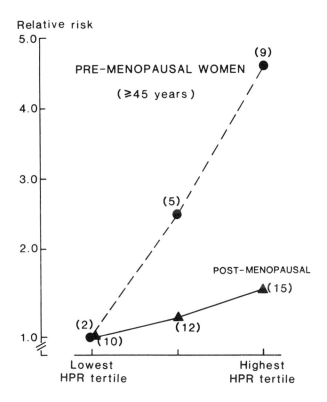

Fig. 4. Relation between prolactin levels and risk of breast cancer in pre- and post-menopausal pre-cancer cases. Risk has been calculated by dividing the number of pre-cancer cases by the number of normal women in each tertile and setting the risk in the lowest tertile to 1. There were 825 pre-menopausal women and 1962 post-menopausal women in the study.

Once the disease is diagnosed, diminished survival is associated with high prolactin levels although the association is weak and is not found in all sub-groups (15). Nevertheless, the concordance between the high risk found in women with high prolactin levels in the silent period and poor prognosis at diagnosis indicates a degree of pre-determination.

Prospective and clinical studies of androgen status

Perhaps the best documented example of events in the silent period having a profound effect on the clinical course of the disease is given by the urinary androgen metabolites. These are low in women at high risk (5) and women with such an abnormal excretion pattern have a rapid rate of recurrence after mastectomy (16) and generally fail to respond to ablative endocrine therapy (7).

The present evidence, therefore, indicates that abnormalites in endocrine function are potent indicators of risk and endocrine stimuli in the silent period do influence the clinical course of the disease following diagnosis.

Breast parenchymal patterns

We may now ask what factors other than anamnestic variables and endocrine function might also be useful prognostic factors in an ostensibly normal population. One that springs to mind is the radiological pattern of the breast parenchyma. While there is a considerable literature on this subject, the majority of reports deal with radiology completely separately from other risk factors. In the prospective studies we have carried out, mammograms were obtained at the same time as blood specimens, together with detailed questionnaires. Wolfe (18) had claimed that various radiological patterns of the breast parenchyma are related to considerable differences in risk of breast cancer. In our own prospective study women with high-risk mammograms (Wolfe classification P_2 or DY) were at approximately twice the risk of those with low risk films (N_1 or P_1). The overall risk level conceals the fact that in some sub-groups, Wolfe grades appear to be useless whereas in others, they appear to be related to high risk (19). What has not been determined is whether the grades are related to clinical course.

What is surprising is that we have so far been unable to correlate endocrine status with the Wolfe grades. The latter appear to be a risk factor in their own right.

265

Discussion and Summary

This preliminary investigation into the effects of host factors on risk and on the clinical course of breast cancer after diagnosis has provided some evidence that the environment during the silent period affects the biological behaviour of overt tumours. A systemmatic attack on this problem might well indicate to what degree recurrence rates after primary therapy, response to endocrinological or chemotherapeutic treatment, and survival are already determined before diagnosis.

As far as risk is concerned, three prognostic factors stand out: these are nulliparity or late age at first child, oestrogenic status, and the radiological appearance of the breast. They appear to be largely (but not entirely) independent of each other, giving 3 dichotomizing variables which should identify women with a risk of 1 in 2. In fact, in 879 women for whom all 3 factors were available, a relative risk of 6 was found in the 11% of the population where all variables were unfavourable. This is high enough to contemplate preventive treatment. Whether assays of prolactin in women approaching the menopause, of androgen metabolites, and sub-groups analysis of the Wolfe gradings would improve this figure remains to be seen. The present data indicate clearly that a substantial high risk group can be identified in the normal population.

REFERENCES

1. Halstead, W.S. Ann Surg. 20,: 497-503, 1894.
2. Fisher, B.F., Carbone, P., Economous, S., et al. N. Engl. J. Med. 292: 117-122, 1975.
3. Bonadonna, G., Brusamolino, E., Valagussa, P., et al. N. Engl. J. Med. 294: 405-410, 1976.
4. Bulbrook, R.D., Eur. J. Cancer Clin Oncol. 19: 1693-1697, 1983.
5. Bulbrook, R.D., Hayward, J.L. and Spicer, C.C. Lancet, ii: 395-398, 1971.
6. De Waard, F., Collette, H.J.A., Rombach, J.J. et al. J. Chron. Dis. 37: 1-44
7. Shore, R.E., Pasternack, B.S., Bulbrook, R.D., et al. In: Commentaries on Research in Breast Cancer, Vol III. (Eds. R.D. Bulbrook & D. Jane Taylor) Alan Liss, Inc., New York, pp. 1-31.
8. Juret, P., Collette, J.E. and Rune, D. Europ. J. Cancer 12: 701-704, 1976.

9. Juret, P. In: Endocrine Relationship in Breast Cancer (Eds. B.A. Stoll) William Heinemann Medical Books Ltd. London 5: 85-106, 1982.
10. Wang, D.Y., Rubens, R.D., Allen, D.S., et al. In Press.
11. Kalish, L.A. J. Clin.Oncol. 2: 287-293, 1984.
12. Moolgavkar, S.H., Day, N.E.,and Stevens, R.G. JNCI, 65: 559-569. 1980.
13. Moore, J.W., Clark, G.M.G., Hoare, S., et al. In Press
14. Kwa, H.G., Cleton, F., Wang, D.Y., et al. Int. J. Cancer 28: 673-676, 1981.
15. Wang, D.Y., Hampson, S., Kwa, H.G., et al. In Press.
16. Thomas, B.S., Bulbrook, R.D., Hayward, J.L., et al. Europ. J. Cancer Clin. Oncol. 18: 447-451, 1982.
17. Wang, D.Y. In: Reviews on Endocrine-related cancer. (Eds. B.A. Stoll). Pharmaceutical Division, I.C.I., Macclesfield, 1979, pp. 19-24.
18. Wolfe, J.N. Cancer, 37: 2486-2492, 1976.
19. Gravelle, I.H., Bulstrode, J.C., Bulbrook, R.D.,and Hayward, J.L. In Press.

23

BASIC AND CLINICAL ASPECTS OF THE STRUCTURE AND FUNCTION OF STEROID RECEPTORS

R. J. B. KING and A. I. COFFER

Hormone Biochemistry Department, Imperial Cancer Research Fund, P.O.Box 123, Lincoln's Inn Fields, London WC2A 3PX, U.K.

INTRODUCTION

The synthesis of high specific activity tritiated oestrogens a quarter of a century ago lead to the identification of intracellular receptor proteins for all classes of steroid hormone. Furthermore, by following the fate of the labelled steroids much information of both a basic and clinical nature has been generated about the receptor machinery. However, it has long been realized that such techniques had the severe limitation of identifying not the receptor protein itself but only the functionality of the ligand binding site; if that was lost, no other way was available for analysing the protein. Major questions that were difficult to answer by using labelled steroids were: 1) How are the various sizes of receptor related to each other? It has still not been determined if multimeric forms such as the 8S or 5S receptors are composed of similar or dissimilar subunits. 2) In so-called receptor-negative tumours, is the protein really lost or merely present in a non-hormone binding form? 3) What is the relationship of the nuclear receptor to the cytosol receptor? 4) What is the distribution of receptor positive cells within a heterogeneous cell population? Autoradiography has been useful but its inherent lack of sensitivity in detecting low levels of binding proteins has limited its use. This has clinical implications in that it has not been possible to determine the proportions of hormone-sensitive and insensitive cells in tumours of the breast.

These and other questions could be probed if antibodies, particularly of the monoclonal variety, were available. Several such antibodies have now been described, the present article will discuss some of the points raised by the immunological work with particular emphasis on the applicability to hormone-sensitive tumours.

Generation of monoclonal antibodies (MAB's).

MAB's generated by immunization with receptor preparations have been described for receptors for oestradiol (RE), progesterone (RP) and glucocorticoids (RG). Their general specificities are summarized in Table 1.

Table 1. Monoclonal antibodies to steroid 'receptors'.

| Receptor | Specificity | | Recognizes Hormone Binding Unit | Reference |
	Species	Cell Type		
Oestradiol	Yes	No	Yes	1
	No	No	Yes	2
	Yes	No	No	3
Glucocorticoid	Yes	No	Yes	4
	Yes	No	Yes/No	5
Progesterone	Yes	?	Yes	6
	Yes	No	No	7
	Yes	No	No	8, 9

? No data presented

With one exception in which only a limited number of species were studied (2), all groups have reported species specificity which unequivocally indicates that not all receptors of a given class (e.g. oestradiol) are the same. However, no one has shown differences in specificity between cell types within a given species. Thus far, only a limited number of antibodies have been tested so the preliminary interpretation could be either that the strongest antigenic determinants on a given class of receptors are similar but that weaker determinants might be different or that there are no major differences between, for example, a glucocorticoid receptor in liver, lymphoma or mammary gland. If the latter proves to be correct, it implies that the type of response elicited by a given steroid is determined not by the receptor itself but by another level of specificity, possibly at the level of acceptor site availability within the genome. Support for this view comes from work showing that liver RG binds to specific regions of chicken lysozyme gene (10) and mouse mammary tumour virus (11, 12). Furthermore, cDNA made against mRNA for liver RG has high homology with the RG genes in lymphoma cells (13).

Receptor structure.

The other interesting feature illustrated in Table 1 is that some MAB's do not react with a hormone binding unit. There is no discernible pattern in the characteristics of this type of MAB (Table 2). Those prepared against chick oviduct RP have broad specificities whereas the human myometrial RE antibody exhibits the specificity expected of RE. The RG case is discussed later. The RP and RG MAB's recognize proteins of the same molecular weights as the relevant hormone binding unit whereas the RE MAB does not. Furthermore, the MAB against the 108K RP protein has been used to identify an oviduct RP gene (14). The significance of these non hormone-binding components remains to be established. They may have physiological relevance but, given the uncertain purity of the immunogens, these MAB's may be directed against contaminating proteins. The answer to this enigma may also be relevant to the question of the structure and function of the 8S cytosol receptor. If, as seems probable, most of the native receptor is in the cell nucleus (15,16,17,18) its release during homogenization may be followed by interaction with a non hormone-binding protein in the cytoplasm. The 8S receptor could therefore be an artefact. However, the 8S form of chick oviduct RP is made up of two progesterone-binding subunits (19) which would argue against its being an artefact. At present the data are too few to make conclusions.

Table 2. Monoclonal antibodies: non-hormone binding 'receptors'.

Immunogen	Size Antigen	Specificity		Quantitative Relationship to Binding Unit	Reference
		Other Receptors	Non-Receptor Cells		
Oviduct RP	90K	Yes	Yes	?	9
	108K	Yes	Yes	?	7
Liver RG	94K	No	?	?	20
Myometrium RE	29K	No	No	Yes	3, 21

? No data presented

Does loss of ligand binding correlate with loss of antigen?

This question is of special importance in relation to the progression of a tumour from the hormone-responsive to unresponsive state. It has been argued that this transition could be due to a change in receptor structure

such that the steroid binding site but not the protein was lost and that
the 'receptor' was fully active   in the absence of steroid. Immunoassay
of RE in human breast tumours indicates that this is not true in the majority
of cases; good correlations between ^{3}H oestradiol binding and both enzyme
linked immunoabsorbent assay (ELISA) (22) and immunoradiometric assay (IRMA)
(21) have been reported. However, there is sufficient scatter of the data
points to allow for the existence of some tumours with non hormone-binding
'receptors'. In the RG/lymphoma system, both antigen (20) and mRNA (13)
related to RG have been found in the unresponsive, receptor-negative cells.
These results, taken together with the uncertain nature of the non hormone-
binding proteins (see above) mean that a definitive answer cannot be provided
yet to the question posed in the title of this section.

Immunoassay of RE: clinical aspects.

The undoubted usefulness of RE assays as a prognostic aid in breast
cancer has been limited by methodological problems related to the use of
^{3}H oestradiol. The major methodological problems have been: 1) Lability
of binding resulting in a difficult assay not widely available outside
specialist centres. 2) Potential blocking of ^{3}H oestradiol binding by
endogenous oestrogen thereby underestimating receptor content. 3) Quantity
and lability of binding makes autoradiography an impractical method for
routine histological assessment of RE.

The generation of antibodies against the oestradiol receptor itself
could circumvent these difficulties. Several polyclonal antibodies have
been described (listed in ref. 3) but have yet to find practical
application at the clinical level. Three groups have been successful with
monoclonal antibodies (1,2,3), two of which have been used in breast
cancer work. Jensen's group, in collaboration with Abbott Pharmaceuticals,
have developed an ELISA that, after the initial cytosol preparation, does
not require low temperatures. The RE values obtained correlate well with
those obtained by oestradiol binding assays (22).

Our own group has produced a different type of MAB to those
described by the Chicago group. RE from human myometrium was partially
purified by oestradiol-affinity chromatography and mouse MAB's produced
by the standard method; antibodies were detected by their ability to
precipitate oestradiol receptor complexes. Despite this property, the
antibody does not recognize the oestradiol-binding unit: the epitope is
on a 29K protein (p29) that, under activating conditions (3) is able to

react with the oestradiol binding unit. This human specific, 29K protein has, with the exception of RE-RP+ breast tumours (see below), only been found in RE positive tissues and is not related to other steroid-binding proteins (3,21). This protein exhibits all the specificities required of a component of the oestradiol receptor machinery except that it does not bind oestradiol. Its biological function is under investigation. Candidate ideas are that p29 may be, 1) a component of the 8S soluble receptor, 2) processed nuclear receptor, 3) related to type II soluble binding sites. However, for this possibility to be relevant, the type II binding protein would have to have the previously undescribed property of reacting with the oestradiol receptor under activating conditions, 4) an oestrogen-induced protein. The lack of correlation with RP content (see below) would argue against that idea.

In collaboration with Amersham International, we have developed an IRMA which requires no refrigeration steps after the cytosol preparation. The correlation between IRMA and conventional oestradiol binding assay is good (Fig. 1) whilst there is no correlation with RP content (Fig. 2 and ref. 21).

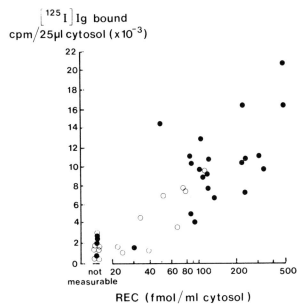

Fig. 1. Relationship between ^{3}H oestradiol-binding assay (REC) and IRMA on a series of human breast tumours. Correlation coefficient r = 0.758, p < 0.001. Patients aged ≥ 50 years (●), < 50 years (0).

An interesting feature of this assay is that positive values are obtained with many of the RE-RP+ tumours (Fig. 2) which fits with their good response rate to hormone therapy (23) and with the view that they may actually be RE positive with blocked oestradiol-binding sites (24). It is interesting to speculate that p29 assay may provide an index of the functionality of the oestradiol receptor machinery and that the discordant cases just mentioned reflect this situation.

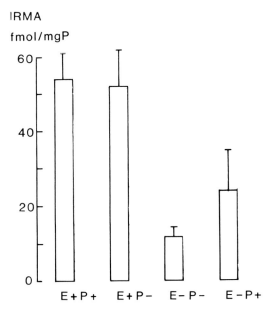

IRMA

fmol/mgP

Fig. 2. Relationship between receptor phenotype and IRMA on human breast tumours. Results are expressed as means ± S.D. Oestradiol (E) and progesterone (P) receptors were assayed by ^{3}H ligand binding. Positive > 10 fmol/mg protein.

Histochemical investigation of breast tumours is also possible with these antibodies and a new facet of receptor usefulness in clinical medicine is already apparent. King et al. (16) and ourselves (25) have noted heterogeneity of staining within many breast tumours. The same observation has been made by autoradiographic localization of ^{3}H oestradiol (26). This raises the possibility of estimating the proportion of hormone sensitive cells within a tumour, something that has not previously been possible on a routine basis. Such information could be useful in deciding whether to give either combined endocrine plus chemo-

therapy or one of the components on its own. Also, on relapse after an
initial response to a first round of hormone therapy, it may be possible
to base the choice between a second round of hormone therapy or chemotherapy
on the histochemical picture.

Semi-quantitative assessment of staining intensity gave similar
results with respect to receptor phenotype (Fig. 3) to those obtained
with IRMA (Fig. 2). Good staining was observed in 9 out of 15 (60%)
RE-RP+ tumours whereas no significant difference was observed between the
RE+RP+ and RE+RP- groups.

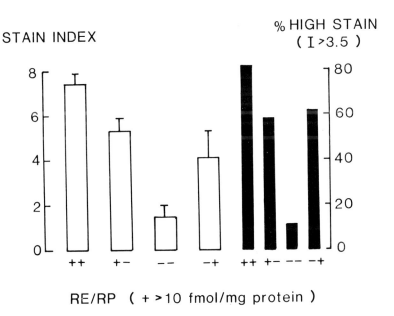

Fig. 3. Relationship between receptor phenotype and histochemical
staining index of human breast tumours. RE and RP phenotypes were
determined by ^{3}H oestradiol and ^{3}H progesterone binding respectively.

The histochemical methods can be used to distinguish between RE
positive and negative tumours but some discordant results are obtained
(Table 3). About 20% of RE negative tumours are positive histochemically
with a smaller proportion of RE positive tumours being negative. It
should be stressed that although the comparative data presented in
Table 3 are broadly similar for the two research groups, the antigens
being detected are different. It remains to be seen if the discordant

results reflect biological or methodological differences.

Table 3. Histochemical analysis of human breast tumours.

| RE phenotype | No. positive tumours/total no. (%). | |
	1*	2*
Negative	5/28 (18%)	16/64 (25%)
Intermediate	15/25 (60%)	-
Positive	137/159 (86%)	52/53 (98%)
Concordance	86% †	85%

* 1. Reference 25 and additional data. Negative $\leq$ 10 fmol/mg protein;
  intermediate 11-20 fmol/mg protein; positive > 20 fmol/mg protein.

† Omitting intermediate group.

* 2. Reference 16. Negative < 300 fmol/g tissue; positive > 300 fmol/mg
  protein.

In our hands, staining was related to differentiation state of the
tumour. Most (87%) grade 1 tumours had a high staining index as compared
to 75% of grade 2 and 53% of grade 3 tumours.

It is thus clear that the immunological methods of RE detection
will both simplify and widen the usefulness of receptor assays in
clinical medicine.

ACKNOWLEDGEMENTS

We thank Amersham International for help with this work,
Dr. Rosemary Millis for supplying the breast tumours and Sarah Murdoch
and Remy Adatia for carrying out the receptor analyses.

REFERENCES

1. Jensen, E.V., Greene, G.L., Closs, L.E., DeSombre, E.R. and Nadji, M.
    Recent Prog. Horm. Res. 38: 1-34, 1982.
2. Moncharmont, B., Su, J.-L. and Parikh, I. Biochemistry 21: 6916-6921,
    1982.
3. Coffer, A.I., Lewis, K.M., Brockas, A.J. and King, R.J.B. Cancer
    Res. in press, 1985.
4. Okret, S., Wikstrom, A.-C., Wrange, O., Andersson, B. and Gustafsson,
    J.-A. Proc. Natl. Acad. Sci. USA, 81: 1609-1613, 1984.

5. Westphal, H.M., Moldenhauer, G. and Beato, M. EMBO J. 1: 1467-1471, 1982.
6. Logeat, F., Hai, M.T.V., Fournier, A., Legrain, P., Buttin, G. and Milgrom, E. Proc. Natl. Acad. Sci. USA, 80: 6456-6459, 1983.
7. Edwards, D.P., Weigel, N.L., Schrader, W.T., O'Malley, B.W. and W.L. McGuire. Biochemistry 23: 4427-4435, 1984.
8. Radanyi, C., Joab, I., Renoir, J.-M., Richard-Foy, H. and Baulieu, E.-E. Proc. Natl. Acad. Sci. USA, 80: 2854-2858, 1983.
9. Joab, I., Radanyi, C., Renoir, M., Buchou, T., Catelli, M.-G., Binart, N., Mester, J. and Baulieu, E.-E. Nature 308: 850-853.
10. Renkawitz, R., Schutz, G., von der Ahe, D. and Beato, M. Cell 37: 503-510, 1984.
11. Payvar, F., DeFranco, D., Firestone, G. L., Edgar, B., Wrange, O., Okret, S., Gustafsson, J.-A. and Yamamoto, K.R. Cell 35: 381-392, 1983.
12. Scheidereit, C. and Beato, M. Proc. Natl. Acad. Sci. USA, 81: 3029-3033, 1984.
13. Miesfeld, R., Okret, S., Wikström, A.-C., Wrange, O., Gustafsson, J.-A. and Yamamoto, K.R. Nature 312: 779-781, 1984.
14. Zarucki-Schulz, T., Kulomaa, M.S., Headon, D.R., Weigel, N.L., Baez, M., Edwards, D.P., McGuire, W.L., Schrader, W.T. and O'Malley, B.W. Proc. Natl. Acad. Sci. USA, 81: 6358-6362, 1984.
15. Gasc, J.-M., Renoir, J.-M., Radanyi, C., Joab, I., Tuohimaa, P. and Baulieu, E.-E. J. Cell Biol. 99: 1193-1201, 1984.
16. King, W.J., DeSombre, E.R., Jensen, E.V. and Greene, G.L. Cancer Res. 45: 293-304, 1985.
17. McClellan, M.C., West, N.B., Tacha, D.E., Greene, G.L. and Brenner, R.M. Endocrinology 114: 2002-2014, 1984.
18. Welshons, W.V., Lieberman, M.E. and Gorski, J. Nature 307: 747-749, 1984.
19. Schrader, W.T., Birnbaumer, M.E., Hughes, M.R., Weigel, N.L., Grody, W.W. and O'Malley, B.W. Recent Prog. Horm. Res. 37: 583-629, 1981.
20. Westphal, H.M., Mugele, K., Beato, M. and Gehring, U. EMBO J. 3: 1493-1498, 1984.
21. Coffer, A.I., Spiller, G.H., Lewis, K.M. and King, R.J.B. Cancer Res. in press, 1985.
22. Symposium on Estrogen Receptor Determination with Monoclonal Antibodies. Abbott Diagnostics, to be published, 1985.
23. King, R.J.B. In: Biochemical and Biological Markers of Neoplastic Transformation (Ed. P. Chandra), Plenum Press, New York, 1983.
24. Sarrif, A.M. and Durant, J.R. Cancer 48: 1215-1220, 1981.
25. King, R.J.B., Coffer, A.I., Gilbert, J., Lewis, K., Nash, R., Millis, R., Raju, S. and Taylor, R.W. Submitted for publication, 1985.
26. Buell, R.H. and Tremblay, G. Cancer 51: 1625-1630, 1983.

ENDOCRINE THERAPY IN PRIMARY AND ADVANCED BREAST CANCER

H.T. Mouridsen

Department of Oncology I, Finsen Institute, 49 Strandboulevarden
49, 2100 Copenhagen 0, Denmark

INTRODUCTION

The various endocrine therapies available in the treatment
of breast cancer can be divided into four groups according to
their demonstrated or suggested mode of biological action. These
include ablative therapy (oophorectomy, adrenalectomy,
hypophysectomy), inhibitive therapy (aminoglutethimide,
trilostane, danazol), additive therapy (estrogen, progestin,
androgen, glucocorticoid) and competitive therapy (antiestrogen).

The rationale for the use of the ablative procedures is that
hormones promote the growth of some mammary tumor cells. Thus a
decrease in the concentration of these hormones is assumed to
induce tumor regression (1-5).

The mechanism of action of aminoglutethimide has recently
been described in detail (6). Briefly it inhibits the production
of the adrenal steroid hormones and the peripheral aromatization
of androstenedione to estrone. Similar mechanisms of action have
been described for the synthetic steroid trilostane (7-8). The
mechanisms of action of danazol, a synthetic testosterone
derivative, probably include binding to progesterone and androgen
receptors (9) and inhibition of the steroid synthesis in the
ovaries as well (10-11).

The mode of action underlying the paradoxical effect of
pharmacological doses of steroid hormones such as estrogens,
androgens, progestins and glucocorticoids on tumor growth is
largely unknown (12-15).

The pharmacodynamics of the non-steroidal antiestrogenic
compound tamoxifen has recently been reviewed in detail (16).
The primary step is the competition with estradiol for binding to
the estrogen receptor. At the chromatin level the mechanism of

action is complex, and ultimately it leads to both partial block of the cell cycle in the early G_1-phase and to an increase in the concentration of the progesterone receptor protein in the tumor cells. Furthermore, recent studies have shown that tamoxifen binds to high-affinity, saturable sites that appear to be different from the estrogen receptor binding sites.

ENDOCRINE THERAPY OF ADVANCED BREAST CANCER. OVERALL RESULTS.

Ablative therapy

The response rates achieved with oophorectomy (17) in premenopausal patients and with hypophysectomy and adrenalectomy (2) are very similar and close to 30%, but with appreciable variation between the different trials, presumably owing to differences in selection criteria and in the definitions of response that were used. The median duration of response is about 12 months and survival is significantly longer in patients who respond compared with those who do not respond.

Additive endocrine therapy

As for ablative therapy a wide range of response rates have been reported for both estrogen (15-38%)(17), androgen (10-38%)(17) and for progestins (9-54%)(15). Apart from various patient selection and response criteria the different dose levels used in the individual trials may also account for some of the discrepancies. Thus, for estrogens the response rate seems to increase with increasing daily dose from 1.5 mg and up to 1500 mg (18), and for androgens one (19) of two randomized trials (19-20) indicated a dose-response relationship. As concerns progestins most of the earlier trials used daily doses of less than 0.5 g, but recent trials appear to demonstrate that the response rate rises when doses of 1-1.5 g per day are used (15). However, the preliminary results of randomized trials have failed to demonstrate significantly different time to progression or survival with the two different dose levels (21-22). Progestins have been administered both orally and intramuscularly but so far randomized trials analyzing the relation between the therapeutic efficacy and route of administration have not been published.

Competitive endocrine therapy

The average response rate with tamoxifen is 32% with a range from 16 to 52% (23). The most frequently used daily doses are 20-40 mg and randomized trials have demonstrated no significant differences in treatment results when comparing 30 mg with 90 mg daily (24) or 20 mg with 40 mg daily (25-26).

Inhibitive endocrine therapy

The average response to treatment with aminoglutethimide supplemented by substitution with glucocorticoids is 31% (range 16-43%)(6). So far no randomized trials of the dose response relationship have been published and also the role of the glucocorticoid substitution needs to be analysed in randomized trials. As of today only very preliminary results have been published for trilostane (27) and danazol (28).

Choice of endocrine therapy

The choice of endocrine therapy will depend on a balance between on the one hand efficacy and on the other hand toxicity of the therapy in question.

For premenopausal patients it is nowadays generally accepted that oophorectomy should be performed when endocrine therapy is indicated. However, preliminary data indicate that tamoxifen may be equally effective but this has yet to be confirmed in larger trials (29-30).

For postmenopausal patients the choice lies between additive, competitive and inhibitive therapy. A number of randomized trials have compared the different endocrine therapies and presented data of the response-toxicity relation. Recent years have also seen the publication of randomized studies comparing single to multiple endocrine modalities.

Trials of different endocrine therapies

Table 1 reviews a number of randomized studies comparing competitive therapy to other forms of endocrine therapy.

Similar response rates were reported for tamoxifen and estrogen, but the side effects were significantly more pronounced in the group treated with estrogen (31-33).

Table 1.   Randomized trials comparing tamoxifen to other
            endocrine therapies.

Reference	Treatment	Number of patients	Response rate
31-33	Tamoxifen	127	33%
	Estrogen	130	35%
34	Tamoxifen	37	30%
	Androgen	42	19%
35-38	Tamoxifen	140	30%
	Progestin	141	27%
39-40	Tamoxifen	99	33%
	Aminoglutethimide +		
	hydrocortisone	93	32%

In the comparative trial of tamoxifen versus androgen a lower response rate and more pronounced side effects were observed in patients treated with androgen (34).

Tamoxifen was compared with a progestin in 4 trials. The response rates were similar but the duration of response was longer and side effects less pronounced in the group treated with tamoxifen (35-38).

More or less the same therapeutic results were obtained in the two trials in which tamoxifen was compared with aminoglutethimide, but the side effects were more pronounced with the latter treatment (39-40).

Trials of combined endocrine therapy

The comparable response rates achieved with the different endocrine therapies do not necessarily mean that the various treatments have the same ultimate mode of action and the considerable degree of cross-sensitivity and the lack of complete cross-resistance (41) suggest that combined methods of endocrine therapy might increase the therapeutic response.

In recent years a number of randomized trials have been published in which tamoxifen alone has been assessed against tamoxifen combined with other endocrine therapy. The results of some of these trials have recently been reviewed (42) and are briefly summarized in Table 2.

Table 2. Randomized trials comparing tamoxifen to tamoxifen
          in combination with other endocrine therapies.

Reference	Treatment	Number of patients	Response rate
43	TAM	65	39%
	TAM + DES	57	37%
44	TAM	52	15%
	TAM + FLU	56	37%
45	TAM	34	35%
	TAM + NAND	44	43%
46	TAM	45	44%
	TAM + MPA	55	26%
47	TAM	57	11%
	TAM + PRED	61	33%
48	TAM	26	19%
	TAM + AG	26	23%
49	TAM	27	26%
	TAM+AG+H	28	39%
50	TAM	23	22%
	TAM + Br	20	20%
51	TAM	99	31%
	TAM+AG+H+D	99	43%

AG   = aminoglutethimide   MEG = megestrol acetate
Br   = bromocriptine   MPA = medroxyprogesterone
D   = danazol   NAND = nandrostelone
DES = diethylstilboestrol   PRED = prednisolone
FLU = fluoxymesterone   TAM = tamixofen
H   = hydrocortisone

No difference was observed when estrogen was added to
tamoxifen (43). When comparing tamoxifen to tamoxifen and
androgen flyoxymesterone, a significant difference in response
rates, 15% versus 37%, was observed (44). It may be argued,
however, that this trial was not conducted as an orthodox phase
III study. Thus different doses of tamoxifen were used, from 2
mg/m to 100 mg/m twice daily, so that the number of patients
who were given the optimum dose of tamoxifen may have been modest.
In Heinonen's trial too (45) the response rate was higher after
the combination therapy, but the difference was not significant.
Tamoxifen combined with medroxyprogesterone acetate (MPA)

produced lower response rate than tamoxifen alone (46), but the dose of MPA was rather low. In one trial tamoxifen was compared to tamoxifen in combination with prednisolone. The combination treatment was significantly more effective that the single-drug therapy, for which the response rate was, in fact, remarkably low (47). In three small trials no significant differences were observed between treatment with tamoxifen alone and tamoxifen in combination with aminoglutethimide (48-49) or bromocriptin (50). In the trial comparing tamoxifen with tamoxifen in combination with aminoglutethimide, hydrocortisone and danazol (51) the response rate was significantly superior with the combination, however, no differences in response durations or survival times were observed.

A number of similar trials of combined endocrine therapy are now in progress. The provisional overall results of these trials are nevertheless disappointing.

From the results of these trials it may be concluded that single agent therapy with tamoxifen should be used as the endocrine therapy of choice in postmenopausal patients, whilst the other forms of treatment may be used as endocrine therapy of second choice, depending on the response to the primary treatment. Thus, in patients who respond to first line therapy the probability of a later response to second line endocrine therapy (cross-sensitivity) is 48% whereas it is only 12% in those who fail to respond to the initial endocrine therapy (non-cross resistance)(41).

Based upon the available clinical data and upon present knowledge about the mechanism of action of endocrine therapy it seems unlikely that overall therapeutic results could be significantly improved. However, for specific subgroups of patients further progress may be obtained through development of improved tests to predict the outcome of endocrine therapy.

ENDOCRINE THERAPY IN PRIMARY BREAST CANCER. OVERALL RESULTS.

Ablative endocrine therapy

The efficacy of primary castration has been investigated in a number of trials (52-56). In these trials no significant reduction in recurrence rate and survival was observed with the exception of a subgroup of premenopausal patients $\geq$ 45 years who in addition received prednisone 7.5 mg daily continued for 5 years (56).

In a randomized trial including 354 premenopausal patients no difference in survival was observed between the groups treated with either ovarian irradiation or tamoxifen for one year (57).

Non-ablative endocrine therapy

Two randomized studies with adjuvant estrogen (58) and aminoglutethimide (59) have been published. In both studies the treated patient groups did better than the non-treated control groups as far as recurrence rate is concerned. Further follow-up is required to determine any survival benefit.

The vast majority of data of adjuvant therapy originates from studies using treatment with tamoxifen. These have recently been analyzed in detail (60) and a summary of the studies who included a non-treated control group is shown in Table 3.

Table 3. Randomized adjuvant studies of tamoxifen versus control.

Reference	Menopausal status	No. of pts.	Median follow-up (months)	Significant improvement of RFS
61-63	PRE	202	77	no (p=0.31)
	POST	94	77	yes (p=0.004)
64-67	POST	865	30	yes (p=0.01)
57	POST	552	NI	NI -
68-69	PRE+ POST	1124	35	yes (p=0.01)
70-72	POST	1647	35	yes (p=0.013)
73	POST	629	36	yes (p=0.001)
74	POST	366	37	yes (p<0.018)

PRE = premenopausal POST = postmenopausal NI = not indicated

When comparing these studies, it should be emphasized that definitions and criteria of eligibility differ with regard to menopausal status, age and node status. Daily dose of tamoxifen varies from study to study and so does treatment duration.

Further it should be noted that the use of postoperative
radiotherapy, which is known to reduce the rate of local
recurrence, differs. In some of the studies (61-63, 70-72) all
patients received postoperative radiotherapy. In one study (73)
none received post operative radiotherapy and in the other
studies some of the patients, predominantly the node positive
ones, received postoperative radiotherapy. Nevertheless all
these 7 trials but on (57) have reported a significant
improvement of recurrence free survival (Table 3). One of the
groups (61-63) specified the results for pre- and postmenopausal
patients and in these trials a significant benefit of tamoxifen
was observed only in the postmenopausal group. Only one of the
trials (68-69) has reported a significant improvement of survival.
It should be emphasized in this connection that times of
observation are still very short and limited to the very early
phase of the course of the clinical disease. Also it should be
mentioned that none of these publications presented information
about the treatment of recurrent disease.

It is evident from the data presented so far that an
improvement of recurrence-free survival can be achieved with
adjuvant tamoxifen but prolonged time of follow-up is required to
conclude about the impact on survival.

COMPARISON OF EFFICACY OF TREATMENT WITH TAMOXIFEN IN PRIMARY AND
ADVANCED DISEASE.
Overall results

Endocrine therapy of advanced disease remains palliative.
Whether this is true also for adjuvant therapy remains to be
established by prolonged follow up of the ongoing trials.

In this connection the question arises what can actually be
expected from adjuvant therapy provided the sensitivity of the
micrometastases is similar to that of overt clinical disease.
Let us assume that 30% of patients with micrometastatic disease
will be cured from adjuvant treatment with tamoxifen
corresponding to the 30% remission rate (PR+CR) in advanced
disease. A 20% survival rate of node positive untreated patients
at 20 years after primary surgery would than be expected to be

increased to 44%. Assuming a 10% cure rate corresponding to the 10% complete remission rate in the advanced disease the survival figures at 20 years would be increased from 20% to 28%. If however, we assume that in the adjuvant situation we just achieve an overall response similar to that reported in the advanced disease one might expect the survival time in patients treated postoperatively with tamoxifen to be delayed to a degree corresponding to time to progression when treating advanced disease, which is approximately 6-12 months. These examples, which are shown in Fig. 1 merely give an impression about the frames within which the adjuvant survival data could be expected provided different assumptions. The time of observation in the ongoing adjuvant trials, however, is still too short to analyze which, if any, of these assumptions is the more likely to be valid.

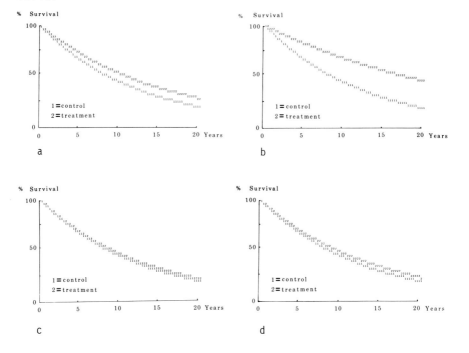

Fig. 1. Constructed survival data with adjuvant treatment provided a) 10% cure rate, b) 30% cure rate, c) 6 months delay of death and d) 12 months delay of death. See text for further explanation.

Results in specific subgroups

Based upon cumulated data the response to tamoxifen seems to increase with increasing age (16). In the adjuvant situation, however, data from the Danish Breast Cancer Cooperative Group (DBCG) demonstrate that the gain achieved with tamoxifen decreases with increasing age (71). This discrepancy cannot be immediately explained and needs further evaluation. In the advanced situation there might well, with increasing age, be an increasing rate of selection of good-prognosis patients, giving rise to a false impression of increasing overall response rate with increasing age. The data presented in the literature are insufficient to enable an analysis of whether this is true.

In advanced disease the response to endocrine therapy is known to be related to the ER-status (42) and some studies have also demonstrated that the rate of response increases with increasing ER-level (75-76). The majority of adjuvant trials have similarly reported the efficacy of adjuvant tamoxifen to be related to the presence of estrogenreceptor in the tumor (60). However, in the DBCG trial it was observed that ER-positive patients with low ER-levels (10-100 fmol/mg cytosol protein) did not benefit from adjuvant tamoxifen, whereas the recurrence free survival was significantly improved with adjuvant tamoxifen in patients with $\geq$ 100 fmol of ER in the tumor. These results should be confirmed in other studies but might be explained by the fact that tamoxifen in the heterogeneous tumor reduces only the hormone sensitive cells and thus possibly permits more rapid growth of the hormone independent cells (77). If this theory is correct one might expect duration of response in advanced disease to be shorter in patients with low ER-levels compared to patients with high levels. Whether this is true is for the moment being analyzed retrospectively in a large danish trial.

The data available so far in the literature do not enable further subgroup comparisons of efficacy in micrometastatic and clinical overt disease.

CONCLUSION

In conclusion endocrine therapy of advanced breast cancer remains palliative and whether cure can be achieved with adjuvant therapy remains to be demonstrated.

When comparing the therapeutic gain achieved with adjuvant and palliative endocrine therapy in some specific subgroups of patients conflicting results seem to be apparent. Future analyses should present more detailed subgroup analyses in both advanced and primary disease in order to improve the prediction of the therapeutic results and to improve our knowledge about the biological behavior of the disease including the biological implications of endocrine adjuvant therapy.

REFERENCES

1. Dao, T.L.: Annu.Rev.Med. 23: 1-18, 1972.
2. Robin, P.E. and Dalton, G.A.: In: Breast cancer management - early and late. (ed. Stoll, B.A.), Chicago Year Book, Chicago 1977, pp. 147-156.
3. Hayward, J.: Hormones and human breast cancer. Springer, Berlin, Heidelberg, New York, Recent Results in Cancer Research, vol 24, 1970.
4. Dao, T.L.: Surg.Clin.North.Am. 58: 801-807, 1978.
5. Hayward, J.L., Atkins, H.J.B., Falconer, M.A.: In: The Clinical Management of Advanced Breast Cancer. (Ed. C.A.F. Joslin, Gleave, E.N.) Alpha Omega, Cardiff, 1970. pp. 50-53.
6. Stuart-Harris, R.C. and Smith, I.E.: Cancer treat. Rev. 11: 189-204, 1984.
7. Jungmann, E. and Althoff, P.H.: Dia 20: 48-50, 1981.
8. Semple, C.G., Thomson, J.A., Stark, A.N., McDonald, M. and Beatstoll, G.H.: Clin. Endocrinol. 17: 569-575, 1982.
9. Chamness, G.C., Asch, R.H. and Paurstein, C.J.: AM.J.Obstec.Gynecol. 136: 426-429, 1980.
10. Menon, M., Azhar, S. and Menon, K.M.J.: Am.J.Obstec.Gynecol. 136: 524-530, 1980.
11. Jenkin, G.: Aust.N.Z.J.Obstet.Gynaec. 20: 113-118, 1980.
12. Lippman, M. Bolan, G. and Hoff, K. Cancer Res. 36: 4595-4601, 1976.
13. Zava, D.T., McGuire, W.L.: Science 199: 787-788, 1978.
14. Nicholson, R.I., Davies, P., Griffiths, K.: Eur.J.Cancer 14: 439-445, 1978.
15. Lober, J., Rose, C., Salimtschik, M. and Mouridsen, H.T.: Acta Ostet.Gynecol.Scand. (suppl.) 101: 39-47, 1981.
16. Furr, B.J.A. and Jordan, V.C.: Pharmca.Ther. 25: 127-205, 1984.
17. Henderson, I.C., Canellos, G.P.: New.Engl.J.Med. 302: 17-30, 1980.
18. Carter, A.C., Sedransk, N., Kelley, R.M.: JAMA 237: 2079-2085, 1977.
19. Volk, H., Deupree, R.H., Goldenberg, I.S., Wilde, R.C., Carabasi, R.A. and Escher: Cancer 9: 33-39, 1974.
20. Talley, R.W., Haines, C.R., Waters, M.N.: Cancer 32: 315-320, 1973.
21. Cavalli, F., Goldhirsch, A., Jungi, W.F., Martz, G., Alberto, P.: Excerpta Medica Intern. Congress. Series no. 64: 224-236, 1982.
22. Kamby, C., Engelman, E., Nooy, M.: 2nd Eur.Conf.Clin.Oncol. 17-29, 1983.
23. Mouridsen, H.T., Palshof, T., Patterson, J. and Battersby, L.: Cancer Treat.Rev. 5: 131-141, 1978.
24. McGuire, W.L.: Semin.Oncol. 5: 428, 1978.
25. Ward, H.W.C.: Br.Med.J. 1: 13-14, 1973.
26. Bratherton, D.G., Brown, C.H., Buchanan, R., Hall, V., Kingsley Pillers, E.M., Wheeler, T.K. and Williams C.J.: Br.J.Cancer 50: 199-205, 1984.
27. Hindley, A.C.: 3rd EORTC Breast Cancer Working Conf. Abstract no. IX, 21, 1983.

28. Coombs, R.C., Dearnaley, D., Humphreys, J., Gazet, J.C., Ford, H.T., Bash, A.G., Mashiter, K. and Powles, T.J.: Cancer Treat. Rep. In press.

29. Pritchard, K.I., Thomson, D.B., Myers, R.E., Sutherland, D.J.A., Mobbs, B.G. and Meakin, J..: Rev.Endocr.Cancer, suppl. 9: 399-408, 1981.

30. Planting, A., Blonk v.d. Mejst, J., Alexiewa-Figusch, J.: 3rd EORTC Breast Cancer Working Conf. Abstract IX, 17, 1983.

31. Stewart, J.F., Forrest, A.P.M., Gunn, J.M.: Eur.J.Cancer, suppl. 1: 83-88, 1980.

32. Beex, L., Pieters, G., Smals, A., Koenders, A., Benraad, T. and Kloppenberg, P.: Cancer Treat. Rep. 65: 179-185, 1981.

33. Ingle, J.N., Ahmann, D.L., Green, S.J., Edmonson, J.H., Bisel, J.H., Kvals, L.K., Nichols, W.C., Creagan, E.T., Hahn, R.G., Rubin, J. and Frytag, S.: New.Eng.J.Med. 304: 16-21, 1981.

34. Westerberg, H.: Cancer Treat. Rep. 64: 117-121, 1980.

35. Ingle, J.N., Creagan, E.T., Ahmann, D.I., Hahn, R.G., Green, S.J., Rubin, J. and Edmonson, J.H.: Am.J.Clin.Oncol. 5: 155-160, 1982.

36. Morgan, L.R. and Donley, P.J.: Rev. Endocr. Rel. Cancer, suppl. 9: 301-310, 1981.

37. Beretta, G., Tabiadon, D., Tedeschi, L. and Luporini, G.: In: The Role of Tamoxifen in Breast Cancer (Ed. S. Iacobelli), Raven Press, 1982, pp. 113-120.

38. Pannuti, F., Martoni, A., Fruet, F., Burroni, P., Canova, N. and Hall, S.: In: The Role of Tamoxifen in Breast Cancer. (Ed. Iacobelli, S., Lippman, M.E. and Robustelli Della Cuna, G.), Raven Press, 1982, pp. 85-92.

39. Lipton, A., Harvey, H.A., Santen, R.J., Boucher, A., White, D., Bernath, A., Dixon, R., Richards, G. and Shafik, A.: Cancer Res. 42: 3434s-3436s, 1982.

40. Smith, I.E., Harris, A.L., Morgan, M., Gazet, J.C., McKinna, J.A.: Cancer Res. 42: 3430s-3433s, 1982.

41. Rose, C. and Mouridsen, H.T.: In: Progress in Cancer Research and Therapy, (Eds. Bresciani, F., King, R.B.J., Lippman, M.E., Namer, M., Raynud, J.P.), Raven Press, New York, 1984. pp. 269-286.

42. Rose, C. and Mouridsen, H.T.: In: Recent Results in Cancer Research. (Eds. Leclercq, G., Toma, S., Paridaens, R., Heuson, J.C.). Springer Veralg, Berlin-Heidelberg, 1984. pp. 230-242.

43. Mouridsen, H.T., Salimtschik, P., Dombernowsky, P., Gelshoj, K., Palshof, T., Rorth, M., Daehnfeldt, J.L. and Rose, C.: Europ.J. Cancer, suppl. 1: 107-110, 1980.

44. Tormey, D.C., Lippman, M.E., Edwards, M.K. and Cassidy: Ann.Intern.Med.: 98: 139-144, 1983.

45. Heinonen, E., Alanko, A., Grohn, P. and Rissanen, P.: Abstract pag. 28. 1st. Scandinavian Breast Cancer Symposium, Aarhus, Denmark, 1982.

46. Mouridsen, H.T., Ellemann, K., Mattsson, W., Palshof, T., Daehnfeldt, J.L. and Rose, C.: Cancer Treat.Rep. 63: 171-175, 1979.

47. Stewart, J.F., Rubens, R.D., King, R.J.B., Minton, M.J., Steiner, R., Tong, D., Winter, P.J., Knoght, R.K. and Hayward, J.L.: Eur.J.Clin.Oncol. 18: 1307-1314, 1982.

48. Milsted, R., Habeshow, T., Sangster, G., Kaye, S. and Calman, K.: Abstract pag. 186. 2nd Eur. Conf. Clin. Oncol. and Cancer Nursing, Amsterdam, 1983.

49. Ingle, J.N., Green, S.J., Ahmann, D.L., Edmonson, J.H., Nichols, W.C., Frytag, S. and Rubin, J.: Cancer Res. suppl. 42: 3461s-3467s, 1982.

50. Settatree, R.S.: Revs. Endocr.Rel.Cancer. Suppl. 5: 63-70, 1980.

51. Powles, T.J., Ashley, S., Ford, H.T.: Lancet 1: 1369-1373, 1984.

52. Nevinny, H.B., Nevinny, D., Rosoff, C.B., Hall, T.C., Mucnek, H.: Am.J.Surg. 117: 531-536, 1969.

53. Ravdin, R.G., Lewison, E.F., Slack, N.H., Gardner, B., State, D., Fischer, B.: Surg.Gynecol.Obstet. 131: 1055-1063, 1970.

54. Cole, M.P.: In: Hormones Breast Cancer. (Eds. Namer, M., Lalanne, C.M.) Inserm, Paris, vol. 55, 1975. pp. 143-150.

55. Nissen-Meyer, R.: In: Hormones and Breast Cancer. (Eds. Names, M, Lalanne, C.M.) Inserm, Paris, vol. 55, 1975. pp. 151-158.

56. Meakin, J.W., Allt, W.E.C., Beale, F.A., Busk, R.S., Clark, R.M., Fitzpatrick, P.J., Hawkins, N.V., Jenkin, R.D.T., Pringle, J.F., Reid, J.G., Riderm, W.O., Hayward, J.L. and Bulbrosch, R.D.: In: Breast Cancer, Experimental and Clinical Aspects. (Eds, Mouridsen, H.T. and Palshof, T.). Pergamon Press, 1980. pp. 179-183.

57. Ribeiro, B. and Palmer M.K.: Br.Med.J. 286: 827-830, 1983.

58. Palshof, T., Mouridsen, H.T. and Daehnfeldt, J.L.: In: Breast Cancer Experimental and Clinical Aspect. (Eds. Mouridsen, H.T. and Palshof, T.). Pergamon Press, Oxford and New York, 1980. pp. 183-189.

59. Coombes, R.C., Chilvers, C., McLelland, R.: J. steroid Biochem. 19: Abstract no. 228, 1983.

60. Mouridsen, H.T.: Rev. in Endocrine Related Cancer 1985. In press.

61. Palshof, T., Mouridsen, H.. and Daehnfeldt, J.L.: In: Breast Cancer Experimental and Clinical Aspect. (Eds. Mouridsen, H.T. and Palshof, T.). Pergamon Press, Oxford and New York, 1980. pp. 183-189.

62. Palshof, T.: Canadian J. Surg. 24: 379-384, 1981.

63. Palshof, T., Carstensen, B., Briand, P. Mouridsen, H.T. and Dombernowsky, P.: Rev.Endocr.Rel.Cancer. 1985. In press.

64. Wallgren, A., Baral, E., Glas, U., Kaigas, M., Karnstrom, L., Nordenskjold, B., Theve, N.O., Wilking, N., Silversward, C.: In: Adjuvant Therapy of Cancer. (Eds. Salmon, S.E. and Jones, S.E.). Grune & Stratton, New York, 1981.

65. Wallgren, A., Glas, U., Gustafsson, S., Skoog, L., Theve, N.O. and Nofdenskjold, B.: Recent Results Cancer Res. 91: 214-219, 1984.

66. Wallgren, A.: Rev.Endocr.Rel.Cancer, suppl. 12: 15-20, 1982.

67. Wallgren, A., Baral, E., Beling, U., Castensen, J., Friberg, S., Glas, U., Kaigas, M. and Skoog, L.: In: Adjuvant Chemotherapy of Breast Cancer. (Ed. Senn, H.J.). Springer Verlag, Berlin, Heidelberg, New York, Tokyo, 1984. pp. 197-203.

68. Baum, M., Brinkley, D.M., Dossett, J.A., McPherson, K., Patterson, J.S., Rubens, R.D., Smidy, F.G., Stoll, B.A., Wilson, A., Lea, J.C., Richards, D. and Ellis, S.H.: Lancel a: 257-261, 1983.
69. Baum, M., Brinkley, D.M., Dossett, J.A., McPherson, K., Patterson, J.S., Rubens, R.D., Smiddy, F.G., Stoll, B.A., Wilson, A., Lea, J.C., Richards, D. and Ellisa, S.H.: Lancet II: 450, 1983.
70. Rose, C., Thorpe, S.M., Mouridsen, H.T., Andersen, J.A., Brincker, H., and Andersen, K.W.: Breast Cancer Res. and treat. 3: 77-84, 1983.
71. Mouridsen, H.T., Rose, C., Brincker, H., Thorpe, S.M., Rank, F., Fischerman, K. and Andersen, K.W.: Recent Results in Cancer Research vol. 96: 117-128, 1984.
72. Rose, C., Thorpe, S.M., Andersen, K.W., Pedersen, B.V., Mouridsen, H.T., Blichert-Toft, M. and Rasmussen, B.B.: Lancet I: 16-19, 1985.
73. Ludwig Breast Cancer Study Group.: Lancet I: 1256-1260, 1984.
74. Pritchard, K.I., Meakin, J.W., Boyd, N.F., Ambus, U., BeBoer, G., Dembo, A.J., Paterson, A.H.G., Sutherland, D.J.A., Wilkinson, R.H., Bassett, A.A., Evans, W.K., Beale, F.A., Clark, R.M., Keane, T.J. In: Adjuvant Therapy of Cancer. (Eds. Salmon, S.E. and Jones, S.E.). Grune & Stratton, New York, 1984. In press.
75. Rose, C., Thorpe, S.M., Lober, J., Daehnfeldt, J.L., Palshof, T. and Mouridsen, H.T.: Rec. Results Cancer Res. 71: 134-141, 1980.
76. Campbell, F.C., Elston, C.W., Blamey, R.W., Morris, A.H., Nicholson, R.I., Griffiths, K., Haybittle, J.L.: Lancet II: 1317-1319, 1981.
77. Noble, R.L.: Cancer Res. 37: 82-94, 1977.

25

New Immunoreagents in Breast Cancer Diagnosis and Experimental Therapy: Report on the Workshop on Markers for Differentiation and Malignancy

Roberto L. Ceriani

John Muir Cancer and Aging Research Institute, 2055 North Broadway, Walnut Creek, California 94596, U.S.A.

The workshop entitled "Markers for Differentiation and Malignancy" comprised sixteen short papers that on hindsight could be divided into three groups: Cell nuclear parameters and breast cancer prognosis; use of breast differentiation and other antigens identified by monoclonal antibodies in histopathology; and the use of anti-breast monoclonal antibodies for sero-diagnostic and therapeutic purposes.

With new molecular immunochemical approaches to breast cancer diagnosis and treatment developed in the last years, the field of markers to be used in breast cancer diagnosis has evolved largely supported by the creation of new reagents and by the availability of very sophisticated and previously not available expensive equipment. In many cases the successful symbiosis between the new reagents and the ultra-sophisticated equipment has been achieved, such as in the case of the use of monoclonal antibodies to immunostain cell populations which are then sorted out with the flow cell cytofluorimeter. Nevertheless, in spite of these new technological approaches, traditional, established ideas for diagnostic approaches in breast cancer have remained extant, and little challenge was presented in this workshop. Now these ideas have been tested at a much higher level of accuracy and sophistication and some of them have stood inquest and remained viable, thus providing valuable guidance for diagnosis and at times for prognosis of breast cancer.

An example of this has been the use of nucleic DNA content for the prognosis of human breast cancer. Two papers, those of Dr. Prop from The Netherlands Cancer Institute, Amsterdam, and of Dr. Spyratos, from the Centre Rene Huguenin, St. Cloud, France, dealt with this established characteristic of tumors. Dr. Prop examined the ploidy of a large number of breast tumors, and then followed their clinical course and, as other investigators have previously shown, he confirmed that euploidy is a good indicator for good prognosis in breast cancer. Determinations were made on nuclei obtained from surgical specimens of breast cancer tumors. To further support these views, Dr. Spyratos applying the recent approach of needle biopsy of the breast, managed to obtain enough nuclear material from these small fragments of tissue, as to be able to obtain a flow cytofluorimetric analysis of the nuclei present in such small sample, and correlate it with the clinical evolution of the patients. This innovative use of very minute biopsy material for use in flow cytofluorimetric analysis with the aim of establishing a prognosis, seems easy to undertake and had satisfactory results in their hands. Most histologically diagnosed breast carcinomas were aneuploid while all benign diseases of the breast were euploid. Procedures of this kind could be very valuable for the establishment of a prognosis even before surgical intervention.

Several papers comprised the group which dealt with differentiation antigens of breast cells. Dr. F. Leoni from the Instituto Nazionale per Studio e La Cura dei Tumori, Milano, Italy, described monoclonal antibodies against the neutral glycolipid antigens produced in Dr. Colnaghi's group (1). These antibodies clearly recognize these cell-surface molecules, which have a characteristic specificity for breast epithelium mainly, and can be used for histopathology as well as for tumor localization studies. These glycolipid saccharide determinants could also be expressed in glycoproteins obtained both from breast epithelial cells and also from human milk fat globule, and also in colon and ovarian carcinomas. In the latter carcinomas, as well as in the breast the oligosaccharide determinant is present in glycoproteins and mucins of varying molecular weight. These cell surface components are found in cells of pleural and peritoneal effusions of patients carrying these tumors and possibly in the serum. Thus, in this paper, and in many of the following ones, again there is an example of an already postulated approach (2), that normal differentiation antigens of epithelial cells used as markers for carcinomas and also in assays aimed at their diagnosis and follow-up is a very valuable approach. In contrast, J. Burchell from the Imperial Cancer Research Fund, London described antibodies to secretory components of breast epithelial cells, namely beta-casein and alpha-lactalbumin. In this work the striking finding was that the same monoclonal antibody will bind to both antigens used. By affinity chromatography experiments, the authors support their view that these two molecules share antigenicity. When the amino acid homology of both proteins had been investigated only four amino acids were shared by alpha-lactalbumin and beta-casein. Thus, the authors surmised that most likely the epitope identified by their monoclonal antibody could be an interrupted epitope. Possibly a study of the binding affinity of the antibody to the two antigens could ascertain whether identical epitopes are involved. Two other interesting papers belonging to this group were devoted to metabolic events of cell-surface antigens of breast epithelial cells identified by monoclonal antibodies against milk fat globule antigens and other cell surface component. Dr. G. Buehring from University of California, Berkeley described conditions for the stimulation of synthesis of the 400,000 approximate molecular weight cell-surface glycoprotein of breast epithelial cells (3,4). Hormones that usually stimulate differentiation in terms of secretory functions in breast epithelium also stimulated MCF-7 cells to increase the synthesis of this antigen. However, two chemicals known to stimulate differentiation in other tumor cells, dimethylsulfoxide and hexamethylenebisacetamide, showed to

have different stimulatory effect on the breast epithelial cells
depending on the hormonal supplement that these cells received.
As a corollary Dr. Buehring suggests that both these promoters of
differentiation interact with the action of mammogenic hormones
in inducing differentiation, or that perhaps they interfere with
the receptor presentation to such hormones. In another paper Dr.
M. Ward from the Ludwig Institute in London reports cell binding
of anti-cell surface monoclonal antibody labeled with radioiodine
or with radioactive indium, using a conjugating arm. After
binding to the cell surface of breast epithelial cells they
became internalized. After internalization of the
antigen-antibody complex Dr. Ward followed the fate of this
complex. He found at the ultrastructural level after tagging the
antibody with colloidal gold, that the incorporation of the
antibody is prompt, using both coated and non-coated vessicles.
After 6 hours it was possible to find the tracer participating in
lysosomal complexes. This proves that the antigen
antibody-complex is fully internalized and then follows a route
of metabolism with defined steps within the cell. Comparisons
are being made now of the antibody's cytoxic action on the target
cells. These last two papers, that study the role of
glycoproteins detected by monoclonal antibodies on the cell
surface of breast epithelial cells, study in fact,
differentiation components of the breast epithelial cell (2)
which share characteristics of cellular metabolism and function
with other cell surface molecules. Thus, they are stimulated in
their expression by mammogenic hormones, and as macromolecules on
the cell surface they participate in membraneous and
trans-membraneous phenomena, such, that after binding to the
corresponding antibody internalization occurs and a definite and
expected sequence of events follows. It can be envisaged that
after these preliminary descriptive findings, monoclonal
antibodies against cell surface components of breast cells will
be used in cell biology experiments in efforts to elucidate cell
membrane architecture and function. This latter area has been a
slowly developing one as a result of the scarce probes available

to identify cell surface components. To aid in the identification of other non-epithelial cells in the breast Dr. S. Dairkee from Peralta Cancer Research Institute, Oakland, California described a monoclonal antibody that binds a 57,000 daltons cytokeratin which apparently is only found on the basal, myoepithelial cells of the breast. In conjunction with antibodies that define the epithelial cells this anti-myoepithelial cell antibody could be useful to the pathologist in assessing the integrity of the myoepithelial network around normal alveoli and ducts. They only drawback of this antibody is its lack of reaction on paraffin embedded sections, a characteristic that has plagued the production of monoclonal antibodies for histopathology studies. Possibly the purification of the identifiable antigen from fresh breast tissue and then preparation of antibodies anew will allow for the selection of those that would bind fixed and embedded tissue.

In the area of comparative studies two interesting papers described the interrelationship of some antigenic markers in different species and humans. Dr. T. Ohno from the Jikei University in Tokyo, Japan described the preparation of monoclonal antibodies against GP52 antigen of mouse mammary tumor virus. It was possible to prepare these antibodies only by immunizing mice which have genetic susceptibility for autoimmune diseases as a source of B-cells for hybridization. The monoclonal antibody created against GP52 reacted with the human mammary epithelial cell lines T47D and MCF-7. The staining was mostly cytoplasmatic, and apparently was also found in human breast tumors. No reaction was found in benign breast lesions, in normal breast tissues, and in lung and testicular carcinomas. This interesting cross reactivity, that has been previously reported (5), will lead the way for studies of the shared expression of products of expression of oncogenetic material. In a similar way, Dr. Hageman from the Netherlands Cancer Institute, Amsterdam, presented evidence that monoclonal antibodies against human milk fat globule (2) cross-reacted with antigens present in feline mammary carcinomas. This finding is a certain significance since not only because it speaks of a maintained antigenic structure for milk fat globule antigens through the higher mammals, but also presents the opportunity for a larger body size model for studies in human breast cancer.

The following papers comprised the group in which monoclonal antibodies against breast epithelial cells and human milk fat globule antigens were used in attempts to develop methodology for histopathology, serum diagnosis and immune therapy.

Two histopathology presentations which made use of cell surface directed anti-breast monoclonal antibodies were discussed first. One of them used the B72.3 monoclonal antibody generated by Dr. Schlom's (6) laboratory. The antigen corresponding to this monoclonal antibody is a prevalent component of epithelial cells, and is also present in colon carcinomas. Using B72.3 Dr. M. Nuti from the Univ. of Pisa, Italy, examined its binding to areas of aprocrine metaplasia in breast tumors. She found that the antibody binds to the apical surface of the clear breast epithelial cells in regions with apocrine metaplasia. The molecular identification of this histological pattern could contribute to establish prognosis for the breast cancer patient. Binding of this monoclonal antibody was not obtained to the surrounding non-apocrine neoplastic breast tissue, neither to the normal ducts, it bound to other apocrine glands of the organism. Apocrine structures share common antigenicity, thus linking antigenicity and morphological features. Interestingly enough, in this case it is shown that even after neoplastic transformation this antigen is expressed. In a similar vein, A. Jonassen from Columbia University in New York City, showed that a monoclonal against a cell surface component of the breast epithelial cell line T47D could be used in its ability to detect breast tissue. These studies were devised to identify, as breast, cutaneous metastases without a carcinoma origin. This antibody stains a large proportion of breast cancers, it also stains normal breast epithelium apically, and in sections of skin, the breast

cancer metastases could be clearly identified as deeply
stained cellular areas. This antibody as well as the
preceding one, will be helpful tools for the histopathologist
in identifying breast cancer patterns with a less desirable
prognosis as well as the sub-cutaneous microdissemination
which also could indicate similar undesirable prognosis. In
addition, in efforts to help derive prognosis, Dr. N. Agnantis
from the Hellenic Anticancer Institute in Athens, studied the
expression of Harvey-ras oncogene expression on breast tumors
and their normal counterpart. She found this oncogene product
was elevated when compared to normal tissue levels, without
finding these increased levels of clear prognostic value.
However, high average values were found for infiltrating and
already metastatic breast tumors, when compared to primaries.
Perhaps full interpretation of these findings will be arrived
at together with a clearer understanding of the role of
oncogene products in neoplasia.

Dr. John Hilkens from the Netherlands Cancer Institute,
Amsterdam discussed studies on levels of a human milk fat globule
antigen in circulation of breast cancer patients. It also
extends it to the antigen of high molecular weight which is under
investigation in many laboratories presently (2,3). Dr. Hilkens
found high levels in the sera of breast, ovarian, cervical and
prostatic cancer. Of particular interest was that 85% of the
breast cancer patients with metastatic dissemination were
positive, while background levels were found in normal subjects
and patients with benign disease of the breast. In view that
upwards and downwards trends of these antigens' levels
corresponded to worsening and improvement, respectively, of the
clinical status of breast cancer patients under therapy, Dr.
Hilkens supports the view that milk fat globule antigens could be
used in the follow-up of breast cancer patients and could add
prognostic indications as previously postulated (7).

The two following papers dealt with the ability of
anti-human milk fat globule antibodies to bind and kill, or at
best arrest growth, of human breast tumors. Dr. A. Griffiths,

from the Imperial Cancer Research Fund in London reported his studies of injection into patients of anti-human milk fat globule antibody and its binding to cutaneous metastases of breast cancer. The cutaneous metastases of human breast cancer bound the antibody in immunoperoxidase stained paraffin-embedded sections. He could also obtain antigen separated from metastases extracts in immunoblots to bind the labeled antibody used in these studies. Further, the antibody also bound pleural effusion cells showing again its ability to label metastatic cells of breast tumors. Once the integrity of the labeled antibody was tested thus, it was injected into the patient. The circulating anti-milk fat globule monoclonal antibody obtained from the serum of the injected subject stained again immunoblots of cell lysates, proving its integrity. In spite of all this convincing evidence for the presence and activity of the antibody in the serum of the patient, possibly due to a low concentration of the antigen on the metastases, or other unidentified factors, imaging could not be obtained. Nevertheless, the antibody could be detected on the tumor metastases that were imaged, once autoradiographs were prepared from the excised tissue. This paper clearly shows the difficulties that are found in the in vivo use of monoclonal antibodies and their uncertain fate once they are injected into the circulation.

To exemplify even further this point Dr. R. Ceriani, from the John Muir Cancer and Aging Research Institute, Walnut Creek, California, described experiments in the experimental immunotherapy of human breast tumors implanted in nude mice. These experiments clearly showed that a mixture or "cocktail" of monoclonal antibodies against human milk fat globule could arrest up to 90% the growth of subcutaneously implanted breast tumors. This effect was obtained by injection of the monoclonal "cocktail" at the same time that the tumor was implanted. This approach was called passive immunization. Once the validity of the "cocktail" approach was proven, each of the components of the monoclonal cocktail was injected separate, or in incomplete mixtures. The results were always inferior to the injection of the full cocktail. It is conceivable that at the root of this need for the use of several monoclonal antibodies simultaneously lies the phenomenon of tumor cell heterogeneity. In further experiments shown by Dr. Ceriani, treatment of already established human breast tumors in nude mice was also proven successful. The growth of these established human breast tumors could be arrested by injection of the "cocktail" of monoclonal antibodies against milk fat globule. However, in either type of approach some tumor tissue survived after antibody treatment in most host mice. By immunohistochemical procedures, the content of antigen of the treatment-surviving tumor could be estimated to be less than 10% the antigen content of the original tumor when grafted. Undoubtedly, tumor cell heterogeneity again in this instance plays an important role in the creation of alternative, treatment-resistant, cell populations, as well as it is well known, it creates newer chemotherapy-resistant cells in breast cancer patients.

Overall the largest contribution to the session was the contingent of presentations where monoclonal antibodies against normal breast cell components were used either for immunohistopathology, sero-diagnosis, therapy of basic cell biology studies. This rapidly enlarging field was initiated with the discovery in the early seventies of antigen-antibody systems in breast epithelia that could be detected by antibodies against milk fat globule (2). Most of the antibodies used by researchers in this session were mainly of this type, thus pointing to the usefulness of these normal breast epithelial determinants with larger or lesser specificity for breast epithelial cells. Among the sources of immunization the human milk fat globule (2,7) represented the most important source of many of the antigens present on the breast epithelial cell. An advantage of the milk fat globule is its easy separation and considerably large availability.

In regards to specificity, most anti-normal breast components, had epithelial specificity within the breast, and secretory epithelia specificity within the organism. Taking these limitations into account it is noticeable their valuable contribution in cell identification, both of metastatic human breast epithelium and interspecies tumors, in the measurement of breast epithelial antigens sera and in immunotherapy and imaging.

As for other presentations related to immuno-histopathological applications this unfolding field will soon be a specialty on its own, considering the number of very valuable immunoreagents continuously being created. They will help pathological diagnosis at a molecular level in the very uncertain area of prognosis. Further, specificity plays a lesser role when these monoclonal antibodies are used in histopathology. In this area, the prognostic importance of the presence, absence or level of a given antigen need not be correlated to its specificity. Establishments of profiles of antigen-binding for breast tumors could lead to valuable prognostic guidelines, however the corroboration of such prognostic capabilities for monoclonal antibodies will imply the performance of important and lengthy anatomo-clinical correlation studies. The main drawback of the present situation is the scarcity of antibodies that would bind fixed breast tissue. Most of them would bind live cells, frozen sections, etc. At this juncture it is most desirable that the often taunted "tailoring" of monoclonal antibodies to its use be taken seriously, and serious efforts should be dedicated to obtain antibodies binding fixed, paraffin-embedded tissues. The immunopathologist will then use them in giving prognostic indications in solid tumors, which are not processed routinely in the pathology laboratory the way hematopoietic malignancies are. The fast application of monoclonal antibodies to the latter in the past was due to the routine handling of unfixed cells of hematopoitic malignancies.

In immunotherapy, imaging and sero-diagnosis it is relevant that many factors other than antigen-antibody binding avidity and specificity will play important roles in their successful use. The studies presented in the session demonstrated the feasibility of these approaches using anti-human milk fat globule monoclonal antibodies, but however pointed out to the role of local tumor conditions, antigenic disposal, tissue permeability, etc. in restricting the applicability of the techniques. Important hope is placed today in efforts conducive to the understanding of all these ancillary tumor biology areas which will help advance the application of these antibodies in the daily clinical practice. In this context, studies presented at the workshop relating to control of the human milk fat globule antigen expression and their cellular metabolism seem like efforts in the right direction.

Thus considering the advancements introduced in the field of markers of breast cancer by the newer technologies, it is possible to look forward to an ever evolving area of studies that will bring to the surgeon-pathologist-oncologist team much more sensitive and specific means for early diagnosis of breast and later ensuring its therapy. The immunopathologist will be able to provide prognosis based on molecular mechanisms in which the antigens detected by the antibodies participate and the oncologist will be armed with more discriminating imaging reagents and newer immunotherapeutic approaches that could play an important role in the management of the breast cancer patient in the near future.

302

REFERENCES

1. Canevair, S., Fossati, G., Balsari, A., Sonnino, S., Colnaghi, M.I., Cancer Res. 43:1301-1305, 1983.
2. Ceriani, R.L., Thompson, K., Peterson, J.A., Abraham, S., Proc. Nat. Acad. Sci., USA, 74:582-586, 1977.
3. Ceriani, R.L., Peterson, J.A., Lee, J.Y., Moncada, F.R., Blank, E.W. Som. Cell Genet. 9:415-421, 1983.
4. Ceriani, R.L., Peterson, J.A., Blank, E.W., Cancer Res. 44:3033-3039, 1984.
5. Mesa-Tejada, R., Spiegelman, S. In: Viruses Associated with Human Cancer (Ed. L.A. Phillips), Marcel Dekker, New York, 1983, pp. 473-500.
6. Colcher, D., Hand, P., Nuti, M., Schlom, J. Proc. Nat. Acad. Sci., USA, 78:3199-3203, 1981.
7. Ceriani, R.L., Sasaki, M., Sussman, H., Wara, W.M., Blank, E.W. Proc. Nat. Acad. Sci., USA, 79:5420-5424, 1982.

26

SYSTEMIC TREATMENT AND SURVIVAL IN CARCINOMA OF THE BREAST

A. HOWELL, G. G. RIBEIRO, D. M. BARNES & M. JONES
Christie Hospital & Holt Radium Institute, Manchester 20, UK

ABSTRACT

The effect of systemic treatment upon survival after mastectomy is reviewed. It is concluded that treatment may have a small effect upon the probability of relapse, it may delay relapse and increase survival after this event. These effects appear to be independent of the major prognostic indicator, axillary node involvement, but are dependent upon the presence of steroid hormone receptors with respect to endocrine therapy.

INTRODUCTION

The aim of this presentation is to assess the impact of systemic treatment on the course of carcinoma of the breast. Such an exercise is fraught with difficulty because of the great variability in the behavior of the disease: patients may relapse and die within months of mastectomy of never have a relapse and die of natural causes many years later.

Systemic treatment may affect the probability of relapse after surgery, it may delay relapse or it may increase the time period between relapse and death. If treatment reduces the probability of relapse it implies that some patients are cured. Relapse is the single most important event affecting the duration of survival for it is almost invariably associated with subsequent death from breast cancer. To illustrate this point we have examined the outcome of a clinical trial of post-operative radiotherapy versus a watch policy conducted at this hospital between 1949 and 1955. Of the 1461 patients randomized after radical mastectomy 916 (63%) had a relapse and 885 (97%) of these subsequently died of breast cancer (figure 1). The median survival of patients who relapsed and died from breast cancer was 3.5 years whereas the median survival of patients who died from other causes was 23 years.

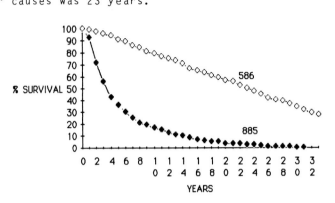

Fig. 1. Survival after mastectomy in patients who died from breast cancer or from other causes.

Because of the long natural history of the disease we can be certain that a particular treatment is curative only after prolonged follow up. In these circumstances cure may be defined as death from other cause in the absence of overt metastatic disease. In many trials of adjuvant systemic treatment there is a delay in relapse in the treated patients compared with the control population. Most of these studies have a follow up period of less than ten years and it is impossible therefore to distinguish, in these studies, between a delay in death from breast cancer and a possible cure from the disease.

An additional problem concerning the interpretation of clinical trials is the possibility that a positive effect of treatment may have been related to an imbalance of prognostic factors within patient groups. For this reason we have chosen to examine the effect on prognosis of axillary lymph node involvement and the presence of steroid hormone receptors within the primary tumour in order to illustrate how these two prognostic factors may or may not affect the interpretation of the results of systemic treatment. There is a complex, but definable, interrelationship between the relapse status of the patient, the two prognostic factors and treatment, which we will discuss in relation to our own data and that of other groups.

AXILLARY LYMPH NODE INVOLVEMENT

Involvement indicates a higher probability of relapse. In the trial mentioned above, at 33 years of follow up, 48% of axillary node negative patients were relapse free and 20% of node positive patients were relapse free. If only relapsed patients were considered those with involved axillary lymph nodes relapsed at a median time of 21 months after mastectomy whereas node negative patients relapsed at a median time of 43 months.

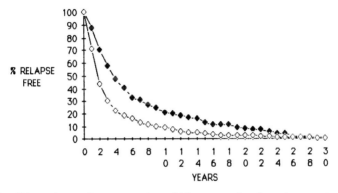

Fig. 2. Time to relapse and axillary node involvement (+ve, -ve).

(Figure 2). After relapse there was little difference in survival between the two groups. Thus, not only does the patient with axillary node involvement have a higher probability of relapse but the relapse is sooner than for the node negative patient.

STEROID HORMONE RECEPTORS

In contrast to axillary node involvement the presence of oestrogen or progesterone receptors in the primary tumour, in our studies, does not indicate the probability of relapse or the time to relapse, but survival after relapse is greater in patients with receptor positive tumours (1). This is demonstrated with

respect to progesterone receptor in Figure 3 for a group of 446
patients followed up after mastectomy. They were treated with
endocrine therapy after relapse but not after surgery. Similar
results were obtained when oestrogen receptors were considered.
These results differ from some other groups who find a delay in
relapse in patients with receptor positive tumours but in many of
these studies adjuvant endocrine therapy was given and would tend
to affect the time of relapse in the receptor positive group (2).

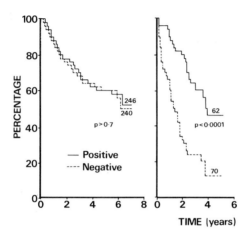

Fig. 3. Time to relapse (left chart) and survival after relapse
(right chart) according to the progesterone receptor status of
the primary tumour. (reprinted with permission from ref. 1).

SYSTEMIC TREATMENT

Systemic treatment with either endocrine therapy or
chemotherapy may be given immediately after surgery, so called
adjuvant therapy, or may be given after relapse for advanced
disease. It is possible for adjuvant therapy to affect the
probability of relapse, time to relapse and survival after
relapse but clearly treatment after relapse will only affect the
latter time period.

Adjuvant Endocrine Therapy

The results of a trial of postoperative adjuvant ovarian irradiation begun here in 1948 and analyzed after fifteen years of follow up showed a small survival advantage for the treated patients throughout the period (3). At fifteen years 76% of node -ve, treated patients were alive compared with 66% controls; the figures for node +ve patients were 40% and 33% respectively (corrected for intercurrent deaths). These differences were significant at a level of p=0.11. The survival curves for treated and control patients are parallel which suggests that a proportion of patients were cured by treatment although thirty year figures are required to confirm this.

A much shorter time of follow up is sufficient to show an effect on the time to relapse. Most of the trials of adjuvant endocrine therapy, using the antioestrogen tamoxifen in postmenopausal women and ovarian ablation in premenopausal women have shown a delay in the time to relapse and in some there has been a significant improvement in survival(2,4-6). It remains to be seen whether a proportion of patients are cured by treatment or whether treatment results in a clinically useful delay in death from breast cancer.

Adjuvant Chemotherapy

The trial performed by Dr. Nissen-Meyer where a 6 day course of cyclophosphamide was given after surgery has now a median follow up of 13 years. 53% of treated patients are alive compared with 47.8% of controls and although this difference is small it may represent a true reduction in the probability of relapse and thus cure (7).

In most other adjuvant chemotherapy trials with a no treatment control arm the follow up is less than ten years. With the exception of some trials using single drugs most of these show a greater time to relapse in treated patients, particularly in premenopausal women. A survival advantage particularly for premenopausal patients was reported in some studies but not others (for review see reference 7). The failure to show a survival advantage after an increase in the time to relapse must indicate that there is a shorter time from relapse to death in some adjuvant treated patients compared with controls.

We and others have shown that patients who develop amenorrhoea during the period of administration of chemotherapy have a longer time to relapse than those who do not (8,9). In addition we have shown that patients with progesterone receptor positive tumours are the group of premenopausal patients who benefit most from adjuvant chemotherapy and suggests that, at least in part, the effectiveness of adjuvant chemotherapy in premenopausal women may be due to the endocrine effect of ovarian suppression.

Therapy for advanced disease

Although dramatic, and by current criteria, complete responses, are seen with both endocrine and chemotherapy no patients are cured of their disease by systemic treatment after relapse. The major effect of these treatments is to, apparently, prolong the period from relapse until death in patients who respond to treatment. This is demonstrated in Fig 4 for a group of 188 patients who relapsed after primary surgery and who were evaluable for response to tamoxifen or ovarian ablation as first endocrine therapy. There was no significant difference in the time to relapse (data not shown), suggesting that the pace of the disease is similar in the two groups, but the responders live for a median time of approximately four years and the non responders for a median of approximately two years after relapse. It is possible that response to treatment selects a good prognosis group who would have done well regardless of treatment but a multivariate analysis of factors which may affect survival including dominant site of disease and receptor status indicated that response was the most important factor with respect to survival. This point is illustrated with respect to receptor status in Fig 5 which shows that although response occurs mainly in patients with receptor positive tumours, patients with

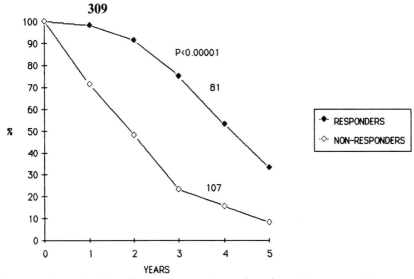

Fig. 4. Survival and response to endocrine therapy after relapse.

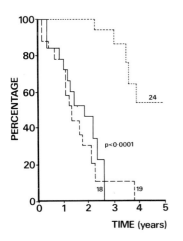

Fig. 5. Survival after relapse related to endocrine therapy and receptor status. (.....) receptor +ve responders, (_____) receptor +ve non-responders and (------) receptor -ve non-responders. (Reprinted with permission from ref. 1).

receptor positive tumours which do not respond, fare as badly as patients with receptor negative tumours.

In a group of 303 patients treated with various combination chemotherapy regimens the picture was similar to the endocrine treated patients in that there was no significant difference between the time to relapse but responders lived on average one year longer than non-responders (data not shown). A multivariate analysis of factors which affect survival after relapse showed response was the most significant variable (10).

Axillary nodes, receptors and response

Axillary node status (at least the comparison between +ve and -ve) appears to be an independent prognostic indicator since there is no apparent relationship of nodal involvement to receptor status or response to endocrine therapy (as an adjuvant or for advanced disease) and chemotherapy for advanced disease (Table 1). Axillary node negative patients are rarely treated by adjuvant chemotherapy.

Table 1. Axillary node involvement, receptors and response to treatment.

	N+ (%)	N- (%)	Total number of patient in population examined
ER+	67	71	398
PR+	46	47	372
Responders+(end*)	46	51	283
Responders+(chem*)	58	65	279

+   includes the "no change" category
*   for advanced disease

In contrast response to endocrine therapy is well known to be dependent upon steroid hormone receptors. When all published studies are taken together it is probable that receptor status does not affect response to chemotherapy (for summary see reference 11).

SUMMARY AND CONCLUSIONS

Some statements can be made concerning the general effectiveness of systemic treatment and its relationship to the two prognostic factors.

1. The probability of relapse is reduced in a small proportion of patients (?5-10%) by adjuvant systemic therapy when studies with long term follow up are considered.

2. Adjuvant therapy delays the <u>time to relapse</u> in most reported studies. A delay in death from breast cancer is being seen and there may be a small effect on cure in the long term.

3. Patients who respond to endocrine and chemotherapy given <u>after relapse</u> live 1-2 years longer than non responders. While it is impossible to be certain that this is a direct antitumour effect of treatment rather than treatment selecting a group of patients with favorable prognostic features, multivariate analyses suggest that the direct antitumour effect is responsible for the survival advantage.

4. The beneficial effects of endocrine therapy at any stage of the disease are seen predominantly in patients with receptor +ve tumours.

5. Axillary node involvement appears to be a prognostic indicator independent of treatment and receptor status.

We have compared the course after mastectomy of patients treated after 1975 with the group from 1949-55 and there appears to be an improvement in survival by a median of two years. Although this is a modest achievement it should not be forgotten that patients who respond to treatment often have symptomatic relief and an improvement in general well being.

The effectiveness of current treatments is thus fairly well mapped. Progress will come by adding new agents and new approaches to this firm foundation.

REFERENCES

1. Howell A. Barnes D M, Harland R N L, et al. Lancet I,
   588-591, 1984.
2. Rose C, Thorpe, S, Anderson K W, et al. Lancet I,
   16-18, 1985
3. Cole M P. Inserm, 55, 143-150, 1975
4. Ribeiro G & Swindell R. Eu J Cancer (in press)
5. Nolvadex Adjuvant Trail Organization. Lancet I,
   257-261, 1983
6. Meakin J W, Allt F A , Beale T C, et al. In: Salmon S
   E & Jones S E (eds) Adjuvant Therapy of Cancer.
   Elsevier, Amsterdam, p. 93, 1984
7. Nissen-Meyer R. Host H, Kjellgren K, et al. In: Senn
   H J (ed) Recent Results in Cancer Research,
   Springerg, Berlin. Vol 96, 48-54, 1984
8. Howell A. Bush H, George D, et al. Lancet II, 307-310,
   1984
9. Tormey D C, as reference 7 p. 184-187.
10. Wagstaff J, Howell A, Mohan P K & Jones M. In
    preparation.

27

BIOLOGICAL IMPLICATIONS OF BREAST CANCER SURGERY[*]

B. FISHER

Department of Surgery, University of Pittsburgh, School of Medicine
3550 Terrace Street, Room 914 Scaife Hall, Pittsburgh, PA   15261

INTRODUCTION

We have recently published findings from two randomized clinical trials carried out by the National Surgical Adjuvant Breast and Bowel Project (NSABP) to determine the efficacy of alternative local and regional treatments of primary operable breast cancer (1,2). Those investigations represent a continuum of effort by us for almost two decades to resolve as definitively as possible existing controversies relative to the local-regional management of primary breast cancer. The first study (Protocol B-04) was begun in 1971 and the specific aims of that trial were to determine (a) whether in patients with clinically negative axillary nodes total mastectomy, followed by delayed axillary dissection in those who subsequently had positive axillary nodes, was as effective as radical mastectomy, (b) whether the outcome of total mastectomy followed by postoperative regional

_____

[*]Presented in part as the Heath Memorial Award Lecture, M.D. Anderson Hospital and Tumor Institute, November 3, 1982and in the Keynote Address presented at the 1983 Annual Symposium on Fundamental Cancer Research, "Cancer Invasion and Metastases" at the M.D. Anderson Hospital & Tumor Institute, Houston, Texas, February 28-March 3, 1983

irradiation was equivalent to that of radical mastectomy, and (c) whether total mastectomy with delayed axillary dissection in patients with subsequently positive nodes was as efficacious as total mastectomy and radiation. For patients with clinically positive nodes the objective was to ascertain whether radical mastectomy and total mastectomy followed by radiation produced an equivalent outcome. When early findings from that trial (Protocol B-04) (3,4) indicated that patients treated by total mastectomy without axillary node dissection and pectoral muscle removal were at no higher risk of distant disease or death than were those undergoing a Halsted radical mastectomy, we considered it clinically and scientifically compelling and justifiable to begin a new study (Protocol B-06) to evaluate the worth of breast conservation by local tumor excision with or without radiation therapy. Beginning in 1976 patients were randomly assigned to one of three treatment groups: total mastectomy, segmental mastectomy, or segmental mastectomy followed by breast irradiation. Women in all the treatment groups had an axillary dissection and those with positive nodes received chemotherapy. The operation employed, lumpectomy, completely abandoned conventional concepts of cancer surgery by removing only enough breast tissue to insure that the margins of the resected surgical specimens were free of tumor. The study was designed to determine (a) the effectiveness of lumpectomy for breast preservation, (b) whether radiation therapy reduces the incidence of tumor in the ipsilateral breast after lumpectomy, (c) whether breast conservation results in a higher risk of distant disease and death than does mastectomy and (d) the clinical significance of multicentricity.

The findings from those two studies have given rise to a multitude of biologic, philosophic and pragmatic clinical considerations. Clinicians in general, particularly surgeons and radiation therapists, have perceived the findings within the framework of their own biases and the perspective of their discipline. Results from the first study were viewed with no special enthusiasm by most surgeons since they were considered to merely reaffirm what has already been "established", i.e., that radical mastectomy need not be employed for the treatment of breast cancer. Moreover, since axillary node dissection is regarded as a necessary requirement for determining prognosis, for making decisions relative to the use of systemic adjuvant therapy and for more effective local-regional disease control, the finding that patients treated by total mastectomy without an axillary dissection are at no survival disadvantage was regarded as having no current clinical relevance. Moreover, since present surgical controversy revolves around the relative merit of breast removal versus breast conservation, the arguments of the 1960's and 1970's, which were confined to the extent of breast removing operations, have been perceived as an anachronism which needs no further debate. Similarly the findings from the second study were perceived as nothing more than "confirmatory" of the efficacy of lumpectomy by surgeons who were already performing breast conserving operations as a result of anecdotal information which had accumulated sporadically over several decades or because of findings obtained from a single prospective randomized trial employing a patient population and an operative approach different from that in our lumpectomy trial (5). Radiation oncologists viewed the study as "rediscovering" the worth of radiation therapy! Those surgeons who have been and remain opponents of breast conserving operations and reluctant acceptors of less radical mastectomies considered the study to be "poorly designed and implemented", having "too short a follow-up time", and having other deficiencies. Such perceptions of the two studies, and the arguments which they engendered have been distressing to me since they indicate a failure to appreciate their true significance.

The biologic relevance of the results of the studies have largely been overlooked, not only by clinicians, but by non-clinical laboratory investigators as well, and there has been singular lack of appreciation of how these studies portray the interrelationship of laboratory and clinical research. The purpose of this commentary is to present my perspective of the interdependence of laboratory and clinical research in the study of metastases and the role which the aforementioned surgical studies have played in furthering knowledge in that area of tumor biology.

COMMENTARY

The gross components of the metastatic process, i.e., tumor cell invasion, dissemination, lodgement, and growth, have long been familiar. Over the last two decades in vitro investigation and animal experimentation have been directed toward dismantling the metastatic "machine" into its more basic constituents and determining how each of them may function as independent variables. With each new methodologic development, the "breakdown" process has proceeded at a more rapid pace. Considerable information, albeit often contradictory, has resulted, providing new insight into the basic components of the metastatic process --at least in the models employed.

Despite what appears to be progress, certain perceptions I have, if they are accurate, cause concern. The position that methodology and animal models have assumed in the study of metastasis justifies comment. Despite the most elegant methodology, the time has not yet arrived when one can assume that findings obtained from in vitro studies are indicative of what takes place in the human being. Extrapolation of the significance and universality of a finding from an in vivo animal model to a patient with cancer is equally precarious, no matter how convinced proponents of a model are that it simulates the human. How each one of those well-characterized functional components becomes modulated when present in an intact environment composed of competing forces cannot possibly be predicted. My concern is intensified by the fact that there is can increasing cadre of investigators who favor the emphasis of in vitro research at the expense of in-vivo animal investigation, and there are those who seek to abolish human clinical trial research because they perceive it to be inefficient, nonproductive, and unjustifiably competitive for research dollars. In my opinion these attitudes are regressive and arise from a lack of appreciation of the interdependence of laboratory and clinical research in the study of cancer.

Another concern relates to the impression I have obtained from comprehensive reviews that despite all of the laboratory research carried out during the last two decades, there has been little or no testing in the human of concepts drived from animal and in vitro studies of metastasis. Perhaps no new hypotheses have been formulated. Perhaps those synthesized have not been worthy of evaluation in humans. Perhaps testing has taken place, but was not recognized as such. Often the only reference to human metastasis in reviews is either observational in nature or consists of a stirring "grant application type" last sentence such as, "Learning more about metastasis and tumor progression in animal tumor systems should lead to the design of more rational therapies for the management of cancer." Moreover, there is no indication that investigations or observations in the human have given rise to concepts that have provided impetus to laboratory investigation. Do reviews reflect the true state of affairs? Have the past two decades been so devoted to experiment-driven research that awareness of purpose has been lost? Are laboratory investigators to blame, or have clinical investigators failed to translocate findings from the laboratory into the clinical setting?

After two decades of effort, there are still facets of metastatic research that have failed to produce findings unifiable into a concept capable of being tested in the human. Tumor cell invasion and penetration exemplifies one such component. Information from a number of models indicates that "...there is a vast indirect (histologic) evidence, but hardly sufficient direct (cinematographic) proof for the occurrence of cell locomotion in tumor penetration in-vivo" (6). Others have considered that a major advance in knowledge of metastasis has been the recognition of the importance of tumor cell surface properties in influencing the invasive process. Investigations have evaluated the capabilities of tumor cells to produce enzymes that enhance their invasiveness by perturbing a normal tissue matrix, and observations from in vitro models have indicated that the cells within a tumor possess variable invasive properties. Can these and other seemingly unrelated phenomena be coordinated into a concept with therapeutic relevance? Since biological events associated with the early stages of the metastatic process have been in operation prior to the discovery of a tumor, even should an intervention be devised to abort the process it could be introduced only after the fact. Perhaps its worth might be to prevent metastases from metastasizing, if this is an event of clinical importance. By discerning properties of human tumor cells that relate to invasiveness, we could make another prognostic marker available to aid in defining a patient population at risk. It is more likely that information on the invasive properties of a tumor has greater relevance to understanding normal cell biology than to the formulation of strategies that can affect the natural history of patients with cancer. These comments are not to be construed as minimizing the importance or worth of such investigations--merely to indicate how I perceive their orientation in the scheme of things.

Redundant as it may seem, it is appropriate to put into focus the purpose of in-vitro and in-vivo research, which is primarily to develop concepts that can be formulated into hypotheses. It is such hypotheses--not individual experiments--that require testing in the human. Clinical benefit is the fringe benefit derived from biological hypothesis testing. The perception held by many that "clinical" trial research is "product testing," i.e., testing of drugs, operations, types of radiation, etc., needs to be changed. Clinical trial research is not only a necessary corollary of laboratory investigation but is an instigator of concept and hypotheses in its own right. Those who would eliminate the testing process provided by clinical trial research may not fully appreciate that they may be supplying an open ticket for laboratory investigators to continue their studies in tangential and repetitive fashion--limited only by urgency in developing new methodology and models and, of course, funding. Without there ever being a day of reckoning, there can be no accountability for their efforts. Sooner or later it becomes necessary to assess what has been and is being done in a field such as metastasis to ascertain whether there are threads in the results capable of being woven into a worthy hypothesis that can be tested in humans. A hypothesis is of value only if it can be evaluated so that it may be rejected, supported, or modified. Otherwise, it assumes the status of armchair philosophy.

There comes a time when hypothesis testing must be undertaken. To continue to look for the "perfect" experiment in the "perfect" model to resolve all doubts and to satisfy all one's peers before instituting such an undertaking is apt to result in investigative stalemate and paralysis. An appropriate hypothesis derived from biological principles tested in a proper human setting will result in information not only of clinical importance but of equal if not greater biological significance. The results will clarify directions for research in metastasis that might be productive and indicate other areas that should be abandoned. Such testing in the human cannot confirm findings obtained from individual laboratory experiments. It is unlikely that more than a few of the experiments carried out in animal model systems will or can ever be duplicated in the human to determine whether findings in the former are valid in the latter.

These remarks are not to be construed as minimizing the importance of nontargeted, non-goal-oriented or fundamental research. There must be increased and unabated support for such effort. There is no conflict between fundamental research and research that may have clinical relevance. Just as one must be cautious about considering all research without a clinical application as fundamental. The term "fundamental" may be considered in a sense akin to a "promissory note."

The remainder of this discussion provides a scenario from our experience to exemplify how a combination of laboratory and clinical research has contributed or may in the future add to the understanding of tumor metastasis and at the same time improve the therapy of cancer. Female breast cancer was the human tumor model used exclusively in these studies. How universally applicable findings from that model are to other human tumors is equally as conjectural as is the relation of findings from in-vivo and in-vitro systems to all or any human tumors.

Halstedian Hypothesis: By the mid 1950s when our laboratory investigations began, little had changed in the perception of the process of metastasis. While by then it was accepted that lymphatic spread occurred by embolization instead of by direct extension, that the bloodstream was an important pathway of tumor dissemination, and that laboratory investigations had clarified certain aspects of the process, the overall concept remained unaltered. The idea prevailed that lymph-borne tumor cells had one destination--lymph nodes, that tumor cells in blood lodged in the first capillary bed they encountered, and that there was an orderly pattern of dissemination based on temporal and mechanical considerations. The only debate related to whether patterns of distant metastases were due to specific properties of various tissues, the "seed-soil" hypothesis first promulgated by Paget in 1889, or to anatomical and mechanical factors.

Intrigued by the possibility that disseminated tumor cells produced metastases only in some individuals, and that the soil concept was somehow related to this occurrence, we began investigations toward obtaining a better comprehension of the biology of metastasis. No convictions or hypothesis directed our efforts; we were entirely involved with experiment-driven research--fact finding. Laboratory studies carried out by us between 1958 and 1968 influenced our own thinking relative to metastatic mechanisms. They revealed that the blood and the lymphatic vascular systems are so interrelated that it is impractical to consider them as independent routes of dissemination (7). Within minutes, viable tumor cells gaining access to the liver via the portal vein could be identified in lymph coming from the liver. Those and other findings led us to conclude as early as 1964 (8) that: "...it would seem obsolete to ascribe either mechanical considerations or soil (host) factors as responsible for tumor distribution. It would seem that patterns of tumor spread are dictated by anatomic considerations as well as intrinsic factors in the tumor cell per se and in the tissue that it reaches."

Using labeled cells, we first obtained quantitative data relative to the deposition and egress of neoplastic cells from organs following their hematogenous dissemination and subcutaneous inoculation. It was observed that the residence of a vast majority of tumor cells gaining access to an organ via the bloodstream was transient (9), confirming and extending the seminal observation of Zeidman (1961) and his associates that tumor cells are not trapped by the first capillary bed they encounter. Such observations permitted us to adopt the thesis that there is no orderly pattern of tumor cell dissemination that could be based on mechanical and temporal factors.

Results from another series of experiments led to the conclusion that RLN are not, as Virchow proposed, effective barriers to tumor spread. Additional studies indicated the biological importance of RLN. They were found to play a role in both initiation (10) and maintenance of tumor immunity (11). We also demonstrated that RLN cells are capable of destroying tumor cells, indicating that the presence of negative nodes may be a result of such a circumstance as well as because tumor cells traverse nodes rather than that a tumor had been removed prior to its dissemination (12). Axillary nodes from patients (13,14) continued to possess immunological capabilities despite the presence of growing tumors. Those qualities vary in nodes within a patient and between patients. The findings indicated that biological rather than anatomical factors might be the reason that certain nodes contained metastases and others did not.

Studies begun in 1958 indicated that host factors are important in the development of metastases and that a tumor is not autonomous of its host as was believed (15). The presence of dormant tumor cells was demonstrated (16), and it was shown that perturbation of the host by a variety of means could produce lethal metastases from those cells (17,18). Our findings led us to consider that local recurrences following operation were apt to be the result of systemically disseminated cells lodging and growing at a site of trauma rather than of inadequate surgical technique (19). We proposed that a tumor is a systemic disease, probably from its inception. That premise never implied that all patients would at some time develop overt metastases; nor did it imply that only those with metastases represent the population with disseminated disease.

In the 1960s, the thesis was formulated that the RLN is an indicator of host-tumor relations. The lymph node that contains tumor cells reflects an inter-relation between host and tumor that permits the development of metastases rather than that the node is an instigator of distant disease.

Concomitant with the laboratory investigations, we obtained information from a series of clinical trials. The results of those studies failed to coincide with expectation. Recurrence and survival were independent of the number of axillary nodes removed and examined (20). Patients having few nodes removed that were all free of tumor had the same prognosis as did those with large numbers removed and free of tumor. Conversely, patients with, for example, two of five nodes positive were at the same risk as those with two of 30 nodes positive. It was also found that despite the fact that cancers of the inner half of the breast metastasize more frequently to internal mammary nodes than do outer quadrant tumors, tumor location failed to influence prognosis (21). In patients who had radical mastectomy, an operation that does not remove internal mammary nodes, the treatment failure and survival was the same whether the tumors were in the inner or outer half of the breast.

Whether the results of all of these laboratory studies and clinical observations were interpreted correctly, were due to the methodologies and models employed rather than to biologic circumstances, could or could not be confirmed in every setting and in every detail, or were obtained from simplistic experiments that did not really provide positive proof for any of our assumptions, they all had the same characteristic. They did not conform to the concepts that provided the principles for the halstedian hypothesis. They provided a matrix on which an alternative thesis could be formulated. That hypothesis, synthesized in 1968, is biological in concept rather than anatomic and mechanistic. Its components are completely antithetical to those in the one attributed to Halsted (Table 1).

TABLE 1. Two divergent hypotheses of tumor biology

Halstedian	Alternative
Tumors spread in an orderly defined manner based upon mechanical considerations.	There is no orderly pattern of tumor dissemination.
Tumor cells traverse lymphatics to lymph nodes by direct extension, supporting en bloc dissection.	Tumors cells traverse lymphatics by embolization, challenging the merit of en bloc dissection.
The positive lymph node is an indicator of tumor spread and is the instigator of disease.	The positive lymph node is an indicator of a host-tumor relationship that permits development of metastases rather the instigator of distant disease.
Regional lymph nodes are barriers to the passage of tumor cells.	Regional lymph nodes are ineffective as barriers to tumor cell spread.
RLN's are of anatomic importance.	RLN's are of biological importance.
The blood stream is of little significance as a route of tumor dissemination.	The blood stream is of considerable importance in tumor dissemination.
A tumor is autonomous of its host.	Complex host-tumor interrelationships affect every facet of the disease.
Operable breast cancer is a local regional disease.	Operable breast cancer is a systemic disease.
The extent and nuances of operation are the dominant factors influencing patient outcome.	Variations in local-regional therapy are unlikely to substantially affect survival.
No consideration was given to tumor multicentricity.	Multicentric foci of tumor are not of necessity a precursor of clinically overt cancer.

Alternative Hypothesis Testing: Opportunity to confirm or deny the tenets of the alternative hypothesis became available in 1971 via a trial involving almost 2,000 women. We fully appreciated that no answers would be obtained from that clinical test that would specifically indicate whether each of our laboratory findings was producible in humans. The aim was to test the hypothesis synthesized from these studies, not to test the studies themselves. After a follow-up of 10 years, the results of that trial have indicated that in patients without clinical evidence of node involvement three distinctly different treatment regimens (radical mastectomy, total mastectomy with local-regional radiation, or total mastectomy without radiation and removal of nodes only if they later became involved) yielded no significant difference in overall treatment failure, distant metastases, or survival (22). In patients having clinical node involvement who were treated by radical mastectomy or total mastectomy followed by local-regional radiation, there was also no significant difference in outcome. The results provide credibility to and confirmation of many of the tenets of the alternative hypothesis.

The similarity of findings in patients with clinically negative nodes was remarkable considering that approximately 40% of women subjected to total mastectomy alone had positive nodes unremoved and untreated. Those nodes should have been expected to serve as a source of further tumor dissemination, resulting in an increase in distant treatment failure and mortality. That such was not so justifies a challenge to temporal considerations in metastatic development and tends to indicate that, even if metastases do metastasize, the consequences, at least in this setting, are clinically irrelevant. Just as not removing nodes was not deleterious, their removal did not adversely affect prognosis, refuting the concept that unremoved regional nodes may provide an immunologic advantage. When considered overall, the findings refute in the human the anatomic and mechanical percepts that have dictated thinking relative to metastases and have influenced therapy. It would thus seem that laboratory research having as its specific goal the obtaining of additional information to confirm or deny the tenets of this hypotheses (which had been evaluated in the human) may not be of high priority.

REFERENCES

1. Fisher, B. et al. N. Engl. J. Med. 312:674-681, 1985.
2. Fisher, B. et al. N. Engl. J. Med. 312:665-673, 1985.
3. Fisher, B. et al. Cancer 39:2827-2839, 1977.
4. Fisher, B. et al. Cancer 46:1009-1025, 1980.
5. Veronesi U. et al. N. Engl. J. Med. 305:6, 1981.
6. Strauli, P. and Weiss, L. Eur. J. Cancer 13:1-12, 1977.
7. Fisher, B. and Fisher, E.R., Surg. Gynecol. Obstet. 122:791-798, 1966.
8. Fisher, B. and Fisher, E.R. In: FIFTH NATIONAL CANCER CONFERENCE PROCEEDINGS (Sponsored by ACS nad NCI, 1964). J.B. Lippincott Co., Philadelphia, pp.105-122, 1965.
9. Fisher, B. and Fisher, E.R. Cancer Res. 27:412-420, 1967.
10. Fisher, B. and Fisher, E.R. Cancer 27:1001-1004, 1971.
11. Fisher, B. and Fisher, E.R. Cancer 29:1496-1501, 1972.
12. Fisher, B. et al. Cancer 33:631-636, 1974.
13. Fisher, B. et al. Cancer 30:1202-1215, 1972.
14. Fisher, B. et al. Cancer 33:271-279, 1974.
15. Fisher E.R. and Fisher, B. In: ENDOGENOUS FACTORS INFLUENCING HOST-TUMOR BALANCE (International Symposium Sponsored by the Argonne Cancer Research Hosp., Univ. of chicago, 1966). (Eds. R.W. Wissler, T.L. Dao, and S. Wood, Jr.) Univ. of Chicago Press, Chicago, pp.149-166, 1967.
16. Fisher, B. and Fisher, E.R. Science 130:918-919, 1959.
17. Fisher, B. and Fisher, E.R. Ann. Surg. 150:731-744, 1959.
18. Fisher, B. et al. Proc. Soc. Exp. Biol. Med. 131:16-18, 1969.
19. Fisher, B. et al. Cancer 20:23-30, 1967.
20. Fisher, B. and Slack, N.H. Surg. Gynecol. Obstet. 131:79-88, 1970.
21. Fisher, B. et al. Surg. Gynecol. Obstet. 129:705-716, 1969.
22. Fisher, B. et al. Cancer 46:1009-1025, 1980.

INDEX